The Treatment of Inherited Metabolic Disease

The Treatment of Inherited Metabolic Disease

Ten Specialist Contributions

Assembled and Edited by
D. N. RAINE

MTP
Medical and Technical Publishing Co. Ltd.

Published by

MTP
MEDICAL AND TECHNICAL
PUBLISHING CO. LTD.
PO Box 55, St. Leonard's House,
St. Leonardgate,
Lancaster, Lancs

Printed and bound in Great Britain by
The Garden City Press Limited, Letchworth Herts SG6 1JS

ISBN 0 852 00078 2

Contents

List of Contributors

W. R. Bergren
Head, Biochemistry Research Laboratory, Childrens Hospital of Los Angeles, California, 90054, USA

Nina A. J. Carson
Research Associate, The Nuffield Department of Child Health, Institute of Clinical Science, Belfast BT12 6BJ

Barbara E. Clayton
Professor of Chemical Pathology, The Hospital for Sick Children, London WC1N 3JH

G. N. Donnell
Professor of Pediatrics, Childrens Hospital of Los Angeles, California 90054, USA

J. Fernandes
Sophia Children's Hospital and Neonatal Unit, Rotterdam 3004, The Netherlands

E. R. Froesch
Professor of Pathophysiology, Kantonsspital, 8006, Zurich, Switzerland

D. Gompertz
Lecturer in Biochemistry and Hon. Consultant in Biochemical Genetics Royal Postgraduate Medical School, London W12 0HS

D. N. Raine
Consultant Chemical Pathologist, The Children's Hospital, Birmingham B16 8ET

Selma E. Snyderman
Professor of Pediatrics, School of Medicine, New York University
Medical Centre, N.Y. 10016, USA

J. M. Walshe
Reader in Metabolic Disease, Department of Investigative Medicine,
University of Cambridge, Cambridge CB2 1QN

Preface

The discovery, in 1953, that the mental retardation associated with untreated phenylketonuria is prevented by rearing the genetically abnormal but, as yet, clinically unaffected infant on a diet low in phenylalanine excited a new interest in metabolic disease which, after 20 years, is in no way diminished. Many excellent centres in all parts of the world now achieve remarkable results in this, and related diseases, but those with experience are the first to admit that success comes more from careful and constant attention to details of management rather than from any magic cure. It is difficult to envisage that there will be, in the near future, any absolute and specific cure for any of the inherited metabolic diseases, and so, for the time being, it is important to achieve the most widespread application of the best methods of management currently available, and it is to this end that the present book has been prepared.

Over the years the most important lesson to have emerged from the management of these disorders is that treatment means much more than keeping the 'blood levels down to normal'. Indeed, an early experience was that this can be harmful, and sometimes fatal, and the concentration of the substance characterising a particular disease often needs to be maintained at something above normal but sufficiently low to avoid its harmful effects. However, much more is involved. The paediatrician has had to learn to interpret arrests and spurts in weight and height, irritability, reluctance to feed, and other subtle clinical observations and has had to define criteria by which to decide whether these reflect the disease, the treatment, or simply the ever-changing normal state of the growing child.

The psychological reaction of parents to their affected child and to the normal siblings presents a fascinating, but constant, challenge and the parents may need substantial help in defining their attitude towards the prospect of having further children. Few clinicians would claim to be even moderately confident that they are able to give the right advice in all these circumstances, and now the opportunity to abort an affected fetus raises questions that require still further careful study and consideration. The risk at which parents would elect to have a potentially affected fetus aborted is given as 1 in 10 for such states as rubella infection during pregnancy, but if this figure is applied to recessively inherited metabolic diseases no parents of an affected child would have any further children. To what extent would their decision be influenced if, instead of stating the chance that their next infant will be abnormal is 1 in 4, they are told that there is a 3 in 4 chance of the child being normal? In fact, parents of affected children are not always deterred from increasing their family and any future work that increases the accuracy of heterozygote detection and the recognition of affected fetuses before birth will ease these decisions for both doctors and parents.

For one whose involvement with inherited metabolic disease began with the evaluation of screening methods for their early detection, while there was still time to treat, the hardest question to answer convincingly has been 'What is the point of looking for them if you can't do anything with them when you have found them?' Many different replies have been given but I have never been in doubt that, within a generation, the treatment of many of these disorders will be found, a view shared by many colleagues in other centres, most of whom pay as much, if not more, attention to the management of the disorders than they do to their early detection. For this reason it is a particular pleasure to be associated with the first book wholly devoted to the Treatment of Inherited Metabolic Disease.

It would be easy for any reader of this book, and even for the several contributors in an idle moment, to take for granted two outstanding contributions to the better understanding and management of inherited metabolic diseases—ones on which we all depend. The first was the publication in 1960 of the first edition of *The Metabolic Basis of Inherited Disease* edited by Stanbury, Wyngaarden and Fredrickson, who have devotedly produced two further editions, the latest in 1972. The academic standard and the comprehensive range of this work has set a standard that is not likely to be exceeded in this subject, and has rarely been achieved in many others.

The second contribution is that of Victor McKusick in producing, in addition to his many other works, the catalogue of human inherited disease *Mendelian Inheritance in Man*, also in its third edition (1971). Without the stimulus created by these two works it is probable that the present book would not have been called for for several years to come.

Finally it is a pleasure to acknowledge my indebtedness for the help

I have received from my colleagues Mrs. Anne Green, M.Sc., of the Department of Clinical Chemistry, Mr. Alan Westwood, M.Sc., and Dr. Susan Terry of the Institute of Mental Subnormality, Lea Castle Hospital, Wolverley. Without the dedicated care Mrs. Judy Pepper, M.Sc., has given to the diseases file the section on the Treatment of Other Inherited Metabolic Diseases could not have been written, and I detect that my secretaries, especially Mrs. Jill Webber, are as pleased to be completing this Preface as the Editor himself!

D. N. RAINE

The Principles of Treatment by Dietary Restriction as Illustrated by Phenylketonuria

Barbara E. Clayton

The rare disorder phenylketonuria (PKU) is one of the few causes of mental retardation for which effective medical treatment is available. When the care of a child with PKU has been good from the early weeks of life, adequate intellectual development takes place[1-5]. Though the mean intelligence quotient of these early-treated patients tends to lie about 10 points below that of the normal population, they are educable at normal schools and differ strikingly from most untreated or late-treated phenylketonuric children whose mean intelligence quotient is about 50. There have been those who have doubted the efficacy of treatment[6,7] but much of the confusion has arisen from a failure to realise that hyperphenylalaninaemia can arise in a variety of ways, and because once a diagnosis of classical PKU has been made, dietary and biochemical care have not been uniformly good. In classical PKU in the untreated infant the phenylalanine concentration in the blood is over 30 mg/100 ml, the plasma tyrosine is normal and metabolites of phenylalanine are present in the urine. With the introduction of more sensitive screening procedures[8], not only are infants with classical PKU detected, but also a whole spectrum of children with hyperphenylalaninaemia, the significance of which is largely unknown[9].

Paediatricians with experience of treating PKU are so convinced of its effectiveness that the performance of a controlled trial is now most unlikely. Since October 1, 1967, a collaborative study of children treated for phenylketonuria has been in progress in the USA[10]. In 1973, it was reported that all the 145 treated children with PKU included in the trial so far were developing normally and it was encouraging to see how closely the intellectual assessment approximated to that of the general population of three- and four-year-olds. The patients did however appear to be slightly lower in intelligence than their normal siblings. An important study by Levy et al. [11] ascertained the prevalence of PKU amongst a quarter of a million teenagers and adults who were being tested for syphilis. Only three subjects with PKU were found and they were all mentally subnormal at least to a mild degree. From the results of newborn screening, 17 cases would have been expected. Further evidence for the efficiency of treatment comes from the PKU register which collects information about the diagnosis and treatment of PKU in the United Kingdom. A recent review of the register[12] showed a decrease in the number of late-diagnosed patients from 1966 onwards and also a decrease in the number of patients presenting with symptoms. These trends are closely linked with improvements in screening methods in the UK and hence with early treatment.

The information given in this chapter emphasises the principles on which a synthetic diet is based and the treatment of PKU is used as a specific example. Where commercial products are named they will usually be those in use in Britain but no attempt has been made to provide complete lists of products, and there is a bias towards the use of products with which I am familiar from personal experience. This does not imply that other products (see p. 253) may not be equally satisfactory.

The dietary treatment of a metabolic disorder such as PKU is highly complex and potentially hazardous. In my view, no doctor should embark on the care of such patients unless he is able to work closely with a dietitian experienced in the treatment of this type of disorder. The dietitian should be responsible for the details of the diet as presented to the parents and child. I therefore consider this chapter to be complementary to the instructions given by my dietetic colleague Miss D. E. M. Francis[13].

Aim of dietary treatment

The cause of mental retardation in PKU is far from understood. There is incomplete myelination of the central nervous system[14], and Menkes[15] has suggested that there may be decreased synthesis of myelin. Certainly animal experiments indicate that high doses of phenylalanine early in life can cause marked changes in the composition of the brain[16,17]. In addition, phenylalanine and its metabolites inhibit the transport and concentration of other amino acids in liver and brain, and they interfere with the activity of enzymes involved in the metabolism of amino acids[18-20]. A variety of other suggestions has been made and these include decreased production of γ-aminobutyric acid[21], impaired synthesis of serotonin[22] and chronic insufficiency of glutamine[23].

The aim of treatment is to lower the circulating level of phenylalanine to a concentration similar to, and a little higher than, that found in normal subjects. There is no general agreement about the level of phenylalanine for which treatment is required. Patients with concentrations below 10 mg/100 ml blood, plasma or serum are not usually treated, and the clinician may or may not decide to treat an infant with concentrations between 10 and 15 mg/100 ml. If the phenylalanine is persistently between 15 and 20 mg/100 ml the clinician may try to reduce the concentration by employing a low protein diet (2·0–3·0 g protein/kg body weight/day with total calories exceeding 115 ± 15/kg during the neonatal period) or he may use a synthetic diet and reassess the infant after 3–6 months. The team at the Hospital for Sick Children in London treats the infant only if the phenylalanine is persistently greater than 15 mg/100 ml and abnormal metabolites are present in the urine when the infant is on a normal diet.

Centres for treatment

For good results these children should be treated in centres where there is a team comprising not only the paediatrician, but a paediatric dietitian, biochemist, psychiatrist and psychologist. In this way the staff gain experience in caring for these children, laboratory facilities can be geared to their needs, and proper dietary supervision can be provided. Where a dietitian looks after numbers of these children she acquires experience in how to adapt the basic principles of the diet to the individual patients and their home environment, and she can provide the recipes and domestic 'know-how' so essential for the mothers. How to bake a low phenylalanine birthday cake is just as important as accurate phenylalanine levels or clinical care! Though there are exceptions, the single patient with PKU at a hospital does not in general get this type of care, and it is in this situation that disastrous effects of poor diet are liable to occur.

In-patient care of the newly diagnosed patient is essential so that the parents come to know the staff well, but the length of admission should be kept as short as possible. The advantages of a centre in my view far outweigh the disadvantages of the journey to the centre. The family doctor will also be intimately involved in the care of the patient, and he will require information and support from the centre since he may never have seen this rare disorder. The local paediatrician may wish to be concerned also and it will then be necessary to be quite certain about the role of each individual in decision making as it affects the patient and his family. There is no doubt too, that new mothers gain confidence and assurance from seeing early-diagnosed treated children at the clinic.

These views on the need for centralisation are in accord with those given by the Department of Health and Social Security, in England and Wales[24], and by many groups of workers[25]. An interesting centralised service in Denmark has been described by Wamberg[26] and is based on a special treatment home and research centre for all newly diagnosed infants. He pointed out both the advantages and disadvantages of such a system.

PRINCIPLES OF A SYNTHETIC DIET

In order to reduce the phenylalanine intake sufficiently in patients with classical PKU it is necessary to use a synthetic substitute for much of the protein in the diet since phenylalanine is a constituent of all animal and vegetable proteins. Such protein substitutes may be mixtures of synthetic amino acids or hydrolysates of whole protein produced by acid or enzymic digestion (see Table 1.1). The manufactured product may or may not contain other ingredients such as fat and carbohydrate, vitamins and minerals.

Hyperaminoaciduria is observed in patients who receive products based on acid-hydrolysed protein and it has been shown[27] that this is due to the excretion of D-amino acids. Acid hydrolysis causes 2–3% of racemisation of the constituent amino acids[28]. The question remains; to what extent might D-amino acids be detrimental to human development, particularly when incorporated in the diet of the newborn? There are marked species differences in the availabilities of the D-amino acids for growth and the maintenance of nitrogen balance, and most of the long-term experimental work relates to animals. Though there is no clear evidence that D-amino acids administered over long periods are detrimental to human development, it would seem advisable to exclude them whenever practical from synthetic diets intended for use with infants and children.

Table 1.1. Composition (per 100 g product) of some synthetic substitutes for protein

	'Protein'*	Phenylalanine (mg)	Calories	Carbohydrate (g)	Fat (g)	Calcium (mg)	Vitamins	Comments
Products based on hydrolysates								
Minafen	12·5	<20	509	47·9	31·0	700	Some added	For infants; acid hydrolysate of casein
Lofenalac	15	80 (average)	460	57	18·0	667	Most added	All ages; enzymic hydrolysate of casein; difficult to give adequate protein to older children
Cymogran	30	<10	400	42·7	9·0	1400	None added	For children; acid hydrolysate of casein; can be adapted for infants
Albumaid XP	33·8	<10	370	50	Nil	800–1000	Some added	All ages, acid hydrolysate of beef serum; needs adapting for infants
Products based on synthetic amino acids								
Aminogran	100	Nil	400	Nil	Nil	In the mineral mixture in the pack	None added	All ages, especially from weaning onwards; needs adapting for infants
PK Aid I & II	100	Nil	400	Nil	Nil	Nil: Metabolic mineral mixture is recommended	None added	I for patients over 2 years, II for those over 5 years

* For products based on hydrolysates this value is the protein equivalent, i.e. total nitrogen in 100 g of product $\times$ 6·25. For products based on synthetic amino acids it is the actual weight of amino acids. The sources of these products are listed on p. 253

In addition to the protein substitute and natural protein to supply the essential requirement of phenylalanine, it is necessary to supply adequate fat and carbohydrate which may or may not be included in the commercial product. Tables 1.2 and 1.3 give details of the daily dietary requirements, using a protein hydrolysate or amino acids as the protein substitute. When using an acid hydrolysate the protein recommended includes the substitute and the natural protein; for amino acid preparations the recommendation is for the substitute only,

Table 1.2. Daily requirements (g/kg body weight) when an hydrolysate-based preparation (Cymogran) is used

Age (years)	Calories	Protein supplied from Cymogran + natural protein	Cymogran*
1–3	90–100	4·2	12·3
4–6	80–100	3·8	11·0
7–9	70–90	3·3	9·3
10+	70–80	2·9	8·0

* This dose of Cymogran will supply the protein supplement required, but additional calories will be needed. It is assumed that 0·5 g natural protein/kg body weight will be added to the diet to supply the essential phenylalanine requirement

Table 1.3. Daily requirements (g/kg body weight) when an amino acid-based preparation (Aminogran) is used

Age (years)	Calories	Aminogran*
0–1	125 ± 25	3
1–3	90–100	2
4–6	80–100	2
7–9	70–90	2
10+	70–80	2

* Assuming natural protein will be added to supply the essential phenylalanine requirement. If the natural protein exceeds 1 g/kg daily in children, or 2 g/kg daily in infants, the intake of Aminogran food supplement should be limited to 3 g and 4 g/kg daily in children and infants respectively

Table 1.4. Requirements (mg/kg/day) for essential amino acids in the healthy human infant

L-Amino acid	Human milk[*] (mg/l)	Requirement calculated from volume of human milk intake			Method of Holt (range)[†]
		<1 month	2–3 months	4–5 months	
Histidine	230	39	33	30	16–34
Isoleucine	860	147	125	115	102–119
Leucine	1610	277	234	212	76–229
Lysine	790	136	115	104	88–103
Methionine	230	39	33	30	33–45 (in presence of cystine)
Phenylalanine	640	110	93	85	47–90 (in presence of tyrosine)
Threonine	620	106	90	82	45–87
Tryptophan	220	38	32	29	15–22
Valine	90	156	130	119	85–105

[*] Macy, I. G. and Kelly, H. J.[86]
[†] Holt, L. E., Jr.[87], from effect of various amino acid mixtures on weight gain and nitrogen retention

Table 1.5. Recommended intake (mg/kg body weight/day) of non-essential amino acids

L-Alanine	37	L-Serine	128
L-Aspartic acid	93	L-Tyrosine	98
L-Cystine	22	L-Arginine[*]	61
L-Glutamic acid	186	L-Proline[†]	65
Glycine	93		

[*] Possibly essential in children
[†] Usually considered non-essential but Harries et al.[88] consider this needs re-examination

Table 1.6. Amino acids in human and cow's milk*
(g/16g nitrogen = average nitrogen/100 g protein)

	Cow's milk	Human breast milk
Arginine	3·7	3·4
Cystine	0·8	1·9
Histidine	2·7	2·2
Isoleucine	6·2	5·6
Leucine	9·9	9·4
Lysine	7·8	6·2
Methionine	2·4	2·1
Phenylalanine	5·1	4·0
Threonine	4·6	4·5
Tryptophan	1·4	1·6
Tyrosine	5·6	4·8
Valine	7·0	6·2
Alanine	3·7	3·8
Aspartic acid	8·2	9·3
Glutamic acid	22·2	19·8
Glycine	1·9	2·2
Proline	9·8	8·6
Serine	5·8	4·8

* Taken from McCance and Widdowson[89]

and natural protein is given in addition. One gram of natural protein provides approximately 50 mg phenylalanine. Vitamins and minerals are required and may be provided separately or be present in the protein substitute.

Essential amino acids and minimal requirements
Certain amino acids are essential since they cannot be synthesised endogenously at rates sufficient to support normal growth. The requirement of protein is also affected by the total nitrogen in the diet. Adequate amounts of non-essential nitrogen and calories from fat and carbohydrate are required to conserve essential amino acids since otherwise they would be degraded in order to supply energy. It is also important that a nutritionally adequate mixture of amino acids should

be ingested, otherwise optimum use of the amino acids cannot be made[29], and a portion of the daily intake of phenylalanine must be given with each helping of protein substitute. The requirements for essential and non-essential amino acids are given in Tables 1.4 and 1.5, and Table 1.6 compares the amino acid composition of human breast and cow's milk. It is essential to realise that marked differences in composition occur amongst milks and foods from different sources.

Phenylalanine requirements
In an elegant study, Snyderman et al.[30] determined the phenylalanine requirements of 6 infants aged 1–9 months. They found that the minimal phenylalanine intake compatible with normal health could be as low as 47 mg or up to about 90 mg/kg/day. Nitrogen in the diet was supplied by a mixture of 18 amino acids, all as the natural isomers. In the normal infant phenylalanine deficiency was associated with failure to gain weight, with impaired nitrogen retention, and the excretion pattern of free amino acids in the urine showed a large decrease in phenylalanine and certain other changes including increased histidinuria.

From the literature and her personal experience Francis[13] takes the daily theoretical requirement of phenylalanine per kg body weight for different age groups to be as follows:

> 70–90 mg at under 1 month
> decreasing to 35 mg at 2 years
> 30 mg at 2–8 years
> 25–27 mg by 10 years

These are only guides; there is considerable variation between different patients and even in any one patient, and in some of the atypical forms the patient may tolerate considerably more.

There is no general agreement about the exact concentration of phenylalanine in blood which is desirable. In recent years, as the dangers of phenylalanine deficiency have been recognised, less strict control of the blood phenylalanine concentration has become accepted in many centres. An important 8-year study has been in progress since 1967 in the USA, with many centres collaborating. Preliminary data show that the children with PKU are developing normally[10]. One group of children received a diet aimed at maintaining the phenylalanine between 1·0 and 5·4 mg/100 ml blood, and in a second group the aim was for levels of 5·5–10·0 mg/100 ml blood. In a paper presented in 1972 Koch and his colleagues stated that preliminary analysis of the data showed no significant differences between those maintained on a 'low' level of phenylalanine intake compared with those maintained on the more 'moderate' level. The final outcome of this trial is awaited with much interest. In the meantime practice varies, for example Hanley et al.[31] have allowed fasting levels of 5–15 mg/100 ml serum since late 1965; Wamberg[26] aims at a therapeutic level of 3–7 mg/100 ml serum; at the Hospital for Sick Children we now aim at concentrations of 3–8 mg/100 ml blood in the non-fasting patient.

In an excellent study Hanley et al.[31] looked at 32 children with PKU in whom dietary therapy was begun prior to 6 months of age. Three patients had shown evidence of severe phenylalanine deficiency during the first year of life. In two of them malnutrition was quickly corrected and the children developed normally. The third patient had prolonged malnutrition and his IQ was subsequently only 56. Signs of less severe but prolonged malnutrition were present in 16 of the patients despite apparently satisfactory diets and adequate serum levels of phenylalanine. Of these children 3 were reported as retarded, 5 were of borderline intelligence, 6 were dull normal, and only 2 were of normal intelligence. In 13 recently diagnosed patients, Hanley et al. allowed more liberal amounts of phenylalanine (50–100 mg phenylalanine/kg/24 hour during the first year of life) and on this regime fasting levels of serum phenylalanine were 5–15 mg/100 ml. Evidence of malnutrition in this group was much less, and when the patients were tested at 25–36 months of age, 9 were of normal intelligence, 4 were dull normal, and there were no borderline or retarded children.

Similar findings were observed by Smith[32] who studied 24 children who had been treated from early infancy at the Hospital for Sick Children since 1955. All of them were over four years of age when she studied them (range 4·25–16·6 years). From the case records she noted symptoms which had been recorded during the first year of life and which could be attributed to nutritional deficiency, i.e. rashes, hair loss, failure to thrive, periods of poor weight gain, diarrhoea, vomiting and recurrent infections. Prior to the performance of intelligence tests, she allocated the children to four groups according to the severity of clinical symptoms attributable to nutritional deficiency in the first year of life. Phenylalanine deficiency was not necessarily the only inadequate dietary factor in these patients but records show it was certainly very important. The results are given in Figure 1.1. The four

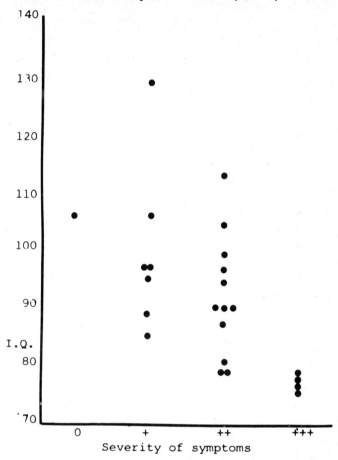

Figure 1.1. The relationship between IQ and symptoms of nutritional deficiency occurring in the first year of life in patients with early treated phenylketonuria (o = no symptoms, +++ = severe symptoms). Taken from Smith *et al*.[32]

patients with severe symptoms had IQ's of 80 or below. They were diagnosed at a time when it was usual to start treatment with diets containing little or no phenylalanine until its concentration in the blood was normal[33], and to continue with daily intakes of phenylalanine of 25 mg/kg or less. For these four patients the total phenylalanine intake was less than 100 mg/day for many weeks during the first year of life. The dietary management was later modified[34] and since 1964 all patients had received over 50 mg phenylalanine/kg from the commencement of diet. Smith found that the mean IQ of patients in whom treatment was started prior to 1964 was 85·9 and for those treated after 1964 it was 97·2 (p <0·05).

In addition to impairing intellectual function, phenylalanine deficiency produces other severe effects and will prove fatal if not recognised and treated. Rouse[35] has described the features of phenylalanine deficiency in two normal infants who were misdiagnosed and treated with a low-phenylalanine diet. They failed to gain weight, developed generalised erythematous rashes refractory to topical therapy, infections were frequent and they were very listless. After resuming normal diet their nutritional status improved but their developmental progress remained slow. Phenylalanine deficiency due to overtreatment of PKU has been fully described[36, 37]. Usually, but not exclusively, infants in the first year of life develop a severe bright red rash starting in the napkin region and intertriginous folds, and possibly spreading to other areas (see Figure 1.2). The baby fails to gain weight, becomes lethargic, refuses food and may vomit and death may ensue. Severe hair loss may be a feature. In addition, one fatal case of megaloblastic anaemia has been described[38]. It was thought that there was a dietary deficiency of folic acid or vitamin B_{12}, or of both superimposed on phenylalanine deficiency.

Smith[32] attempted to assess the importance of episodes of hyperphenylalaninaemia during treatment by studying the relationship between IQ and the duration of phenylalanine concentrations greater than 10 mg/100 ml in the first two years of life. She found that if a series of 24 patients at the Hospital for Sick Children was divided into two according to whether the total duration of phenylalanine concentrations above 10 mg/100 ml in the first two years was longer or shorter than 0·02 years, there was a significant difference in IQ (p < 0·01). Twelve children with a shorter period of hyperphenylalaninaemia had

---

Figure 1.2. Rash due to phenylalanine deficiency in a treated phenylketonuria infant

Figure 1.3. The vitamin deficiency state (a, b), Infant in severe deficiency with emaciation, pallor, scabbed external nares, fissured lips, skin lesions at the outer canthi of the eyelids and severe eruption on the buttocks; (c), psoriasiform patches in occipital region in a milder deficiency state; (d, e), typical facies in milder deficiency states. Taken from Mann et al. [48]

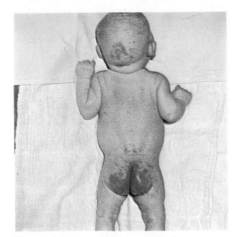

Figure 1.2

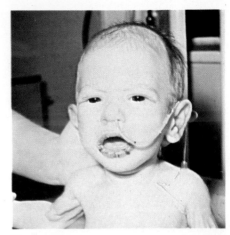

Figure 1.3a

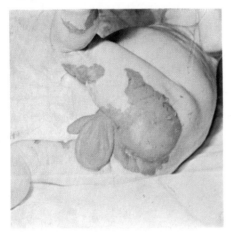

Figure 1.3b

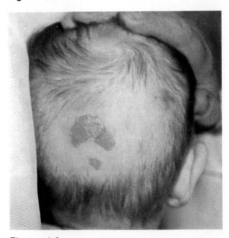

Figure 1.3c

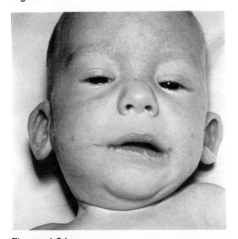

Figure 1.3d

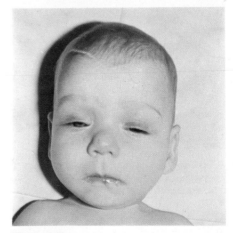

Figure 1.3e

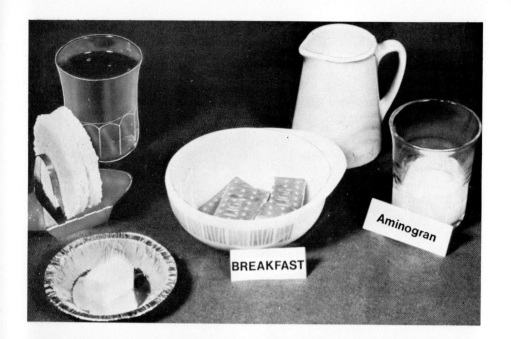

BREAKFAST

Aminogran

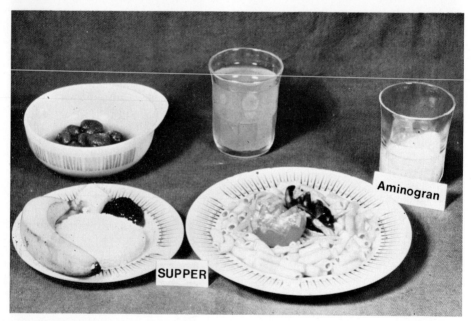

SUPPER

Aminogran

Figure 1.4 Typical meals. The amount of Aminogran at each meal is one third of the total daily intake. Each meal must contain one third of the total daily measured phenylalanine, usually in the form of milk, cereals, potato or crisps.

a mean IQ of 99·7 (SD 12·6) and 12 with a longer period had a mean IQ of 86·2 (SD 9·3). If the period before the start of treatment was omitted from the calculation, there was still a significant negative correlation between the duration of high phenylalanine concentrations and IQ. Long periods of hyperphenylalaninaemia during the treatment of classical PKU may therefore be an important cause of intellectual impairment.

Monitoring treatment

Because the effects of both under and overtreatment may be serious it is essential to monitor the diet by the determination of phenylalanine in blood, and the service must be prompt, regular and employ a micro method.

At the Hospital for Sick Children the practice is to use capillary samples of blood collected by heel or finger-prick on to special filter paper so that the level can be determined by a modification of the Guthrie test[39,40]. Additional standards are placed on the culture plates namely 1, 2, 4, 6, 8, 10, 12, 15 and 20 mg/100 ml, and very low levels can be recorded as 'less than 1 mg/100 ml'. Such a monitoring service is conveniently incorporated into a screening service. This ensures that positive results are continually being obtained and increases the interest of the technical staff. Unlike the experience of Belton et al.[41] the determination of lower concentrations has not been a problem, and correlation with liquid samples of blood determined on an amino acid analyser has been excellent.

The collection of the blood spots must be performed correctly[42] and the technique is usually taught to one of the infant's parents so that blood spots can be collected at home and the papers sent by post to the laboratory. If the patient is receiving antibiotics the Guthrie blood spot is eluted with acetone and the phenylalanine level determined by thin-layer chromatography[43]. Other methods for determining phenylalanine are satisfactory provided they use micro quantities of blood, for example a fluorimetric method[44] or a chromatographic method.

Phenylalanine concentrations should be determined regularly and a suitable regime is: –

(1) Twice weekly during stabilisation
(2) Weekly in infants
(3) At 2–3 week intervals in toddlers
(4) Monthly thereafter for the duration of the diet

During treatment *low phenylalanine* may occur for the following reasons:–

(1) The requirement for phenylalanine may have increased in association with an increased rate of growth

(2) The child may not be consuming the allowed amount of phenylalanine because he is refusing his food or vomiting. The measurement of the concentrated sources of phenylalanine may be inaccurate

(3) Determination of phenylalanine in the blood may be too infrequent

(4) The diagnosis may not be sufficiently precise and the patient may have a variant form of hyperphenylalaninaemia

High phenylalanine concentrations in the blood also arise from several causes:–

(1) From infections or any illness causing catabolism

(2) From lack of protein and calories in the diet

(3) There may be a reduced requirement in association with a reduced growth rate

(4) The child may have taken food from the larder or a friend

(5) The phenylalanine allowance may not be divided equally between meals. The blood test is most helpful if taken $3\frac{1}{2}$–4 hours after a meal

Vitamins

When substituting man-made products for natural foods and where natural food intake is greatly restricted, correct supplementation with vitamins becomes essential especially in infants and toddlers.

Severe and extensive skin eruptions in infants receiving a low phenylalanine preparation for the treatment of PKU were formerly seen not infrequently[45−47]. Though some of these rashes were undoubtedly due to phenylalanine deficiency it is most unlikely that this was the sole cause. A deficiency state characterised by disseminated lesions of a distinctive kind coupled with failure to thrive was described in 5 infants receiving synthetic milks[48]. Two deaths occurred before the nature of the disturbance was appreciated. These infants, who had metabolic disorders but not PKU, were receiving synthetic milks low in lactose, sodium or calcium.

The clinical picture found in the babies with this deficiency state is a striking one (see Figure 1.3). Most distinctive are the various skin lesions which, in the florid case may be itemised as follows:-

(1) A well-demarcated pink psoriaiform eruption affecting particularly the buttocks. The rash may extend forwards to involve the perineum and the external genitalia and posteriorly to the natal cleft and sacral region. Similar lesions may occur elsewhere, e.g. over the scalp and the lower limbs. The rash could be moist at first, with blistering on occasions, later becoming dry, scaly and glazed

(2) A pink, moist, or dry intertrigo of the groins

(3) Cracking of the lips often associated with exudation and bleeding

(4) Fissuring at the angles of the mouth and the outer canthi of the eyelids, again with exudation and sometimes bleeding

(5) Pink exudative lesions over the external ears especially the helices, with a tendency to crusting. The retro-auricular reflection of skin may be particularly affected

(6) In one fatal case crusting of the external nares was a persistent feature and assumed to be part of the generalised eruption

Other recurring features noted in the three severe cases were skin pallor, emaciation, anorexia and fatigue while feeding. Vomiting occurred frequently, coughing was troublesome, and irritability and restlessness occurred, especially at night. Abdominal distension was a constant development as the patient's condition slowly deteriorated. There was a striking tendency for septic lesions to be a late complication.

The unusual and distinctive lesions affecting the lips and eyes are a feature of these nutritionally disturbed infants. While lip fissuring alone has been described in cases of riboflavine deficiency[49], our patients were not only receiving adequate amounts of this vitamin but failed to respond to additional large supplements.

A series of studies on young rats supported the clinical impression that the 2 infant deaths were due to a deficiency state. This was subsequently shown to be likely when complete vitamin supplements were given to 3 other similarly affected infants and led to rapid clinical improvement. I have never observed this particular syndrome subsequently in any patient receiving the complete vitamin supplement. The vitamins may be present in the synthetic manufactured protein substitute or may need to be given separately. The total daily intake should be:-

1	Aneurine hydrochloride	3·0	mg
2	Riboflavine	3·0	mg
3	Pyridoxine hydrochloride	0·99	mg
4	Nicotinamide	9·9	mg
5	Calcium pantothenate	3·48	mg
6	Ascorbic acid	49·8	mg
7	α-Tocopheryl acetate	15·0	mg
8	Inositol	150·0	mg
9	Biotin	0·51	mg
10	Folic acid	0·75	mg
11	Acetomenaphthone	1·5	mg
12	Vitamin A	2500	units
13	Vitamin D	400	units
14	Choline chloride	150·0	mg
15	Cyancobalamin	12·5	μg

1–11 are provided by 3 Ketovite tablets daily and 12–15 by 5 ml Ketovite (supplement) liquid daily (Paines and Byrne Ltd).

It appears that high levels of vitamins may be necessary for optimal growth in the early months of life when metabolism is proceeding at a very rapid rate. Mann et al.[48] compared the age at which the synthetic foods together with the inadequate vitamin supplements were first given, and the time taken for the rash to appear thereafter. Although it was impossible to assess the part played by the primary disease under treatment in the time taken for the rash to develop, it is of interest that the most rapid appearance of the eruption was in the oldest babies (see Table 1.7) whose vitamin reserves may have been by this time less plentiful.

Every patient receiving dietary treatment for PKU must therefore receive a complete vitamin supplement, and the diet of each patient should be considered most carefully from this point of view. For example: Minafen (Cow and Gate) does not contain vitamins A, D, C, B_{12} and choline and Ketovite tablets and liquid should be given; Aminogran (Allen and Hanburys) contains no added vitamins and it is essential to give the complete supplement each day.

Minerals and trace metals
Synthetic diets such as those used in the treatment of PKU may lack

Table 1.7. Time of appearance of rash in infants receiving synthetic diets and incomplete vitamin supplements

Patient	1	2	A	B	C
Age when synthetic food and incomplete vitamin supplement was given	7 days	15 days	10 weeks	5 months	6 months
Period on diet before rash appeared	10 weeks	7 weeks	10 weeks	2 weeks	4 weeks

essential trace metals to varying extents and therefore may require supplementation. The daily intakes of copper, magnesium, manganese and zinc recommended by different authors differ widely[50-52], and the requirements of cobalt, chromium and molybdenum have not been established with any certainty[52]. Nickel has been regarded as a contaminant in human metabolism but recent workers[53, 54] have suggested that it may come to be regarded as an essential trace metal; there is no recommended intake.

Mineral and trace metal supplements used in Britain are based on a mixture originally devised by Dent and Westall[55], and later modified [56, 57] in the light of the trace metal content of one litre of cow's milk. Examples of some minerals and trace metals in, or used in conjunction with, synthetic diets in the treatment of patients with PKU are shown in Table 1.8.

Recent studies[58] comprising metabolic balances in healthy children eating normal food and patients receiving synthetic diets, have provided some more data. They have shown that Aminogran mineral mixture (Allen and Hanburys) and Metabolic Mineral Mixture (Scientific Hospital Supplies) (see Table 1.8) are low in zinc, iron, copper and manganese and require adjusting in the following ways:– zinc, a 4-fold increase: copper, a 2-fold increase, iron, increased by 25%: and manganese, to provide 60 μg/kg body weight daily. The patients' diets also contained other items contributing to the intake of trace elements e.g. cow's milk, protein-free bread and fruit. On the other hand, Minafen (see Table 1.8) appeared to be adequate for the young infant with regard to trace elements.

Table 1.8. Minerals and trace metals contained (per 100 g product) by two protein substitutes and by two mineral mixtures intended for use in synthetic diets

	Aminogran[*] mineral mixture	Metabolic[†] mineral mixture	Minafen[‡] powder	Albumaid[§] XP
Calcium	8·20 g	8·20 g	0·5 g	0·8–1·0 g
Potassium	8·30 g	8·30 g	0·32 g	1·0–1·3 g
Sodium	4·00 g	3·96 g	0·32 g	1·0–1·3 g
Magnesium	0·97 g	0·97 g	11·00 mg	150 mg
Iron	50·30 mg	50·00 mg	5·8 mg	20 mg
Copper	6·30 mg	6·30 mg	0·4 mg	2 mg
Zinc	12·00 mg	10·50 mg	0·16 mg	1·2 mg
Manganese	5·70 mg	5·70 mg	0·16 mg	2·2 mg
Iodine	0·765 mg	0·76 mg	100·0 μg	0·08 mg
Aluminium	30 μg	20 μg	Not added	0·002 mg
Cobalt	105 μg	80 μg	Not added	0·008 mg
Molybdenum	198 μg	150 μg	Not added	0·015 mg
Phosphate	17·85 g	18·10 g	0·555 g	1·0 g

[*] Allen and Hanburys: used with Aminogran food supplement
[†] Scientific Hospital Supplies: used with P.K. Aid I and II food supplements
[‡] Allen and Hanburys: used in infants
[§] Scientific Hospital Supplies: used in infants and children

In the healthy children[58] the intake of calcium was 900 mg daily at three months, falling to 550 mg at one year and then rising to 700 mg at 8·5 years; these are similar to the findings of Beal[59] though Macy[50] recorded a somewhat higher intake. Excretion and retention agreed well with Macy's figures taking into account the greater number of children under 4 years of age in the studies of Alexander et al.[58]. The ratio of calcium to phosphorus was 0·76 for the diet of the healthy children which agrees with Macy's value of 0·77[50].

From their studies on the healthy children, Alexander et al.[58] have formulated a new mineral and trace metal mixture. It is sufficient to provide patients receiving synthetic diets in which few or no additional foods are allowed, with adequate amounts of all the essential minerals and trace metals. It is necessary to have two preparations so that the intakes of minerals and trace elements can be adjusted to the weight of the infant or child (see Table 1.9).

Hazards of the diet

A synthetic diet presents several serious problems and in PKU they are:–

(1) The diet, although as satisfactory as present knowledge permits, may nonetheless not be ideal for the growth and development of the infant and child

(2) Phenylalanine deficiency can of itself lead to intellectual impairment and must be avoided

(3) A strict diet causes emotional problems in the patient and in his family

The first two points are dealt with elsewhere in this chapter. The diet is usually accepted without much difficulty in infancy, but during the toddler stage and later years of childhood many children grow to dislike the food, especially the protein substitute, and as a result tensions and anxieties occur in the families[60]. The emotional problems were studied in some detail in 12 children who had PKU when an amino acid mixture (Aminogran) was used instead of an hydrolysate-based preparation (Cymogran)[61]. All the parents reported that problems began at the toddler age; finickiness, fussiness and periods of refusal lead to real battles at mealtimes, and sometimes there was a need for forced feeding. Many children showed such features as a dislike of dirty hands or clothes, and some of them particularly liked savoury foods such as salad cream on spaghetti and curry sauce. Some showed temper tantrums, anxiety, dependent clinging and night terrors. Bentovim et al.[60] found that the impact on family life varied and in some instances social life for the parents was restricted and there was a tendency to overprotection and over-involvement with the child. These emotional problems and hence the quality of the family life improved when Cymogran was replaced by Aminogran since the children accepted the latter easily and fed it to themselves instead of having to be spooned or force-fed. It was apparent from these studies that efforts to improve the palatability of these diets should continue.

Termination of dietary restrictions

The optimal age at which the low phenylalanine diet may be stopped is

Table 1.9. A mineral and trace metal mixture recommended for use with severely restricted diets*

Element	Daily intake from Mixture A	Daily intake/kg body weight from Mixture B	Calculated total daily intake from Mixtures A and B at three given body weights (observed values from actual balance data on children are in parentheses)		
			10 kg	20 kg	30 kg
Na	0	78 mg	780 mg (793)	1560 mg (1572)	2340 mg (2340)
K	880 mg	18·8 mg	1075 mg (1066)	1255 mg (1250)	1445 mg (1448)
Ca	20 mg	4 mg	560 mg (558)	600 mg (600)	640 mg (640)
Mg	50 mg	4·2 mg	92 mg (92·5)	134 mg (135)	176 mg (176)
Fe	2 mg	0·166 mg	3·66 mg (3·6)	5·32 mg (5·3)	6·98 mg (6·95)
Cu	100 µg	220 µg	300 µg (302)	500 µg (510)	700 µg (715)
Zn	3·2 µg	50 µg	3·7 mg (3·65)	4·2 mg (4·2)	4·7 mg (4·7)
Mn	0	60 µg	0·6 mg (0·51)	1·20 mg (1·50)	1·8 mg
Mo	13 µg	2 µg	33 µg (32·5)	53 µg (52)	73 µg (71)
Co	33 µg	2 µg	53 µg (52·5)	73 µg (73)	93 µg (95)
Cr	23 µg	0·5 µg	28 µg (27·5)	33 µg (32·5)	38 µg (37)
I†	300 µg				

* Taken from Alexander et al.[57]. This recommendation has not yet been used in a clinical trial. Two mixtures are necessary: A is given in constant amount and B is given in relation to body weight

† Alexander et al.[57] did not include iodine in their study, but it should be included in Mixture A

not known and opinions vary so that some workers feel it is safe at three years, others that it is never safe and yet others who compromise at some age in between. As Parker[62] has pointed out, even within the same clinic at Los Angeles, clinicians hold differing opinions. His own preference was the age of ten years since he felt this allowed for maximum brain development.

Although Murphy[63,64] returned two children to a low phenylalanine diet after they had shown deterioration in IQ and behaviour on a normal diet, this appears to be an unusual happening. The major worry is that deterioration may occur so slowly that it escapes clinical detection until it has proceeded for many years. However, the psychological effects of such a strict diet particularly in adolescence, are so overwhelming that most clinicians do in fact advise stopping the diet at some stage prior to this age.

Kang, Sallee and Gerald[5] stopped the diet in all patients treated from an early age when the mean age of the group was 51 months. When they reported after the group had been off the diet for a mean period of 26·8 months, there had been no detectable clinical changes. They also stopped treatment in 15 late-treated children and after a mean period of 45 months off the diet there was no significant change. Hudson and Hawcroft[65] described five early treated children who had been taking normal diet for 15 months to nearly 10 years, having stopped treatment at ages between 3 and 6 years. Repeated IQ testing showed some variation in results but though the changes were generally small they were all in a downward direction. These workers felt however that the psychological advantages of freeing the patients from the diet far outweighed any other disadvantage.

In our clinic's practice diet has been stopped for as long as $5\frac{1}{2}$ years, at first in older children of 10 and 12 but now routinely in patients of 7 or 8 years. There has been no evidence of any deterioration, but it is not uncommon for parents to complain of behaviour problems and these tend to occur when the blood phenylalanine rises above 35 mg/ 100 ml[66]. Parents may become very worried at the time of stopping the diet as they have been obsessed with it for so long and they need much support. The patient is of course delighted, and life for the whole family is greatly eased and improved. A normal intake of phenylalanine may be introduced in hospital with the change from a low intake to a normal intake being made in one step. The patient is likely to show disturbed behaviour with swings of mood for about three weeks and then settles down. Alternatively, phenylalanine intake may be increased gradually and then no behaviour changes are observed[67].

It has been suggested that the decreased myelin synthesis seen in the presence of raised phenylalanine may be due to alteration of the free amino acid pool in the brain during the vulnerable period of brain development. Much of the wet weight of the adult brain is accounted for by myelin which is not in a dynamic state and therefore cannot be early drawn upon to meet a metabolic need. Thus early in life is the time when myelin formation is vulnerable. Davison[69] concluded that in the human infant the vulnerable time for impaired myelination is the seventh gestational month to the first few months of postnatal life. However, more recent studies on 139 complete human brains ranging in age from 10 weeks gestation to 7 years led Dobbing and Sands[70] to conclude that the growth-spurt complex, including myelination, may possibly continue into the fourth or fifth postnatal year. Thereafter the human brain increases in weight until adolescence, and it is likely that deposition of myelin continues until the age of 15–20 years[71].

In view of these experimental findings it is easy to see why the clinician is perturbed about the best course to adopt with his patients. I think it is probable that in the future, early treated patients taken off diet may be advised to limit their intake of first-class protein so that blood phenylalanine concentrations do not rise above about 25–35 mg/100 ml.

TREATMENT OF MATERNAL PHENYLKETONURIA

The children of mothers with untreated phenylketonuria have a very high incidence of congenital abnormalities[72, 73], including mental retardation, intrauterine and postnatal retardation of growth, microcephaly, skeletal, cardiac and ocular malformations. There is also an increased miscarriage rate. Patients treated from early life are now reaching reproductive age and it has been suggested[74] that planned pregnancies with dietary restriction during the fertile period and during any subsequent pregnancies is the only way of avoiding the teratogenic effect of phenylalanine.

Recent work[75] has shown that the activities of phenylalanine: pyruvate and tyrosine:α-ketoglutarate aminotransferases are much lower in the foetus than in the child. It has been known for some time that amino acid concentrations in the foetal liver[76] and circulation[77–80] are much higher than those in the maternal liver and circulation, and this could well be a reflection of the relative inability of the foetal aminotransferases to metabolise the amino acids further. Foetal rat liver is also deficient in tyrosine aminotransferase activity[81]. It is possible that a number of the aminotransferases in foetal liver are also somewhat inactive, although the tyrosine enzyme does appear to be particularly late maturing. Also serum concentrations of phenylalanine are higher in pregnant heterozygous women than in non-pregnant heterozygous women or non-pregnant controls[82].

The diet during pregnancy presents many problems and is potentially hazardous since under-nutrition and malnutrition in the prenatal period can affect brain development[83]. It has been made a little easier perhaps now that amino acids may be used instead of a hydrolysate. Such information as there is suggests that 10–30 mg phenylalanine/kg body weight is the requirement, and the daily intake of protein should be 1·0 g/kg body weight daily and not less than 50 g total made up of natural foods and amino acids. A low phenylalanine diet has been used successfully for varying periods during several pregnancies. For example Allan and Brown[84] maintained a patient on a low phenyla-lanine diet (Albumaid) during the last 5 months of pregnancy using a daily intake of phenylalanine of 10 mg/kg body weight. At the time of reporting when the infant was 9 months old, he appeared physically and mentally normal, though he may have had a mild microcephaly. Farquhar, Miller and Lindsay[85] treated a patient from the twentieth week of pregnancy. They used Aminogran and when the infant was 17 weeks old there was no evidence of damage.

I wish to acknowledge the help and teaching I have received from the dietitians at the Hospital for Sick Children and especially from Miss D. E. M. Francis, who has provided some examples of actual diets.

EXAMPLES OF TYPICAL DIETS

Regime for an infant of 3 kg fed 4 hourly × 5 feeds daily using a hydrolysate-based preparation (Minafen) as the protein substitute

	Protein (g)	Calories	Phenyl-alanine (mg)
(1) 30 ml milk/kg/day = 90 ml (3 oz) ÷ 15 ml (½ oz) at 4 feeds + 30 ml (1 oz) at 1 feed Give before each Minafen feed (Replace if rejected or vomited)	3·0	60	150
(2) 30 g Minafen/kg/day = 90 g (3 oz) Boiled water to 450 ml (12 oz) = 20% solution ÷ 90 ml (3 oz) at 5 feeds × 4 hourly Give after milk supplement	11·25	458	<18
Total/day	14·25	518	168
Total/kg/day	4·8	173	56
Theoretical total/kg/day	4·5	125 ± 25	Initially 50–60

NOTE:

(i) If the infant wakes at night (e.g. 2 a.m.) fruit juice or 5% dextrose can be given

(ii) If the infant cannot consume all the milk plus at least ¾ of the Minafen daily, a more frequent feeding schedule, e.g. 3 hourly × 6, 7 or 8 feeds daily may be indicated. Extra Minafen can be given according to appetite in a fast growing infant

(iii) 5 ml Ketovite liquid together with 50 mg ascorbic acid or 3 crushed Ketovite tablets should be given daily

Regime for an infant of 3 kg fed 4 hourly × 5 feeds daily using an amino acid based preparation (Aminogran) as the protein substitute

	Protein + amino acid (g)	Calories	Phenyl-alanine (mg)
(1) 30 ml milk/kg/day = 90 ml ÷ 15 ml (½ oz) at 4 feeds + 30 ml (1 oz) at 1 feed. Give before each Aminogran feed (Replace if rejected or vomited)	3·0	60	150
(2) 150 ml Aminogran recipe/kg/day			
i.e. 9 g Aminogran food supplement	9·0	36	Nil
4·5 g Mineral Mixture (Allen & Hanburys)	–	–	–
22·5 g glucose and/or sugar	–	90	–
40 ml Prosparol (BDH)	–	180	–
14 ml rosehip or black-currant juice	–	30	–
Boiled water to 450 ml ÷ 90 ml at 5 feeds × 4 hourly Give after milk supplement			
Total/day	12·0	390	150
Total/kg/day	4·0	130	50
Theoretical total/kg/day	3 from amino acids + natural protein	125 ± 25	Initially 50–60

NOTE:

(i) If the infant wakes at night (e.g. 2 a.m.) fruit juice or 5% dextrose can be given

(ii) If the infant cannot consume all the milk plus at least 90% of the Aminogran daily, a more frequent feeding schedule, e.g. 3 hourly × 6, 7 or 8 feeds daily may be indicated

(iii) 3 Ketovite tablets (crushed) + 5 ml Ketovite liquid daily are essential with this regime, as vitamin supplements

(iv) Natural fruit juice is used as a flavouring and source of natural trace minerals

Girl of 20 kg aged 5 years, using an amino acid based preparation (Aminogran) as the protein substitute

	Protein + amino acids (g)	Calories	Phenyl-alanine (mg)
DAILY			
40 g Aminogran food supplement	40	160	Nil
8 g mineral mixture (Allen and Hanburys)	Nil	Nil	Nil
30 g sugar and/or flavouring	Nil	120	Nil
Add water to mix to the desired consistency; divide into 3 portions and give one before each main meal			
3 Ketovite tablets			
5 ml Ketovite liquid			
BREAKFAST			
(Aminogran mixture)			
1 Weetabix (20 g)	2·0	50	100
30 ml milk	1·0	20	50
1 slice (30 g) Rite Diet protein-free bread	0·2	100	3·6
2 small tomatoes	1·0	30	20
Fruit juice	Trace	50	Trace
MID-MORNING			
Fruit juice	Trace	50	Trace
1 Aminex biscuit	0·1	50	2·9

	Protein + amino acids (g)	Calories	Phenyl- alanine (mg)
LUNCH			
(Aminogran mixture)			
40 g potato crisps	2·0	224	100
4 slices (120 g) Rite Diet protein- free bread	0·8	312	14·4
Tomar margarine (20 g)	Nil	150	Nil
Jam	Nil	40	Nil
1 orange	0·4	50	20
1 banana	0·8	50	40
TEA			
Cup of tea with 'no-protein milk'*	Nil	20	Nil
Sugar	Nil	20	Nil
1 Aminex biscuit	0·1	50	2·9
SUPPER			
(Aminogran mixture)			
20 g baked beans	1·0	25	50
60 g potato chips	2·0	140	100
Fried onion (1 medium)	0·9	14	20
Runner beans (2 large tablespoons)	0·6	4	20
Tinned peaches (3 halves) ⎱ made	0·6	115	30
2 Aminex biscuits ⎬ into a	0·3	100	5·8
Tomar margarine ⎰ crumble	Nil	36	Nil
Total/day	53·8	1980	579·6
Total/kg/day	2·7	99	29
Theoretical total/kg/day	2 from Aminogran + natural protein	80–100	†

* No-protein milk; 30 g sugar, 30 ml prosparol, water to 300 ml
† As individually tolerated according to blood test. If food is not eaten it must be replaced by an equivalent amount of phenylalanine

REFERENCES

1. Clayton, B. E., Moncrieff, A. and Roberts, G. E. (1967). Dietetic treatment of phenylketonuria. A follow-up study. *Brit. Med. J.*, **iii**, 133
2. Baumeister, A. A. (1967). The effects of dietary control on intelligence in phenylketonuria. *Amer. J. Ment. Def.*, **71**, 840
3. Fuller, R. N. and Shuman, J. B. (1969). Phenylketonuria and intelligence: trimodal response to dietary treatment. *Nature (London)*, **221**, 639
4. Hudson, F. P., Mordaunt, V. L. and Leahy, I. (1970). Evaluation of treatment begun in first three months of life in 184 cases of phenylketonuria. *Arch. Dis. Childh.*, **45**, 5
5. Kang, E. S., Sollee, N. D. and Gerald, P. S. (1970). Results of treatment and termination of the diet in phenylketonuria (PKU). *Pediatrics*, **46**, 881
6. Bessman, S. P. (1966). Legislation and advances in medical knowledge—acceleration or inhibition? *J. Pediatrics*, **69**, 334
7. Birch, H. G. and Tizard, J. (1967). The dietary treatment of phenylketonuria: Not proven? *Devel. Med. and Child Neurol*, **9**, 9
8. Medical Research Council Working Party on Phenylketonuria. (1968). Present status of different mass screening procedures for phenylketonuria. *Brit. Med. J.*, **iv**, 7
9. Bickel, H. (1970). Phenylalaninaemia or classical phenylketonuria (PKU). *Neuropädiatrie*, **I**, 379
10. Koch, R., Dobson, J. C., Blaskovics, M., Williamson, M. L., Ernest, A. E., Friedman, E. G. and Parker, C. E. (1973). Collaborative study of children treated for phenylketonuria. *Treatment of Inborn Errors of Metabolism*, p. 3. (J. W. T. Seakins, R. A. Saunders and C. Toothill, editors). (London: Churchill Livingstone)
11. Levy, H. L., Karolkewicz, V., Houghton, S. A. and MacCready, R. A. (1970). Screening the normal population in Massachusetts for phenylketonuria. *New Eng. J. Med.*, **282**, 1455
12. MRC/DHSS Phenylketonuria Register. Newsletter No. 1. April 1973
13. Francis, D. E. M. (1974). *Diets for Sick Children.* (In press). (Oxford: Blackwell Scientific Publications)
14. Malamud, N. (1966). Neuropathology of phenylketonuria. *J. Neuropath. Exp. Neurol.*, **25**, 254
15. Menkes, J. H. (1968). Cerebral proteolipids in phenylketonuria. *Neurology*, **18**, 1003
16. Agrawal, H. C., Bone, A. H. and Davison, A. N. (1969). Inhibition of brain protein synthesis by phenylalanine. *Biochem. J.*, **112**, 27P
17. Chase, H. P. and O'Brien, D. (1970). Effect of excess phenylalanine and of other amino acids on brain development in the infant rat. *Ped. Res.*, **4**, 96
18. Neame, K. D. (1961). Phenylalanine as inhibitor of transport of amino acids in brain. *Nature (London)*, **192**, 173

19. Tashian, R. E. (1961). Inhibition of brain glutamic acid decarboxylase by phenylalanine, valine and leucine derivatives; a suggestion concerning the aetiology of the neurological defects in phenylketonuria and branched-chain ketonuria. *Metabolism*, **10**, 393

20. Gruemer, H. D., Grannis, G. F., Hetland, L. B. and Costantini, M. L. (1971). Amino acid transport and mental retardation. *Clin. Chem.*, **17**, 1129

21. Hanson, A. (1958). Inhibition of brain glutamic acid decarboxylase by phenylalanine metabolites. *Naturwissenschaften*, **45**, 423

22. Woolley, D. W. and van der Hoeven, T. (1964). Serotonin deficiency in infancy as one cause of a mental defect in phenylketonuria. *Science*, **144**, 883

23. Perry, T. L., Hansen, S., Tishchler, B., Bunting, R. and Diamond, S. (1970). Glutamine depletion in phenylketonuria. *New Eng. J. Med.*, **282**, 761

24. H.M. (69) 72. National Health Service. Screening for early detection of phenylketonuria

25. O'Grady, D. J., Berry, H. K. and Sutherland, B. S. (1970). Phenylketonuria: Intellectual development and early treatment. *Dev. Med. Child. Neurol.*, **12**, 343

26. Wamberg, E. (1973). A survey of centralised treatment of phenylketonuria in Denmark. *Treatment of Inborn Errors of Metabolism*, p. 35. (J. W. T. Seakins, R. A. Saunders and C. Toothill, editors). (London: Churchill Livingstone)

27. Clayton, B. E., Heeley, A. F. and Heeley, M. (1970). An investigation of the hyperaminoaciduria in phenylketonuria associated with the feeding of certain commercial low-phenylalanine preparations. *Br. J. Nutr.*, **24**, 573

28. Martin, A. J. P. and Synge, R. L. M. (1945). Analytical chemistry of the proteins. *Adv. Protein Chem.*, **2**, 1

29. Cannon, P. R., Steffee, C. H., Frazier, L. J., Rowley, D. A. and Stepto, R. C. (1947). The influence of time of ingestion of essential amino acids upon utilization in tissue synthesis. *Fed. Proc.*, **6**, 390

30. Snyderman, S. E., Pratt, E. L., Cheung, M. W., Norton, P., Holt, E. L. Jr., Hansen, A. E. and Panos, T. C. (1955). The phenylalanine requirement of the normal infant. *J. Nurt.*, **56**, 253

31. Hanley, W. B., Linsao, L., Davidson, W. and Moes, C. A. F. (1970). Malnutrition with early treatment of phenylketonuria. *Pediat. Res.*, **4**, 318

32. Smith, I., Lobascher, M. and Wolff, O. H. (1973). Factors influencing outcome in early treated phenylketonuria. *Treatment of Inborn Errors of Metabolism*, p. 41. (J. W. T. Seakins, R. A. Saunders and C. Toothill, editors). (London: Churchill Livingstone)

33. Woolf, L. I., Griffiths, R. and Moncrieff, A. (1955). Treatment of phenyl-ketonuria with a diet low in phenylalanine. *Brit. Med. J.*, **i**, 57

34. Clayton, B. E., Francis, D. and Moncrieff, A. (1965). A method of feeding the phenylketonuric infant. *Brit. Med. J.*, **i**, 54

35. Rouse, B. M. (1966). Phenylalanine deficiency syndrome. *J. Ped.*, **69**, 246

36. Report to the Medical Research Council of the Conference on Phenyl-ketonuria (1963). Treatment of phenylketonuria. *Brit. Med. J.*, **i**, 1691
37. Pitt, D. (1967). Phenylalanine maintenance in phenylketonuria. *Aust. Pediat. J.*, **3**, 161
38. Royston, N. J. W. and Parry, T. E. (1962). Megaloblastic anaemia com-plicating dietary treatment of phenylketonuria in infancy. *Arch. Dis. Childh.*, **37**, 430
39. Guthrie, R. and Susi, A. (1963). A simple phenylalanine method of detect-ing phenylketonuria in large populations of newborn infants. *Pediatrics*, **32**, 338
40. Lemag Working Party (1971). Estimation of blood phenylalanine from a dried blood spot using the Guthrie test. *J. Clin. Path.*, **24**, 576
41. Belton, N. R., Crombie, J. D., Robins, S. P., Stephen, R. and Farquhar, J. W. (1973). Measurement of phenylalanine in routine care of phenyl-ketonuric children. *Arch. Dis. Childh.*, **48**, 472
42. Clayton, B. E. and Jenkins, P. (1970). Collection of Blood for the Guthrie Test. *Midwife and Health Visitor*, **6**, 170
43. Ersser, R. (1971). *Chromatography in Clinical Biochemistry using Flexible Thin Layers.* (Koch-Light-Laboratories Ltd., England)
44. McCaman, M. W. and Robins, E. (1962). Fluorimetric method for the determination of phenylalanine in serum. *J. Lab. Clin. Med.*, **59**, 885
45. Moncrieff, A. and Wilkinson, R. H. (1961). Further experience in the treatment of phenylketonuria. *Brit. Med. J.*, **i**, 763
46. Brimblecombe, F. S. W., Blainey, J. D., Stoneman, M. E. R. and Wood, B. S. B. (1961). Dietary and biochemical control of phenylketonuria. *Brit. Med. J.*, **ii**, 793
47. Wilson, K. M. and Clayton, B. E. (1962). Importance of choline during growth with particular reference to synthetic diets in phenylketonuria. *Arch. Dis. Childh.*, **37**, 565
48. Mann, T. P., Wilson, K. M. and Clayton, B. E. (1965). A deficiency state arising in infants on synthetic foods. *Arch. Dis. Childh.*, **40**, 364
49. Spies, T. D., Vilter, R. W. and Ashe, W. F. (1939). Pellagra, beriberi and riboflavin deficiency in human beings. *J. Amer. Med. Ass.*, **113**, 931
50. Macy, I. G. (1942). *Nutrition and Chemical Growth in Childhood.* Vols I and II. (Springfield, Illinois: Thomas)
51. Berfenstram, R. (1952). Studies on Blood Zinc. A clinical and experi-mental investigation into the zinc content of plasma and blood corpuscles with special reference to infancy. *Acta Paed. Scand.*, **41**, Suppl, 87, 389
52. Engel, R. W., Price, N. O. and Miller, R. F. (1967). Copper, Manganese, Cobalt and Molybdenum in Pre-adolescent girls. *J. Nutr.*, **92**, 197
53. McNeeley, M. D., Sunderman, F. W., Nechay, M. W. and Levine, H. (1971). Abnormal concentrations of nickel in serum in cases of myocardial infarction, stroke, burns, hepatic cirrhosis and uremia. *Clin. Chem.*, **17**, 1123

54. Schroeder, H. A. and Nason, A. P. (1971). Trace-element analysis in clinical chemistry. *Clin. Chem.*, **17**, 461

55. Dent, C. E. and Westall, R. G. (1961). Studies in maple syrup urine disease. *Arch. Dis. Childh.*, **36**, 259

56. Westall, R. G. (1963). Dietary treatment of a child with maple syrup urine disease (branched chain ketoaciduria). *Arch. Dis. Childh.*, **38**, 485

57. Francis, D. E. M. and Dixon, D. J. W. (1970). *Diets for sick children*, pp. 220–2, 258–61, 293–6, (Oxford: Blackwell Scientific Publications)

58. Alexander, F. W., Clayton, B. E. and Delves, H. T. (1974). Mineral and trace metal balances in children. *Quart. J. Med.*, **43**, 89

59. Beal, V. A. (1957). On the acceptance of solid foods, and other food patterns of infants and children. *Pediatrics*, **20**, 448

60. Bentovim, A. (1968). Controlled observations of phenylketonuric children on and during withdrawal from low phenylalanine diet. *Arch. Dis. Childh.*, **43**, 745

61. Bentovim, A., Clayton, B. E., Francis, D. E. M., Shepherd, J. and Wolff, O. H. (1960). Use of an amino acid mixture in treatment of phenylketonuria. *Arch. Dis. Childh.*, **45**, 640

62. Parker, C. E. (1973). Remarks on the long term aspects of phenylketonuria. *Treatment of Inborn Errors of Metabolism*, p. 19. (J. W. T. Seakins, R. A. Saunders and C. Toothill, editors). (London: Churchill Livingstone)

63. Murphy, D. (1963). Termination of dietary treatment of phenylketonuria. *Irish. J. Med. Sci.*, **6**, 355

64. Murphy, D. (1969). Termination of dietary treatment of phenylketonuria. *Irish J. Med. Sci.*, **2** (7), 177

65. Hudson, F. P. and Hawcroft, J. (1973). Duration of treatment in phenylketonuria. *Treatment of Inborn Errors of Metabolism*, p. 51 (J. W. T. Seakins, R. A. Saunders and C. Toothill, editors). (London: Churchill Livingstone)

66. Smith, I. Personal communication

67. Holtzman, N. A. (1973). Personal communication

68. Agrawal, H. C., Bone, A. H. and Davison, A. N. (1970). Effect of phenylalanine on protein synthesis in the developing rat brain. *Biochem. J.*, **117**, 325

69. Davison, A. N. (1970). *Myelination*, p. 100–43. (Illinois: Charles C. Thomas)

70. Dobbing, J. and Sands, J. (1973). Quantitative growth and development of human brain. *Arch. Dis. Childh*, **48**, 757

71. Davison, A. N. (1970). *Myelination*, pp. 166–70. (Illinois: Charles C. Thomas)

72. Yu, J. S. and O'Halloran, M. T. (1970). Children of mothers with phenylketonuria. *Lancet*, **i**, 210

73. Leader (1970). Maternal phenylketonuria. *Brit. Med. J.*, **iv**, 192

74. Yu, J. and O'Halloran, M. (1970). Children of mothers with phenylketonuria. *Aust. Paed. J.*, **6**, 157

75. McLean, A., Marwick, M. J. and Clayton, B. E. (1973). Enzymes involved in phenylalanine metabolism in the human foetus and child. *J. Clin. Path.*, **26**, 678

76. Ryan, W. L. and Carver, M. J. (1966). Free amino acids of human foetal and adult liver. *Nature (London)*, **212**, 292

77. Crumpler, H. R., Dent, C. E. and Lindan, O. (1950). Amino Acid pattern in human foetal and maternal plasma at delivery. *Biochem, J.*, **47**, 223

78. Kerr, G. R. and Waisman, H. A. (1966). Phenylalanine transplacental concentrations in Rhesus monkeys. *Science*, **151**, 824

79. Ghadimi, H. and Pecora, P. (1964). Free amino acids of cord plasma as compared with maternal plasma during pregnancy. *Pediatrics*, **33**, 500

80. Schain, R. J., Carver, M. J. and Copenhaver, J. H. (1967). Protein metabolism in the developing brain: Influence of birth and gestational age. *Science*, **156**, 984

81. Sereni, F., Kenney, F. T. and Kretchmer, N. (1959). Factors influencing the development of tyrosine –α–ketoglutarate transaminase activity in rat liver. *J. Biol. Chem.*, **234**, 609

82. Kang, E. and Paine, R. S. (1963). Elevation of plasma phenylalanine levels during pregnancies of women heterozygous for phenylketonuria. *J. Pediat*, **63**, 283

83. Dobbing, J. (1968). Vulnerable periods in developing brain. *Applied Neurochemistry*, p. 28 (A. N. Davison and J. Dobbing, editors). (Oxford: Blackwell Scientific Publications)

84. Allan, J. D. and Brown, J. K. (1968). *Some Recent Advances in Inborn Errors of Metabolism*, p. 14. (K. S. Holt and V. P. Coffey, editors). (London and Edinburgh: E. S. Livingstone)

85. Farquhar, J. W., Miller, M. C. and Lindsay, G. (1971). Maternal phenylketonuria. *Brit. Med. J.*, **i**, 46

86. Macy, F. G. and Kelly, H. J. (1961). *Milk: The mammary gland and its secretion*, pp. 265–304. (H. S. K. Kon and A. T. Cowie, editors). (New York: Academic Press)

87. Holt, L. E. Jr. (1967). Amino acid requirements of infants. *Curr. Therap. Res.*, **9**, 149

88. Harries, J. T., Piesowicz, A. T., Seakins, J. W. T., Francis D. E. M. and Wolff, O. H. (1971). Low protein diet in type 1 hyperproteinaemia. *Arch. Dis. Childh.*, **46**, 72

89. McCance, R. A. and Widdowson, E. M. (1960). The Composition of Foods. *Med. Res. Counc. Spec. Rep.* Ser. No. 297. (London: HMSO)

CHAPTER 2

Homocystinuria

Nina A. J. Carson

Homocystinuria, an inborn error of methionine metabolism was discovered in 1962 independently in Northern Ireland by Carson and Neill[1] and in the United States by Gerritsen et al.[2]. The basic defect was defined by Mudd[3] and his co-workers in 1964 as a deficiency of the hepatic enzyme cystathionine synthase.

Clinical picture
A classical clinical picture has emerged in severely affected individuals. They tend to have fair hair and skin, a malar flush and lividoreticularis, often well marked, in the lower limbs. Ectopia lentis is present but may not be detected until the age of 6 years. Eye complications are common, pupil block occurs as a result of the complete dislocation of the lens into the anterior chamber resulting in glaucoma. Many of the older patients are first diagnosed in eye hospitals. Mental retardation is common, but unlike phenylketonuria, is slowly progressive often without noticeable delay in developmental milestones over the first year and a half of life. Fits are common in the first few years sometimes accompanied by abnormal EEG records. A connective tissue defect is present with a typical Marfan-like skeletal picture appearing in the older patients with long limbs and chest deformities, high arched palate and scoliosis or kyphosis or both. Unlike the Marfan syndrome osteoporosis is present.

The most life-threatening feature of homocystinuria is the occurrence of thrombotic episodes affecting all ages. As these are found in both arteries and veins, a biochemical rather than an anatomical reason must be sought.

Biochemical defect
More than one reason exists for the presence of homocystine in the urine, only that due to the inactivity of cystathionine synthase will be considered here.

Methionine is the essential sulphur-containing amino acid in man. The first step in the main catabolic pathway is conversion to S-adenosyl-methionine, and there appears to be only one enzyme involved in this reaction, S-adenosylmethionine synthase. S-adenosy-methionine is the primary biological methyl group donor and it is mainly trans-methylated to S-adenosyl homocysteine and adenosine, this reaction is known to be reversible (Figure 2.1). Although the main metabolic flow is from methionine through homocysteine to cystathionine and cysteine, homocysteine also acts as substrate to two other specific enzymes which resynthesise methionine with the aid of methyl group donors thus producing a methionine-homocysteine cycle.

In the normal course of events homocysteine unites with serine to form cystathionine, this reaction is catalysed by the specific enzyme cystathionine synthase, and is a unidirectional reaction. Cystathionine

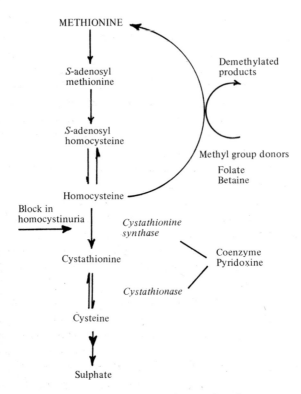

Figure 2.1. The main metabolic pathway of methionine

is acted upon by cystathionase with the formation of cysteine and homoserine (homoserine is not free but is deaminated to α-ketobutyrate), both these latter reactions require vitamin B_6 as a co-enzyme.

The further metabolism of cysteine takes place through several intermediate steps with final oxidation of the sulphydryl group to inorganic sulphate. Homocysteine and cysteine are converted to their oxidised forms, both enzymatically, and non–enzymatically, and unless specific precautions are taken at the time of venepuncture to protect the SH groups, these amino acids are quickly converted to the S – S form. Therefore, plasma and urinary concentrations of these amino acids will be referred to as their oxidised forms—homocystine and cystine.

TREATMENT

The treatment of specific inborn errors of metabolism is still a question of environmental modification. Depending on the site of the metabolic block, there may be more than one way of correcting the biochemical imbalance resulting from the deficiency or dysfunction of the mutant enzyme protein. The cause of the brain damage and the other pathological sequelae in homocystinuria is unknown, therefore, we can only deal with the abnormal biochemical findings as we know them, that is, accumulation in the body of homocysteine accompanied by a secondary rise in methionine and a lack of cystathionine and cysteine. There is also present in plasma and urine of homocystinuric subjects a mixed disulphide of homocysteine and cysteine.

In general there are two main approaches to therapy in disorders due to single gene defects, restriction of substrate accompanied by product replacement and co-enzyme supplementation. The former approach is generally only successful in situations where the substrate cannot be synthesised, e.g. phenylalanine in phenylketonuria. In disorders of non-essential amino acids, e.g. prolinaemia or glycinaemia, substrate restriction is of limited value and a natural restricted protein intake is the only dietary means of dealing with the situation. Co-enzyme supplementation is only likely to be of benefit in situations where the basic enzyme defect involves the apoenzyme at the binding site preventing the formation of the active holoenzyme, instability of either apoenzyme or co-enzyme, or a defect in the biosynthesis of the co-enzyme, or its vitamin precursor.

Co-enzyme supplementation

Homocystinuria is one of 5 inborn errors of metabolism influenced by supplementation with vitamin B_6. Pyridoxal phosphate is the most important active form of the vitamin which as co-enzyme takes part in a wide variety of enzymatic reactions involving amino acids. The other pyridoxine-dependent disorders so far reported include pyridoxine-dependent convulsions[4], pyridoxine-responsive anaemia[5], cystathioninuria[6], and pyridoxine-dependent xanthurenic aciduria[7]. Co-enzyme supplementation in the treatment of homocystinuria was first reported in 1967 by Barber and Spaeth[8] who recorded the biochemically successful treatment of 3 patients with homocystinuria in 2 families receiving an unrestricted diet. Other workers have reported their experience with pyridoxine therapy, some with success[9] some without success[10-12]. It became apparent from the results of Carson and Carré[13] and of Cusworth and Dent[14], who studied a series of 11 patients and 13 patients respectively, that 2 basic defects existed causing the clinical picture in homocystinuria; one was unresponsive to pyridoxine and presumably due to deficiency of the apoenzyme cystathionine synthase, while the other was a further example of a pyridoxine-dependent syndrome.

There has been so far, no report in the literature of any deleterious effect of high doses of pyridoxine given over prolonged periods either to children or during pregnancy[15]. Because this form of therapy is simple and apparently safe with no restrictions on the patients' diet it is obviously the method of choice. Therefore, on diagnosis of a patient with homocystinuria a trial of pyridoxine should be given irrespective of age. The dose of pyridoxine in the first instance should be approximately 150 mg daily in the young infant, 300 mg in the older child and 500 mg daily in the adult given in divided doses throughout the day. The simplest way to judge the effectiveness or otherwise of this form of treatment is to examine daily samples of urine preferably collected at the same time each day, e.g. 1 hour after the midday meal, and testing for homocystine by the use of the nitroprusside-cyanide test[16] or the ammonia-silver-nitroprusside-cyanide test[17]. The first will detect homocysteine and cysteine and the latter will distinguish between the 2 amino acids since it is positive for homcysteine only. Techniques for these tests are given in Appendix 1.

During the trial, where possible, plasma methionine, homocystine and cystine should be determined twice weekly. The most important criterion in blood is a rise in the cystine level as sometimes there is a temporary fall in homocystine which returns to the previous high concentration at a later stage. Trials of pyridoxine given to 9 patients unresponsive to this form of therapy have not shown a rise in plasma cystine. If, after 4–5 days' therapy, there is no change in the amount of homocystine excreted in the urine, as shown by the nitroprusside test, then the dose should be doubled for a further 4–5 days. The highest dose necessary to restore the plasma amino acids to normal in our series of pyridoxine-responsive patients has been 600 mg daily. Gaull[18] however, reports a patient in whom 1200 mg together with reduction of the methionine intake was necessary before a response was achieved. Although in the earlier patients pyridoxine was given for a period of up to 6 weeks our overall experience has been that prolonged trials are unnecessary and it is generally known within 3 weeks if a patient is responding, allowing for time to try increased dosage. The patient should be permitted a normal diet with an average as opposed to a high protein content for the age group, with not too much variation in the quantity of protein from day to day.

In the young homocystinuric infant plasma methionine tends to be high over the first few months and in the neonate it is advisable in the presence of these very high levels to combine a low methionine intake with pyridoxine therapy. Our experience in treating one such infant will serve to illustrate this point. This affected infant was born into a family known to be pyridoxine responsive and was expected to follow the same genetic pattern of homocystinuria. Diagnosis was made at 4 days when plasma methionine was 0·14 mmol/l (normal: 0·01–0·04 mmol/l), homocystine 0·07 mmol/l, there was no plasma cystine and the nitroprusside test applied to urine was strongly positive. Pyridoxine therapy (50 mg daily) was started at 4 days of age. After 6 days the nitroprusside test on the urine was still weakly positive and the pyridoxine was increased to 100 and then to 150 mg daily. It was noted at this time that the plasma methionine was further elevated to 0·36 mmol/l, and at 5 weeks the baby was placed on a low methionine diet, the pyridoxine therapy being continued at 150 mg daily. One week after starting the methionine-restricted diet plasma methionine was normal, and plasma and urinary homocystine were absent. At the age of 5 months the infant was given an unrestricted diet while pyridoxine therapy was continued, and apart from an initial rise in plasma methionine to 0·08 mmol/l accompanied by a plasma homocystine concentration of 0·02 mmol/l, the methionine level has remained below 0·045 mmol/l. At 9 months it was necessary to increase the pyridoxine to 200 mg daily where it has remained since—the child is now 4·5 years old. Having established that the patient is responsive to pyridoxine, the correct dose can be determined by monitoring the plasma methionine, homocystine and cystine levels in this way.

Plasma folic acid concentrations in untreated homocystinuric patients tend to be at the lower limits of normal, and it has been noted[13,19] that in patients receiving pyridoxine therapy these levels are further reduced. Morrow and Barnes[20] have reported one patient who only responded to pyridoxine after administration of folic acid, thus supporting the fact that the reverse reaction from homocysteine to methionine is a functionally important metabolic step.

As can be seen from Figure 2.2, two different enzymes can remethylate homocysteine back to methionine. Of these the most important is N^5-methyltetrahydrofolate-homocysteine methyltransferase (MTHF methyltransferase), and of lesser significance is betaine-homocysteine methyltransferase (BH methyltransferase). By giving supplements of folate or betaine (the methyl group donors of the 2 reactions respectively) plasma homocysteine is reduced and plasma methionine increased. Work by two authors[20,21] has shown that there is increased utilisation of folate in homocystinuric patients. Therefore, plasma folate should be monitored in patients receiving pyridoxine therapy and either courses of folate given as required, or they can be given

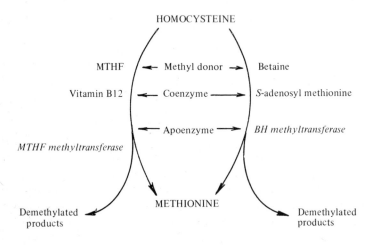

Figure 2.2. Transmethylation of homocysteine
BH = betaine-homocysteine; MTHF = N^5-methyltetrahydrofolate

continuously in small doses daily or on alternate days. It is difficult to obtain folic acid tablets containing amounts of folate suitable for this form of therapy (0·5 mg daily is more than sufficient to keep plasma folate levels greater than 24 μg/ml), and multivitamin preparations are unnecessary as these patients are receiving a normal diet, unlike those on low-methionine diets where vitamin supplements are essential.

In the event of the patient being unresponsive to pyridoxine, a methionine-restricted diet should be given.

Substrate restriction and product replacement
By lowering the intake of dietary methionine one hopes to reduce the amount of methionine, homocysteine and the mixed disulphide of homocysteine and cysteine in the body tissues and fluids. It is important to remember that, in the homocystinuric individual, cysteine is an essential amino acid and should be available either in natural food or as a supplement of the pure amino acid.

A review of the literature shows that there is marked variation in methionine requirement at different ages and from one homocystinuric to another, a situation similar to that found with respect to phenyl-alanine in phenylketonuric patients. The requirement of methionine in the healthy young infant is given as 33–35 mg/kg/day[22], and more recently[23] 24–31 mg/kg/day. In adults, in the presence of cystine, the requirement has been estimated at 1·2–3·3 mg/kg/day[24]. In homo-cystinuric patients various workers have reported intakes of 30–40 mg/kg/day in the newborn period gradually reducing to 20 mg by the end of the first year. In the second year intakes varying from 23–16 mg/kg/day are reported, and in the older child and adolescent as little as 10 mg/kg/day are required in order to reduce plasma methionine to acceptable levels. Brenton and Cusworth[25] state that plasma methionine should be reduced to less than twice the normal value in order to eliminate homocystine from plasma and urine. The above methionine intakes are given as a guide but the actual amount in an individual patient can only be found by monitoring blood methionine and homocystine concentrations.

The high methionine levels in homocystinuric infants, even if untreated, tend to decrease after a few months. One can postulate the reason for this is that at birth either methionine activating enzyme is depressed or that the activity of MTHF methyltransferase or BH methyltransferase is increased (Figure 2.2.). No enzyme studies have yet been reported in the livers of affected infants with these high methionine levels. However, it has been reported[26] that in human foetal liver the activity of MTHF methyltransferase is 4 times higher whereas that of BH methyltransferase is 4 times lower than in mature liver. These findings, together with the fact that cystathionase is virtually absent from the liver and brain of the human foetus[27] suggests that the methionine-homocysteine cycle in the newborn favours remethylation of homocysteine to methionine rather than the formation of cystathionine. This might account for the high levels of methionine in newborn infants and the raised levels of plasma homocystine will only act as a further stimulus in this direction.

Low methionine diet in infancy
Because of the relatively high protein requirement in the newborn period and during the first year of life it is difficult to construct a diet supplying adequate protein, and yet sufficiently low in methionine from natural sources. There is a semi-synthetic low-methionine food available from Scientific Hospital Supplies Ltd, Liverpool, England, called Albumaid Methionine Low (Metinaid in North America). The protein consists of bovine albumin hydrolysate (methionine content 0·04 g/100 g of amino acids). It also contains maize starch, minerals, electrolytes and some vitamins. Full details of its composition are given in Appendix 2. Ten grammes/kg body weight/day of Albumaid Methionine Low will provide approximately 3 g protein/kg body weight/day. It is necessary to add fat which may be given as double cream or as a vegetable oil, one such suitable preparation being Prosparol (BDH Pharmaceuticals Ltd, London E2 6LA) consisting of 50% arachis oil in water. Additional vitamins are necessary as supplied for instance by Ketovite tablets and liquid. This complete vitamin preparation (details in Appendix 3) was specially made for use with synthetic diets and is particularly useful in homocystinuria as it contains folic acid and vitamin B_{12}. When using Albumaid Methionine Low the essential methionine requirement can be conveniently met by giving a small quantity of cows milk. There is a seasonal variation in the protein content and therefore in the methionine content of cows milk, with a range of 50–140 mg/100 ml but in practice it is most convenient to use an approximate figure of say 70 mg/100 ml. The initial amount of methionine prescribed for the newborn is 30–40 mg/kg body weight/day, the precise requirement being determined by monitoring the plasma concentrations of methionine and homocystine.

An alternative to the above low-methionine preparation would be the use of low-methionine proteins such as gelatine and soy-bean protein. Compared with protein of high biological value gelatine is low in methionine, leucine, isoleucine, valine, phenylalanine and tryptophan and contains more lysine and threonine. A diet using a gelatine base with added amino acids, vitamins, minerals, etc has been described in detail[28,29]. However, great care is required in the preparation of such a diet with close co-operation between pharmacist, dietitian and paediatrician.

The soya bean is rich in protein of high biological value and, compared with milk proteins, is relatively low in methionine. Soy-protein formulae are available as proprietary preparations and are convenient to use. One such product universely available is Sobee, manufactured by Mead Johnson, Evansville, Indiana. This is a balanced formula originally designed for the adequate nutrition of infants who cannot tolerate cows milk. When using Sobee no methionine or vitamin supplements are required. Its formula is given in Appendix 2. The latest figures available from the manufacturers give the methionine content as 240 mg/100 g Sobee powder. When made up in the recommended dilution of 1 packed level scoop (9·5 g) to 2 USA fl oz (62 ml) the methionine content is 11·4 mg/USA fl oz (31 ml) or 10·2 mg/British fl oz (28·4 ml) of reconstituted Sobee. The protein content is 22% w/w of the dry powder. Therefore if feeding a newborn infant of 3·5 kg with 3·5 g protein/kg body weight, 57 g of Sobee would be required. This will supply 12·6 g protein and 140 mg methionine. This amount of Sobee will be rather low in calories and more carbohydrate should be supplied (see Appendix 2). However, in later infancy when the methionine requirement approaches 20 mg/kg/day the use of Sobee is not so satisfactory, for example in a child of one year weighing 10 kg the methionine required would be approximately 200 mg which would be contained in 83 g of Sobee, giving the equivalent of only 1·8 g protein per kg body weight per day. Fomon et al.[30,31] have shown that when using a soy protein formula with added methionine infants from 8 days to 6·5 months of age thrived on a protein intake of approximately 1·7 g/kg/day. Nevertheless for the older infant and toddler, Sobee by itself is not a suitable preparation and Albumaid Methionine Low is the formula of choice.

The possibility of using Sobee and giving the extra protein as Albumaid Methionine Low should be considered in those infants who do not readily accept the Albumaid mixture.

Irrespective of which low-methionine formula is used mixed feeding is introduced at about 6–8 weeks of age by the addition of low-protein rusks such as Aminex (Liga Infant Food Ltd) and puree of fruits and low-methionine vegetables. In later infancy mothers are provided with methionine exchange lists. When using Albumaid Methionine Low part of the milk ration may be exchanged for other foods of equal methionine content. Chase et al.[32] recommended that one-third of the methionine derived from Sobee may be replaced by items from the methionine exchange list.

Low methionine intake in older children and adults
Young infants accept special formulae such as hydrolysate and soy-protein mixtures very well, the trouble arises when trying to introduce them to the toddler and older child. One way of achieving this is by offering the special mixture in liquid form in small amounts at the beginning of each meal and gradually increasing the quantity to the prescribed amount. Food preferences of the patient constitute the central point in compiling diets for older children and adults and if they can be persuaded to take an amino acid supplement low in methionine such as Albumaid Methionine Low a greater variety of natural foods can be given. The methionine requirement of the older children and adult is approximately 10 mg/kg body weight/day. Foods of a normal diet are classified into those forbidden, those allowed in permitted amounts, and those unrestricted. In order to provide variety in the diet lists of portions of the restricted foods containing 20 mg methionine are supplied, together with recipes for bread, cakes and puddings using low-protein flour and a vegetable oil such as Prosparol. Baking with low protein flour is difficult and demonstrations should be given to the mother in the diet kitchen. Methionine exchange lists and recipes are given in Appendices 4 and 5.

Cystine supplementation
Nitrogen balance studies in homocystinuric patients show that cyst(e)ine is an essential amino acid, whereas a matched control study confirmed that cyst(e)ine is not an essential amino acid for healthy individuals[33]. In association with a low-methionine diet it is usual to give added cyst(e)ine if dietary cysteine proves insufficient to provide normal plasma cystine levels. Cystine supplements may be given as cystine, cysteine, or as the more soluble calcium cystinate. The dosage given varies throughout the literature from 1–3 g daily depending on the age and weight of the patient. It has been noted[34] that the effect of

supplemental cystine is to increase the plasma concentration of the mixed disulphide of homocysteine and cysteine rather than free cystine and to increase the urinary excretion of taurine and inorganic sulphate[11]. Komrower and Sardharwalla[35] have stated that cystine levels only show improvement when plasma homocystine and the mixed disulphide are significantly reduced. Cystine supplements are often well accepted by adding to dinners or soups.

It is of the greatest importance that parents understand the reason for the special diet and what the paediatrician is trying to achieve by its use. Successful parental management is generally related to the intelligence of the parents, their understanding of the disorder and of the dietary restrictions. It is sometimes difficult for a parent to understand the importance of the diet when their infant appears to be normal, and one has to continuously reinforce its importance and encourage the parents at every opportunity to persevere with dietary control.

Management of the diet
Treatment is monitored by determining plasma methionine, homocystine, cystine and the mixed disulphide of homocystine and cystine: this is best achieved by the use of an ion-exchange amino acid analyser. Venous blood should be obtained ideally after an overnight fast but if this is not possible then at least 3 hours after the previous meal. Special precautions should be taken to see that there is no delay in separating the cells from the plasma and deproteinising the latter as otherwise disulphide binding of homocyst(e)ine and cyst(e)ine to sulphydryl groups of plasma proteins occurs with resulting loss of the disulphide amino acids. Urine, as already mentioned, is also examined for excess homocystine by the use of one of the nitroprusside tests. The optimal frequency of the tests depends on the age of the patient and how well the diet is controlled. As the methionine can vary so much in the first 6 weeks of life weekly determinations are advisable but at a few months of age these can be made fortnightly and by a year, monthly in a well controlled child. It is important to keep blood letting and visits to hospital down to the necessary minimum.

At each visit height, weight and head circumference are measured and this, in association with the plasma amino acid concentrations, will reassure the physician that there is no danger of over-treatment with the possibility of negative nitrogen balance. Chase, Goodman and O'Brien[32] found raised levels of plasma methionine, alkaline phosphatase, SGOT and DHL in a patient who was deprived of methionine.

These enzyme changes have also been described in phenylketonuria patients on too low a protein intake[36]. During routine visits the mother is interviewed by the dietitian. The importance of the role played by the dietitian cannot be emphasised too strongly. A good liaison with the mother is particularly important during the preschool years. The successful introduction of mixed feeding graduating to the use of methionine exchange lists necessitates constant supervision and support. After the first year of life the artificial nature of the diet calls for the preparation of unusual dishes in the home in order to provide a varied and balanced diet adequate in calorie value.

Ophthalmological examination and intelligence tests are undertaken routinely once yearly and where possible the same ophthalmologist and psychologist should examine the patient. Radiological examination of long bones and vertebrae are also undertaken yearly.

From early childhood the parents are warned about the possibility of eye complications and advised to inform the ophthalmologist immediately if the child complains of sore eyes. It is difficult to warn about thrombotic episodes without causing alarm but if they have confidence in the paediatrician they will alert him to any untoward symptoms which might appear.

Reasons for hypomethioninaemia
(1) Too little prescribed in diet
(2) Prescribed amount adequate but child refusing the formula, or formula presented in too great a volume for child to manage, or misunderstanding of exchange values by parents

Reasons for hypermethioninaemia
(1) Prescribed intake too high
(2) Prescribed intake correct but high methionine levels found due to:–
    (a) misunderstanding of exchange values by parents
    (b) forbidden foods being given by other siblings, friends, etc. or child pilfering extra food unknown to mother
    (c) infections resulting in increased metabolism. The best course to take in this situation is to increase the fluids and carbohydrates, it is generally difficult, if not impossible, to get patients to eat special formulae when feeling ill
(3) High methionine levels have been described due to too low

44

an intake of methionine and protein. In these circumstances there will be poor weight gain and the child will be irritable and anorexic

Precautions to be taken in the management of homocystinuric patients

(1) Surgical procedures. Many patients have suffered thrombotic episodes after surgical procedures especially those associated with eye operations. It is recommended that patients who are resistant to pyridoxine therapy when subjected to surgical procedures should be given a strict low methionine intake prior to and for at least three weeks after the operation. In the past anticoagulants have been given after operations but these are hazardous in themselves with the possibility of haemorrhage an ever-present threat. The immobility imposed after surgical procedures should be reduced to an absolute minimum as this may contribute to the thrombotic tendency

(2) Drugs likely to cause an increase in the clotting mechanism, such as contraceptives, should be avoided

(3) The possibility of folic acid deficiency should be kept in mind and treated if necessary

(4) Pregnancy. There appears to be a tendency for some homo-cystinuric women to miscarry. In one patient studied throughout pregnancy the cervix was found to be effaced and dilated at 30 weeks gestation. This may have been due to a connective tissue weakness in the cervix—although this was not proven. As with surgical procedures patients should be encouraged to be mobile as quickly as possible after parturition

Results of therapy

As with all treatable genetic diseases the sooner after birth the diagnosis is made and the treatment started the better the outlook. Unlike phenylketonuria, homocystinuria is a slowly progressive disease and as such one hopes at least to stop the progression of the disease and prevent the sequelae even if treatment is not commenced in infancy; this especially applies to the occurrence of thrombotic episodes.

Perry *et al.*[11] have reported an infant treated from the 16th day of life with a low-methionine diet who at 5 years had average intelligence, normal skeletal development and no lens abnormality. Komrower *et al*[35] likewise treated a patient with a low-methionine diet from the 9th day of life who at 6y 4m, apart from an IQ of 80 has not so far suffered from any of the sequelae of homocystinuria. The low IQ in this patient was thought to be due in part to very bad home conditions.

In Northern Ireland 2 siblings received pyridoxine therapy commencing at age 4 days and age 11 months. They have now been treated for 5 and 6 years respectively. Both have the classical appearance of other homocystinuric patients from Northern Ireland with fair hair and high malar flush but so far no skeletal or eye changes are present and no thrombotic episodes have occurred. Intelligence tests have shown the youngest (the earliest treated) to have low average intelligence and the second child to have an IQ of 107.

Five other patients have received pyridoxine therapy for periods of 5–6 years. The age at commencement of treatment varied from 5–23 years. These patients all had ectopia lentis, skeletal manifestations and were mildly to severely mentally retarded with IQ varying from 50 to 70. Since therapy started no thrombotic episodes have occurred. Stiffness of the small joints of the hands and feet present in 2 patients has disappeared, and the parents of 2 other patients have stated that they are much easier to handle in the home situation.

McKusick, Hall and Char[37] have reported 'dramatic improvement in behaviour, including school performance, darkening of the hair and reduction in flushing' in 12 homocystinuric patients treated with a low-methionine diet and in 7 of 10 patients given pyridoxine therapy. Perry[11] reported a child of 9 years whom he had treated with a low-methionine diet for 3 years. Before therapy she had suffered repeated cerebral and other thrombotic episodes and fractures after trivial falls, she was mentally retarded: since therapy commenced no further thromboses or fractures have occurred. A second patient of 19·5 years was placed on a diet after several cerebrovascular accidents: he has been under dietary control for 3 years and has not suffered any further thromboses.

In Northern Ireland 5 patients are receiving a low-methionine diet of which only 2 are well controlled, these patients commenced dietary treatment from 2 months to 6 years of age and diets have been given for 1·5–4 years. The youngest child is now 3 years of age, is under good dietary control and appears to be normal physically and mentally. His sibling started treatment at 1y 9m and has lowered intelligence, mild skeletal defects but no eye changes to date; he is under poor dietary control. Two children started dietary treatment at ages 4 and 6 years they have lowered intelligence, skeletal and eye defects and are poorly controlled on their diets. The fifth child had convulsive episodes followed by hemiplegia at age 7 months, and at 19 months when being investigated for salaam type fits was diagnosed and placed on a low-methionine diet. He has been well controlled for 3 years and has had no further thrombotic episodes or fits.

It appears from the natural history of homocystinuria that some patients have a greater tendency to recurrent thrombotic episodes than others, and in such patients the first thrombotic episode may occur as early as 7 months of age.

Although it is much too early to predict the final outcome of therapy, nevertheless, treatment in the form of pyridoxine or low-methionine diets appears to prevent, or at least delay, the sequelae of homocystinuria especially with regard to thrombotic episodes.

Duration of treatment

In phenylketonuria many feel that after age 6 years it is possible to give a normal diet without causing intellectual deterioration. However, one cannot follow this argument through to homocystinuria as clinically it causes a wider variety of physical and biochemical defects with the ever-present threat of thrombosis. The personal view of the author is that in pyridoxine responsive patients treatment should be continuous. In the unresponsive patients, where it is very difficult to continue the monotonous diet into adulthood, at least these patients should be encouraged to continue with a diet restricted in natural protein.

Other methods of environmental manipulation in the treatment of homocystinuria

Although pyridoxine therapy or a low-methionine diet are the methods of choice in the treatment of homocystinuria, it is of interest to consider other therapeutic approaches which may be of value.

Remethylation of homocysteine to methionine

As already mentioned, two different enzymes can transmethylate homocysteine back to methionine (Figure 2.2) therefore by giving supplements of folate or betaine, plasma homocystine may be reduced and plasma methionine increased. This might be a helpful adjunct to dietary therapy provided the plasma methionine is not markedly elevated.

Komrower and Sardharwalla[35] reported the use of betaine hydrochloride supplements in association with a low-methionine diet in an 18-month-old patient. At the time of the trial the patient's plasma methionine was normal, homocystine virtually absent but the mixed disulphide of homocysteine and cysteine was still present. A progressive fall in the level of the mixed disulphide occurred and was reversed on cessation of betaine supplements. In a further patient in whom the plasma methionine, homocystine and mixed disulphide were moderately elevated, supplemental betaine therapy for one week resulted in the disappearance of both homocystine and the mixed disulphide but produced a marked rise in plasma methionine. Two other patients given a trial of betaine while moderately controlled by a reduced methionine intake also responded by showing a marked elevation in plasma methionine.

Using choline dihydrogen citrate—a precursor of betaine, Perry[34] reported similar results in a homocystinuric patient receiving a normal diet: plasma methionine fell and homocystine increased when choline was discontinued. Restarting choline produced a rise in methionine, but this time no decrease in homocystine. The patient was then placed on a low-methionine diet while choline therapy continued: this caused a decrease in plasma methionine and homocystine. One patient aged 5 years in Northern Ireland was given a trial of folate therapy commencing at 10 mg daily while on an unrestricted diet. Initially this resulted in a decrease in plasma homocystine and a rise in methionine, but the homocystine became elevated again in spite of increasing the dose of folate to 20 mg daily.

It would appear that administration of folate or betaine might be useful if used in conjunction with a restricted methionine intake but they are only of limited value when patients are receiving a free diet.

Penicillamine
Penicillamine forms a stable disulphide complex with cysteine and homocysteine[38] and its use has been reported in cystinuric patients[39]. Chase *et al.*[32] reported that treatment of homocystinuria with penicillamine resulted in a decrease in urinary homocysteine accompanied by a corresponding increase in the mixed disulphides of homocysteine and cysteine, and homocysteine and penicillamine respectively. No changes were observed in plasma or urinary methionine but therapy was only carried out for a period of seven days.

In view of the potential nephrotoxicity of pencillamine and the availability of less hazardous therapy this treatment is not recommended.

Increased renal excretion of homocystine by lysine and arginine
It has been shown[40] that rats injected intra-peritonealy with homocystine and lysine excrete homocystine as well as cystine and lysine.

Similarly when homocystine and arginine are injected, homocystine, arginine and cystine are excreted. A homocystinuric patient given an intravenous infusion of arginine glutamate excreted increased amounts of homocystine, mixed disulphide of homocysteine and cysteine, cystine, arginine, lysine, ornithine and glutamic acid. The authors suggest that oral therapy with arginine glutamate or lysine might aid the reduction of plasma homocystine by inhibiting its renal tubular reabsorption.

More studies are required before this method of treatment could be adopted even as a secondary measure.

Homoserine and cysteine supplementation

Cystathionine is present in the human and primate brain in higher concentration than in any other species[41], and has been found to be absent or markedly deficient in the brain of untreated homocystinurics[42]. If cystathionine is essential for the normal functioning of the human brain then lack of its formation in homocystinuria may contribute to the brain damage found in many of these patients. On the other hand homocystinuric subjects are described with normal intellect and presumably they also are lacking in cystathionine. However, cystathionine is very expensive, it has a high renal clearance, little is known about its transport across the blood-brain barrier and its use in the treatment of homocystinuria has not so far been reported.

In mice[43,44] the conversion of cystathionine to cysteine is reversible, and by feeding homoserine and cysteine it is possible to increase the cystathionine content of the brain and liver of these animals. In 1968 Wong[45] demonstrated *in vitro* in a liver homogenate from a homocystinuric patient the formation of labelled cystathionine from ^{14}C labelled cysteine and homoserine. Moreover oral loading of a homocystinuric patient with cysteine and homoserine resulted in the excretion of cystathionine in the urine.

It is not yet proven that cystathionine can be synthesised from homoserine and cysteine in the brain but work reported in animals suggests that this may be so[46,47].

To date, no trials have been undertaken in homocystinuric patients with oral homoserine and cysteine but Professor Wong and his group are proposing to undertake such a trial[48].

Supplementation with serine

Decreased urinary homocystine has been noted in an homocystinuric patient when given a methionine load with 1 g L-serine compared with when methionine was given alone[49]. A trial of serine supplements was given for a period of 7 days in 4 homocystinuric subjects by other workers[32] without any decrease in plasma methionine being noted: urine was not examined for homocystine.

No other reports of this form of therapy are known to the author.

Supplementation with cyst(e)ine
After the discovery of homocystinuria one of the first suggestions for therapy was oral supplementation with cyst(e)ine[50], the rationale being that cyst(e)ine deficiency might contribute to the pathogenesis of the disease. One patient was given 3 g daily for a total of 9·5 months without there being any evidence of clinical improvement.

Genetic counselling

Cystathionine synthase is present in fibroblasts derived from skin and amniotic fluid and individuals may be classified into homozygotes and heterozygotes by quantitative enzyme assay of fibroblast homogenates[51]. In a family at risk amniotic fluid obtained early in pregnancy could allow an affected offspring to be anticipated by finding a lack of cystathionine synthase in the cultured amnion cells[52]. However, these cultures are difficult to establish and it is a slow process to grow sufficient cells in order to carry out the enzyme assay. Insufficient pregnancies in individuals at risk have so far been studied for the value of this procedure to be ascertained. One can appreciate that with improved techniques examination of amnion fibroblasts for cystathionine synthase would be of great assistance in the prevention of homocystinuria in individuals at risk.

Summary

Homocystinuria is a very rare disease. Figures from Northern Ireland show its incidence to be approximately one-fifth that of phenylketonuria in this geographical area. It is unique among the inherited amino acid disorders in presenting with such a wide diversity of clinical and pathological sequelae with the basic reason for the pathological processes being largely unknown.

Attempts at treatment with a low-methionine diet were first published in 1966 and 1968 by Komrower and his co-workers and by Perry's group respectively. Pyridoxine therapy has been on trial since

1968 with the results in the largest groups of patients being published by Cusworth and Dent, and Carson and Carré in 1969.

From the results of both forms of therapy so far documented, it would appear that in the late-treated cases the thrombotic episodes can be prevented and the eye changes at least delayed if they were not already present when treatment was started. Some workers report a positive change in the behaviour and general well-being of the patients. Only a few patients have been reported whose treatment was started in infancy and the results in these children are promising. No thrombotic episodes have occurred and to date no connective tissue defects have appeared. Intelligence tests to date show them to have low-average to average intelligence.

Because of the rarity of this disorder and the fact that it is less than a decade since attempts at therapy have been undertaken, it is not surprising that insufficient data has accumulated so far to assess the eventual success or otherwise of the above two modes of therapy or for how long it should be continued.

I am indebted to Miss May E. Beck, Senior Therapeutic Dietitian, Royal Belfast Hospital for Sick Children, Belfast, for the dietetic section of this chapter.

APPENDIX I

Sodium cyanide-nitroprusside test. (Brand, Harris and Biloon 1930) To 1·0 ml of urine add 0·6 ml of 5% sodium cyanide. Stand at room temperature for 10 minutes, add a few drops of freshly prepared 5% sodium nitroprusside. The development of a bright magenta colour denotes a positive reaction.

NB. In the presence of a generalised aminoaciduria a brown/pink colour may be apparent.

Ammonia-silver-nitroprusside test (Spaeth and Barber 1967) This is a modification of the original cyanide-nitroprusside test. Homocystine, penicillamine, some disulphides and thiolesters give a positive result but a negative result is given by cystine.

Saturate the urine with solid sodium chloride. To a 5·0 ml sample add 0·5 ml of ammoniacal silver nitrate (1% silver nitrate in 3% ammonium hydroxide). To a control sample add 0·5 ml of 3%

ammonia (no silver) leave for one minute. Add 0·5 ml of freshly prepared 1% sodium nitroprusside followed by 0·5 ml of 0·7% sodium cyanide. The development of an immediate deep pink or purple colour in the test sample only, represents a positive reaction.

APPENDIX 2

Composition of Albumaid Methionine Low

Amino acids g/100 g)

L-Alanine	3·2
L-Arginine	2·4
L-Aspartic acid	5·3
L-Cystine	2·0
L-Glutamic acid	6·0
Glycine	2·4
L-Histidine	1·6
L-Isoleucine	0·8
L-Leucine	1·8
L-Lysine	3·7
L-Phenylalanine	2·4
L-Proline	0·9
L-Serine	1·0
L-Threonine	1·8
L-Tryptophan	0·4
L-Tyrosine	2·4
L-Valine	1·9
	——
	40·0
	——
L-Methionine	0·04

Minerals (g/100 g)

Sodium as Na^+	0·75
Potassium as K^+	0·75
Calcium as Ca^{++}	0·70
Magnesium as Mg^{++}	0·08
Phosphorus as PO_4^{3-}	1·50

Trace minerals (mg/100 g)

Iron	4·0
Zinc	0·9
Copper	0·5
Manganese	0·5
Iodine	0·06
Molybdenum	0·01
Cobalt	0·006
Aluminium	0·002

Vitamins (mg/100 g)

Meso-inositol	100
Nicotinamide	10
Calcium pantothenate	4
Thiamine hydro-chloride	2
Riboflavine	2
Pyridoxine hydro-chloride	1
Folic acid	0·2
Biotin	0·05
B_{12} (Cyanocobal-amin)	0·02

Carbohydrate (g/100 g)

Maize starch (pre-gelatinised)	50

Moisture (g/100 g) (approx) 4

Composition of Sobee

Amino acids (g/100 g)

Methionine	0·242
Isoleucine	0·88
Leucine	1·58
Lysine	1·30
Phenylalanine	1·03
Threonine	0·79
Tryptophan	0·22
Valine	0·90
Arginine	1·3
Histidine	0·51
Alanine	0·95
Aspartic acid	2·68
Cystine	0·20
Glutamic acid	3·78
Glycine	0·88
Proline	1·08
Serine	0·95
Tyrosine	0·79

Carbohydrate

53 g/100 g Sobee

Corn syrup solids with added sucrose

Fat

18 g/100 g Sobee

Soy-bean oil (46% linoleic, 4% linolenic) + added coconut oil

Minerals

4·5 g/100 g Sobee

The electrolyte content is almost identical with that of the typical cow's milk-carbohydrate formula. The calcium content is similar to that of the typical modified milk formula and contains about five times as much iron as the usual milk formula

Vitamins (per 100 g Sobee)

Vitamin A	987	USP units
Vitamin D	263	USP units
Vitamin E	3·3	INT units
Ascorbic acid	33	mg
Thiamine	0·33	mg
Riboflavine	0·66	mg
Nicotinamide	4·6	mg
Pyridoxine	0·26	mg
Cyanocobal-amin	1·32	mg

APPENDIX 3

Composition of Ketovite Tablets and Ketovite (Supplement) Liquid
(Manufactured by Paines & Byrne Ltd, Pabyrn Laboratories, Greenford, England)

Ketovite tablets each contain:

Aneurine hydrochloride	1·0 mg
Riboflavine	1·0 mg
Pyridoxine hydrochloride	0·33 mg
Nicotinamide	3·3 mg
Calcium pantothenate	1·16 mg
Ascorbic acid	16·6 mg
α-Tocopheryl acetate	5·0 mg
Inositol	50·0 mg
Biotin	0·17 mg
Folic acid	0·25 mg
Acetomenaphthone	0·5 mg

Ketovite (Supplement) liquid contains in each 5 ml dose:

Vitamin A	2500 units
Vitamin D	400 units
Choline chloride	150 mg
Cyanocobalamin	12·5 µg

Both preparations are lactose and sucrose free.

Dosage. As a complete vitamin supplement for infants and young children on restricted diets: 1 Ketovite tablet three times a day plus 5 ml Ketovite (Supplement) liquid daily.

APPENDIX 4

Classification of Foods for Low-Methionine Diets

LIST A: The following lists are merely intended to offer a practicable scheme, sufficiently accurate for dietary purposes. In many instances precise information is lacking as to methionine content of individual foods. There are indications that wide variations sometimes occur in different specimens of the same item.

Methionine exchanges. Each portion supplies approximately 20 mg methionine.

Food, edible portion	Size of portion
Asparagus	75 g
Beans, broad, boiled	100 g
Beans, haricot, soaked and boiled	25 g
Beetroot	60 g
Brussel sprouts boiled	90 g
Cauliflower, boiled	70 g
Lentils	15 g
Lentils, soaked and boiled	50 g
Onion	130 g
Peas, fresh, boiled	40 g
Peas, dried	10 g
Peas, dried, soaked and boiled	30 g
Potato	60 g
boiled	100 g
chips	30 g
crisps	20 g
Spinach, boiled	25 g
Avocado	70 g
Banana	100 g
Marcaroni	10 g
Macaroni, boiled	35 g

Food, edible portion	Size of portion
Oatmeal	10 g
Rice, white	15 g
Rice, white, boiled	40 g
Cream, 50% fat	50 ml
Milk	25 ml

LIST B:– The following foods may be given in unweighed average helpings, an estimate being made of their contribution to the methionine intake in each individual case:

Food, edible portion	mg/100 g	Size of portion	mg/portion
Cabbage	26	60 g	15
boiled	10	100 g	10
Carrot	8	40 g	3
boiled	7	70 g	5
Celery	25	60 g	15
Cucumber	8	40 g	3
Lettuce	24	20 g	5
Tomato	7	70 g	5
Turnip	10	70 g	7
Apple	3	100 g	3
Apricot	4	50 g	2
Melon	2	120 g	2
Orange	3	100 g	3
Pear	3	100 g	3
Pineapple	1	120 g	1

Most fruits are low in protein and can be given in unrestricted amounts

Butter	15	10 g	1·5
Margarine	8	10 g	0·8
Sweet loaf		30 mg/loaf	
Rock buns		20 mg/batch	
Shortbread		10 mg/batch	

Food, edible portion	Size of portion
Biscuits	20 mg/batch
Shortcrust pastry	10 mg/batch
Loaf ★—yeast recipe	27 mg/batch

LIST C:– The following contain little or no methionine and are unrestricted:

Cornflower	Sago	Tapioca
Margarine	Sugar	Syrup
Cooking fats and oils	Honey	Jam
Fruit flavoured iced lollipops	Boiled sweets	Marmalade
	Vinegar	Salt
Minerals and squashes	Spices	Pepper
Black tea	Black coffee	Curry powder

Examples of suitable low-protein proprietary foods which may be taken in unrestricted amounts

Nutregen Wheat Starch (Amylum B.P. Pulv.), Energen Foods Co, Ashford, Kent, England

Rite-Diet protein-free flour and bread. Welfare Foods (Stockport) Ltd, 63–65 Higher Hillgate, Stockport, Cheshire, England

Tritamyl protein-free, self raising flour. Procea Ltd, Alexandra Road, Dublin 1, Eire

Aproten flour and crispbread. Aproten pasta and semolina. Carlo-Erba (UK) Ltd, 28–30 Great Peter Street, London, SW1P 2BX. Distributors for Carlo-Erba, Milan, Italy

Azeta low-protein biscuits and wafers. Carlosta Ltd, 33 Ermine Road, London, SE13 7JY. Agents for Ditta Federico Salza, Piza, Italy

Aminex low-protein biscuits. Liga Food Products (UK) Ltd, Liga House, 23 Saxby Street, Leicester, England. Distributors for Liga Fabriekden, N.V., Roosendaal, Holland

★ There is uncertainty as to the correct figure for the methionine content of bakers yeast and the figure given here can only be approximate.

LIST D:– The following foods are forbidden unless specifically prescribed to provide the methionine allowance:

Meat	Fish	Eggs
Cheese	Milk	Ordinary bread

Biscuits and baked products

APPENDIX 4: DIETS

Specimen diet for a newborn using Albumaid Low Methionine

Weight of infant 3·5 kg

Requirements:

Protein 4 g/kg body weight	= 14 g
Calories 125/kg body weight	= 437
Methionine 40 mg/kg body weight	= 140 mg
Fluid 150 ml/kg body weight	= 525 ml

Diet	Protein g	Carb. g	Fat g	Methionine mg
Milk 160 ml	5·4	7·7	5·9	128
Add 370 ml boiling water — Albumaid Low Methionine* 30 g	9·0	15·0	–	12
Prosparol† 30 ml	–	–	15·0	–
Sugar 25 g	–	25·0	–	–
	14·4	47·7	20·9	140

Calories—436

Vitamin supplements as prescribed, e.g. Ketovite 3 tablets and 1 teaspoon liquid.

The daily milk allowance must be finished in the course of 24 hours. To make certain of this it should be presented separately, spread out over the day, a little being given before each Albumaid feed.

* Albumaid Low Methionine is 50% carbohydrate and 40% amino acids, equivalent to 30% protein

† The same amount of fat could be provided by 30 ml of cream of 50% fat content. This would provide also methionine equivalent to a half portion of List A

Commencement of spoon feeding

This is best effected by introducing foods which will not make a
significant contribution to the methionine intake: for instance strained
fruits and vegetables selected from List B, also low-protein bread and
biscuits moistened with water or fruit juice, or with a little of the
Albumaid mixture. When the child has become accustomed to spoon
feeding, foods from the methionine exchange list can be introduced.

Specimen menu for a child aged 9 months

Body weight 9 kg
Estimated requirements:

Protein 3 g/kg   =   27 g
Methionine 20 mg/kg   = 180 mg
Calories—1000

	Portions List A
Early morning	
Juice of one orange, with water and sugar added	
Breakfast	
Albumaid Low Methionine mixture	
Porridge (10 g oatmeal)	I
Milk 25 ml	I
Sugar	
Mid-day:	
Albumaid Low Methionine mixture	
Boiled potato mashed 50 g	$\frac{1}{2}$
Vegetable from List B, mashed or sieved	
I teaspoon butter	
Vegetable cooking water to moisten	
Milk 50 ml	2
Low-protein biscuit	
Evening meal:	
Albumaid Low Methionine mixture	
Cornflour pudding (milk thickened with corn-flour) 2 level tablespoons (30 ml)	I
Fruit, e.g. stewed apple	
Low protein biscuit	
Bed-time:	
Albumaid Low Methionine mixture	
Milk 25 ml	I

	Portions List A
Estimated methionine intake from unrestricted foods	1
Methionine intake from Albumaid	$1\frac{1}{2}$
Total	9

Albumaid mixture
  Albumaid Low Methionine 70 g
  Prosparol* 30 ml
  Sugar 40 g
  Water to a total of 700 ml
  Vitamin supplements as prescribed
To drink between meals:
  Water, which may be flavoured with fruit
  squash, if desired

Specimen menu for a child aged 4 years
Body weight 16·5 kg
Estimated requirements:
  Protein 2·5 g/kg   = 40 g
  Methionine 10 mg/kg   = 165 mg

	Portions List A
Breakfast:	
Albumaid Low Methionine	
Porridge (10 g oatmeal)	1
Milk 25 ml	1
Low-protein bread as desired, butter and jam	
Mid-morning:	
Fruit from List B, or low-protein biscuit as required	
Mid-day:	
Albumaid Low Methionine	
Potato chips 50 g	$1\frac{1}{2}$
Vegetable from List B, e.g. grilled tomato	
Low-protein fruit crumble—see recipe (Appendix 5)	
Water to drink—or see List C	

* 30 ml cream, 50% fat content, may be given instead of Prosparol in which case methionine equivalent to a half portion List A would be supplied by the cream.

Portions List A

Evening meal:
Albumaid Low Methionine
Vegetable salad—see List B or;
Low protein soup—see recipe (Appendix 5)
20 g plain potato crisps   1
Low protein bread as desired, butter and jam
Estimated methionine intake from unrestricted
foods   1
Methionine intake from Albumaid Low Methi-
onine $2\frac{1}{2}$

Total   8

Albumaid Low Methionine 120 g daily. This can be mixed with water and flavoured with sugar, fruit squash, vegetable cooking water, tomato or fruit juices. It could also be incorporated in dishes such as the low-protein vegetable soup, or tomato and onion savoury. Provided butter and other fats are included in the diet where appropriate, it is unnecessary to include a source of fat with the Albumaid. Vitamin supplements should be given as prescribed.

Specimen diet for a newborn using Sobee
Weight of infant 3·5 kg
Requirements:
Protein 12·25 g (3·5 g/kg body weight)
Calories 440
Methionine 140 mg
Fluid 525 ml

	Protein g	Carb. g	Fat g	Methionine mg
To a total of 550 ml with water { Sobee 6 packed level scoops (57 g)	12·6	30	10·2	140
Sugar 45 g	–	45	–	–
Totals	12·6	75	10·2	140
Calories—442				

APPENDIX 5: LOW PROTEIN RECIPES
(For list of manufacturers of low protein flours and products see page 57
and the table on p. 253)

BREAD, BISCUITS AND CAKES

Loaf
Special flour 340 g
Lard or other fat 15 g
Baker's yeast 15 g
Sugar 1 teaspoon
Salt 1 level teaspoon
Warm water 300 ml approx. (The amount of water required will
depend upon which flour is used. For example Rite-Diet flour
requires less than half the above amount)

Add the salt to the flour and rub in the fat. Cream the yeast and
sugar. Warm the water and add to the yeast and sugar mixture. Add
this to the flour and mix well. The mixture should be a thick batter.
Pour into a greased loaf tin and leave in a warm place until almost
twice its original size. Bake in a hot oven 450 °F (230 °C) until firm
(about 20 minutes). Lower the heat a little and cook until a skewer
comes out clean. The loaf will probably not brown very much on top.
Remove from the tin and cool.

Sweet loaf
Special flour 230 g
Sugar 60 g
Margarine 60 g
Baking powder 3 heaped teaspoons
Water 200–280 ml

Rub the margarine into the flour and add sugar and baking powder.
Make a well in the centre and pour in most of the water all at once.
Mix lightly with a spoon and stir in the remaining water to make a
soft, lumpy dough. Mix quickly and as little as possible and put the
mixture, while still lumpy, into a well-greased tin. Too much stirring,
or too little water, will make the loaf heavy. Bake in a hot oven
450 °F (230 °C) for 10 minutes, then reduce the heat slightly for a
further twenty minutes approximately. When firm turn out to cool.

Rock buns
Special flour 140 g
Sugar 60 g
Margarine 85 g
Baking powder 1 heaped and 1 level teaspoon
Glacé cherries 6
Water to mix
Spices such as ground ginger, cinnamon and allspice, and essences
   such as vanilla and almond, may be used as desired
Rub the margarine into the flour, mix in the other dry ingredients,
including the cherries cut into halves. Add enough water to make a
firm dough. Put out on to a greased baking sheet in small heaps. Cook in
a moderately hot oven 375 °F (190 °C) until firm—about 20–30 minutes.

Shortbread
Special flour 140 g
Sugar 85 g
Margarine 60 g
Put the margarine and sugar into a bowl and cream them together
with the back of a wooden spoon. The mixture may be warmed a little
if necessary. Add the flour and mix well. Press into small sandwich tin
about 18 cm across. Bake in a moderate oven, 350 °F (180 °C) until
slightly coloured—about 25 minutes. Cut into sections while hot but
do not remove from the tin until cold.

Biscuits
Special flour 140 g
Sugar 60 g
Margarine 85 g
Milk 1 tablespoon (15 ml)
Rub the margarine into the flour and mix in the sugar. Add the
milk and press firmly against the side of the bowl, adding a few drops
of water if necessary to make a ball of dough. Roll out, cut into biscuit
shapes, place on a greased tin and bake slowly in a moderate oven until
lightly browned. These can be sandwiched together with jam and
coated on top with water icing.

Shortcrust pastry
Special flour 100 g
Margarine or cooking fat 50 g

Pinch of salt
Water to mix
Rub the fat into the flour and mix with a little water to a firm consistency. Roll out and use as required, e.g. for a jam tart, or for fruit or savoury pies, using permitted fruits and vegetables.

SAVOURIES

Tomato and onion savoury
Tomato 1
Water $\frac{1}{2}$ teacup
Onion, $\frac{1}{2}$ medium-sized
Cornflour $\frac{1}{2}$ teaspoon
Cooking fat
Seasoning
Fry the chopped onion in a little cooking fat until tender, add the chopped tomato and some salt and pepper. Cook for 2 minutes. Blend the cornflour with the water and stir this into the onion and tomato mixture. Bring to the boil. Serve with low-protein bread toasted or with the potato ration.

Tomato soup
Tomato juice and vegetable cooking water mixed, 200 ml
Sago, or Aproten semolina, 1 dessertspoon
Butter $\frac{1}{2}$ teaspoon
Seasoning
Mix together the tomato juice and water and bring to the boil. Add the sago or special semolina slowly, stirring all the time. Simmer slowly, stirring at intervals, until cooked. Stir in a small knob of butter. Check seasoning before serving.

Vegetable soup
Vegetable cooking water, e.g. water kept after cooking cabbage, cauliflower, celery, etc, 400 ml
Some pieces of carrot, turnip, onion, celery, cabbage, etc as available cut into pieces
Cooking fat or margarine
Melt the fat in a saucepan and fry the onion. Add the other vegetables and stir all together. Add the vegetable cooking water and some salt

and pepper and simmer slowly until the vegetables are tender. Add chopped parsley at the end.

Sago or Aproten semolina can be used to thicken this soup.

A pinch of curry powder can be added along with the vegetables.

Low-protein pasta

Boil in salted water, following the manufacturer's instructions carefully. It is easy to over-cook the pasta. Drain into a strainer and hold the strainer under running water for a few moments to prevent stickiness.

Suggestions for serving:

(1) Fry some onion in a little margarine. Add the cooked pasta, with more margarine if necessary. Heat thoroughly and add chopped parsley at the end before serving.

(2) Prepare as for (1) but add either a chopped tomato or some tomato puree to the onions while they are frying.

(3) Prepare as for (1) adding 2 mushrooms cut up roughly to fry along with the onions.

(4) Add curry powder to taste ($\frac{1}{4}$ teaspoon or less) and fry this along with the onions. Add salt and pepper and 1 cup of water or vegetable cooking water, blended with 1 rounded teaspoon cornflour. Bring to the boil and cook very slowly for a few minutes. This sauce may be added to the cooked pasta. Some bottled sauces and ketchups are low in protein and can be used in savoury dishes.

PUDDINGS

Protein-free milk

Water 1 teacup

Sugar 1 dessertspoon

Prosparol 2 dessertspoons

Dissolve the sugar in the water and add the Prosparol. This mixture can be added to tea or coffee instead of milk.

Milk pudding

Prepare water, sugar and Prosparol as in the above recipe. Gradually blend in 2 teaspoons cornflour. Bring to the boil. This can be served instead of milk pudding, or with fruit or a spoonful of jam.

Apple crumble
Special flour 60 g
Sugar 30 g
Margarine 30 g
Stewed apple, sweetened

Put the stewed apple into a small dish which can be put into the oven, such as an individual pie-dish. Rub the margarine into the special flour and add the sugar. Sprinkle the crumble lightly on top of the apple and cook in a moderate oven until the top is crusty and brown.

Amber pudding
Stewed fruit such as apple or gooseberries, pureed or crushed pine-
   apple, 2 teacups
Cornflour 2 teaspoons
Knob of butter or margarine
Sugar to sweeten

Blend the cornflour with the fruit and bring to the boil, add the sugar and butter. Serve hot or cold. Culinary colouring such as cochineal may be added as required.

Lemon sago
Sago 30 g
Water 300 ml
Juice of 1 lemon
Syrup 1 tablespoon
Sugar as required
Butter 1 teaspoon

Boil sago and water until it thickens and the sago is clear. Add lemon juice, syrup and some sugar if required. Add the butter. Pour into a mould and turn out when cold.

REFERENCES

1. Carson, N. A. J. and Neill, D. W. (1962). Metabolic abnormalities detected in a survey of mentally backward individuals in Northern Ireland. *Arch. Dis. Childh.*, **37**, 505
2. Gerritsen, T., Vaughn, J. G. and Waisman, H. A. (1962). The identification of homocystine in the urine. *Biochem. Biophys. Res. Commun.*, **9**, 493
3. Mudd, S. H., Finkelstein, J. D., Irreverre, F. and Laster, L. (1964). Homo-cystinuria: an enzymatic defect. *Science*, **143**, 1443

4. Hunt, A. D. Jr., Stokes, J. Jr., McCrory, W. W. and Stroud, H. H. (1954). Pyridoxine dependency. A report of a case of intractable convulsions in an infant controlled by pyridoxine. *Pediatrics*, **13**, 140

5. Harris, J. W., Whittington, R. M., Weisman, R. Jr. and Horrigan, D. L. (1956). Pyridoxine responsive anemia in the human adult. *Proc. Soc. Exp. Biol., N.Y.*, **91**, 427

6. Frimpter, G. W., Haymovitz, A. and Horwith, M. (1963). Cystathioninuria. *New Engl. J. Med.*, **268**, 333

7. Tada, K., Yokayama, Y., Nakagawa, H., Yoshida, T. and Arakawa, T. (1967). Vitamin B_6 dependent xanthurenic aciduria. *Tohoku J. Exp. Med.*, **93**, 115

8. Barber, G. W. and Spaeth, G. L. (1967). Pyridoxine therapy in homocystinuria. *Lancet*, **i**, 337

9. Hooft, C., Carton, D. and Samyn, W. (1967). Pyridoxine treatment in homocystinuria. *Lancet*, **i**, 1384

10. Turner, B. (1967). Pyridoxine treatment in homocystinuria. *Lancet*, **i**, 1151

11. Perry, T. L. (1971). Treatment of homocystinuria with a low methionine diet and supplemental L-cystine. *Inherited Disorders of Sulphur Metabolism: Proc. 8th Symposium of the Society for the Study of Inborn Errors of Metabolism. Belfast, 1970*, p. 245. (Carson and Raine, editors) (London: Livingstone)

12. Hambraeus, L., Wranne, L. and Lorentsson, Rosa. (1968). Biochemical and therapeutic studies in two cases of homocystinuria. *Clin. Sci.*, **35**, 457

13. Carson, N. A. J. and Carré, I. J. (1969). Treatment of homocystinuria with pyridoxine. *Arch. Dis. Childh.*, **44**, 387

14. Cusworth, D. C. and Dent, C. E. (1969). Homocystinuria. *Brit. Med. Bull.*, **25**, 42

15. Ritchie, J. W. K. and Carson, N. A. J. (1973). Homocystinuria and pregnancy. *J. Obstet. Gynaec. Brit. Cwlth.*, **80**, 664

16. Brand, E., Harris, M. M. and Biloon, S. (1930). Cystinuria; excretion of cystine complex which decomposes in urine with liberation of free cystine. *J. Biol. Chem.*, **86**, 315

17. Spaeth, G. W. and Barber, G. L. (1967). Prevalence of homocystinuria among the mentally retarded: evaluation of a specific screening test. *Pediatrics*, **40**, 586

18. Gaull, G. E., Sturman, J. A., Rassin, D. K. and Schaffner, F. (1971). Biochemical and ultrastructural studies in homocystinuria: effects of vitamin B_6. *Inherited Disorders of Sulphur Metabolism: Proc. 8th Symposium of the Society for the Study of Inborn Errors of Metabolism. Belfast, 1970*, p. 289. (Carson and Raine, editors) (London: Livingstone)

19. Wilcken, Bridget and Turner, B. (1973). Homocystinuria: reduced folate levels during pyridoxine treatment. *Arch. Dis. Childh.*, **48**, 58

20. Morrow, G. and Barness, L. A. (1972). Combined vitamin responsiveness in homocystinuria. *J. Pediat.*, **81**, 946

21. Carey, M. C., Fennelly, J. J. and Fitzgerald, O. (1968). Subnormal serum folate levels, increased folate clearance and effects of folic acid therapy. *Amer. J. Med.*, **45**, 26

22. Holt, L. E. Jr. and Snyderman, S. E. (1967). The amino acid requirements of children. *Amino Acid Metabolism and Genetic Variation*, p. 381. (W. L. Nyhan, editor). (New York: McGraw Hill)

23. Fomon, S. J., Thomas, L. N., Filer, L. J. Jr., Anderson, T. A. and Bergmann, K. E. (1973). Requirements for protein and essential amino acids in early infancy. *Acta Paediat. Scand.*, **62**, 33

24. Rose, W. C. and Nixom, R. L. (1955). The amino acid requirements of man XIII. The sparing effect of cystine on the methionine requirement. *J. Biol. Chem.*, **216**, 763

25. Brenton, D. P. and Cusworth, D. C. (1971). The response of patients with cystathionine synthase deficiency to pyridoxine. *Inherited Disorders of Sulphur Metabolism: Proc. 8th Symposium of the Society for the Study of Inborn Errors of Metabolism. Belfast, 1970*, p. 264. (Carson and Raine, editors) (London: Livingstone)

26. Gaull, G. E. (1972). Homocystinuria, vitamin B_6 and folate; metabolic interrelationships and clinical significance. *J. Pediat.*, **81**, 1014

27. Sturman, J. A., Gaull, G. E. and Raiha, N. C. (1970). Absence of cystathionase in human fetal liver. Is cystine essential? *Science*, **169**, 74

28. Komrower, G. M., Lambert, A. M., Cusworth, D. C. and Westall, R. G. (1966). The dietary treatment of homocystinuria. *Arch. Dis. Childh.*, **41**, 666

29. Coutts, J. M. J. and Fowler, B. (1967). Low methionine diets for homocystinuria with reference to two cases. *Nutrition*, 35

30. Fomon, S. J. (1959). Comparative study of human milk and a soya bean formula in promoting growth and nitrogen retention by infants. *Pediatrics*, **24**, 577

31. Fomon, S. J., Thomas, L. N., Filer, L. J. Jr., Anderson, T. A. and Bergman, K. E. (1973). Requirements for protein and essential amino acids in early infancy. Studies with a soy isolate formula. *Acta Paediat. Scand.*, **62**, 33

32. Chase, H. P., Goodman, S. I. and O'Brien, D. (1967). Treatment of homocystinuria. *Arch. Dis. Childh.*, **42**, 514

33. Brenton, D. P., Cusworth, D. C., Dent, C. E. and Jones, E. E. (1966). Homocystinuria. Clinical and dietary study. *Quart. J. Med.*, **35**, 325

34. Perry, T. L., Hansen, S., Love, D. L., Crawford, L. E. and Tischler, B. (1968). Treatment of homocystinuria with a low methionine diet, supplemental cystine and a methyl donor. *Lancet*, **ii**, 474

35. Komrower, G. M. and Sardharwalla, I. B. (1971). The dietary treatment of homocystinuria. *Inherited Disorders of Sulphur Metabolism: Proc. 8th Symposium of the Society for the Study of Inborn Errors of Metabolism. Belfast, 1970*, p. 254. (Carson and Raine, editors) (London: Livingstone)

36. Umbarger, B. (1960). Phenylketonuria: treating the disease and feeding the child. *Amer. J. Dis. Child.*, **100**, 908

37. McKusick, V. A., Hall, J. G. and Char, F. (1971). The clinical and genetic characteristics of homocystinuria. *Inherited Disorders of Sulphur Metabolism: Proc. 8th Symposium of the Society for the Study of Inborn Errors of Metabolism. Belfast, 1970*, p. 179. (Carson and Raine, editors) (London: Livingstone)

38. Milne, M. D. (1964). Disorders of amino acid transport. *Brit. Med. J.*, **i**, 327

39. Crawhall, J. C., Scowen, E. F. and Watts, R. W. E. (1963). Effect of penicillamine on cystinuria. *Brit. Med. J.*, **i**, 588

40. Cusworth, D. C. and Gatterau, A. (1968). Inhibition of renal tubular reabsorption of homocystine by lysine and arginine. *Lancet*, **ii**, 916

41. Tallan, H. H., Moore, S. and Stein, W. H. (1958). L-cystathionine in human brain. *J. biol. Chem.*, **230**, 707

42. Brenton, D. P., Cusworth, D. C. and Gaull, G. E. (1965). Homocystinuria: biochemical studies of tissues including a comparison with cystathioninuria. *Pediatrics*, **35**, 50

43. Wong, P. W. K. and Fresco, R. (1972). Tissue cystathionine in mice treated with cysteine and homoserine. *Pediat. Res.*, **6**, 172

44. Sturman, J. A., Schneidman, K. and Gaull, G. E. (1971). Cystathionine synthesis in brain: implications for treatment of homocystinuria. *Biochem. Med.*, **5**, 404

45. Wong, P. W. K., Schwarz, V. and Komrower, G. M. (1968). The biosynthesis of cystathionine in patients with homocystinuria. *Pediat. Res.*, **2**, 149

46. Hope, D. B. (1958). Studies of taurine and cystathionine in brain. *Proc. 4th International Congress of Biochemistry, Vienna, 1958*, **XIII**, 63. (London: (Pergamon Press)

47. Mudd, S. H., Finkelstein, J. D., Irreverre, F. and Laster, L. (1965). Transsulfuration in mammals. *J. biol. Chem.*, **240**, 4382

48. Wong, P. W. K. Personal communication

49. Gerritsen, T. and Waisman, H. (1964). Homocystinuria: an error in the metabolism of methionine. *Pediatrics*, **33**, 413

50. Carson, N. A. J., Cusworth, D. C., Dent, C. E., Field, C. M. B., Neill, D. W. and Westall, R. G. (1963). Homocystinuria: a new inborn error of metabolism associated with mental deficiency. *Arch. Dis. Childh.*, **38**, 425

51. Uhlendorf, B. W., Conerly, E. B. and Mudd, S. H. (1973). Homocystinuria: studies in tissue culture. *Pediat. Res.*, **7**, 645

52. Bittles, A. H. and Carson, N. A. J. (1973). Tissue culture techniques as an aid to prenatal diagnosis and genetic counselling in homocystinuria. *J. med. Genet.*, **10**, 120

CHAPTER 3

Maple Syrup Urine Disease

Selma E. Snyderman

Maple syrup urine disease—branched chain ketoaciduria—was first described as a clinical entity in 1954[1]. The original report contained all the salient clinical features: it described 4 children in one family, all of whom succumbed in the first weeks of life to a rapidly progressive neurological disorder. Of particular interest was the description of the odour of the children's urine, which was very similar to that of maple syrup. In the intervening years the site of the biochemical defect has been located, the pattern of inheritance studied, some features of the pathologic process documented and an effective treatment has been developed. In addition, several variants of what now should be called 'classical maple syrup urine disease' have been described.

Clinical features
These infants appear normal at birth, clinically there is no reason to believe that there is any problem. The first symptoms usually appear at about 3–5 days of age. The child seems listless and difficult to feed. A high pitched incessant cry is also an early feature. Neurological manifestations soon appear. These include loss of the Moro and the tendon reflexes, and abnormalities of eye movement; ophthalmoplegia has been recorded on a number of occasions. Alternating periods of flaccidity and hypertonicity are quite striking and are often followed by an opisthotonic position. Convulsions often appear at this stage in the the clinical progression of the disease. Coma and the onset of disturbances in respiration which include a very slow rate and periods of apnoea usually occur next. Once the disease has progressed to this stage, there is usually a steady downhill fatal course unless intensive therapy is instituted immediately. A rare infant has survived this initial phase but has suffered severe neurologic sequelae and profound mental retardation.

The characteristic odour of this malady frequently makes its appearance about the time that the neurological manifestations are apparent.

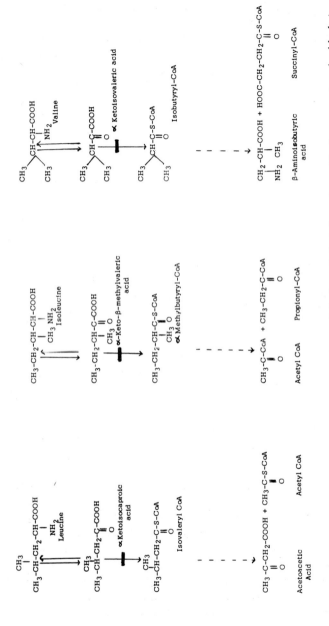

Figure 3.1. A simplified version of the metabolism of the branched chain amino acids demonstrating the block in maple syrup urine disease

It has been described as sweet, malty, caramel-like, or resembling that of maple syrup. It is usually noted first in the urine, but may also occur in the perspiration and ear cerumen. At times it may be so permeating that it is readily apparent when one enters the room of an affected infant.

The disease does not affect any one racial group predominantly. It has been observed in the United States, Great Britain, France, Switzerland, Norway, Germany, Italy, Morocco, Syria, India, Israel, Turkey and Japan. We have also observed it in the Negro, in several Jewish families originating in Central Europe, and in a Chinese family who emigrated from Hong Kong. Inheritance as Mendelian recessive is strongly suggested by the pattern of familial distribution. However, attempts to identify the carrier state have not been completely successful. Such attempts have included both amino acid loading tests and direct enzyme determination. Three variations of the load test have been studied; a leucine load and the observation of the rate of its disappearance from the plasma[2]: a similar procedure with the keto acid derivative of leucine: and a load of all 3 amino acids with observation of the formation of alloisoleucine[3]. We have not been able to demonstrate any clear-cut differences between heterozygotes and normal homozygotes, either with the use of a leucine load or the appearance of alloisoleucine after a load of isoleucine[4]. The ability of the leukocyte to metabolise sodium α-ketoisocaproate-2-[14]C *in-vitro* seems to be a somewhat better indicator of the carrier state. Cells obtained from fathers of affected children demonstrated significantly less activity, but the reduction in activity of cells obtained from the mothers could not be considered to be significant[5].

Biochemical features

The relationship of this disorder to the branched chain amino acids was first appreciated when Westall[6] found elevated levels of these in the plasma and urine of an affected infant. Subsequently the site of the metabolic block was demonstrated to be in the second step in the degradation of these amino acids; transamination procedes in a normal fashion, but oxidative decarboxylation is impaired[7-9] (Figure 3.1). It was originally presumed that these 3 keto acids shared a single decarboxylase, but subsequent work has demonstrated that at least 2 occur in the normal individual[10]. In bovine liver, the decarboxylation of α-ketoisocaproic acid (derived from leucine) and of α-ketomethylvaleric acid (from isoleucine) is catalysed by a single enzymatic agent while a second enzyme is active in the decarboxylation of the valine derivative[11], α-ketoisovaleric acid. The exact situation in the human is not at present clear. Since the alteration of 2 enzymes by a single gene defect has been questioned, an alternate explanation has been offered: that the accumulation of α-ketoisocaproic acid inhibits the decarboxylation of the other 2 keto acid derivatives. Since defective decarboxylation of each keto acid has been demonstrated in individual tissue culture studies, such inhibition cannot be solely responsible for this accumulation, but it is quite possible that it may aggravate the situation.

The enzyme defect results in the accumulation of both the keto acid derivatives and the branched chain amino acids in the child with the classical form of the disease. Elevated levels have been demonstrated in the plasma, urine, erythrocytes and the cerebrospinal fluid. The leucine concentration is usually much more abnormal than that of the other two amino acids; the reason for this is still not clear (Table 3.1). This is observed both at the time of the original diagnosis and whenever there is a biochemical relapse after the initiation of therapy.

In addition to elevation of the concentrations of the branched chain amino acids which normally occur in the plasma, a fourth branched chain amino acid, alloisoleucine, is also observed[12]. Its appearance there can be attributed to the enolisation of α-keto methylvaleric acid and its subsequent reamination (Figure 3.2). This is a consequence of the elevation of the plasma isoleucine level; in fact, if one loads a normal individual with isoleucine, alloisoleucine may appear in the plasma after a lag of several hours.

The only other alteration in plasma amino acid concentration observed with any degree of regularity is a depression of that of alanine: this may be in the range of $\frac{1}{4}$–$\frac{1}{3}$ of the normal. This reduction

Table 3.1. Plasma amino acid concentrations (mg/100 ml) in 18 cases of maple syrup urine disease, 5 days to 8 months old, at time of diagnosis

	Mean	Range	Normal subjects mean (SD)
Valine	11·8	7·1 –23·2	2·27 (0·57)
Isoleucine	8·1	4·1 –14·1	0·78 (0·19)
Leucine	39·5	24·6 –60·6	1·37 (0·40)
Alloisoleucine	3·1	1·96– 5·42	0
Alanine	0·58	0·24– 0·81	2·45 (0·63)

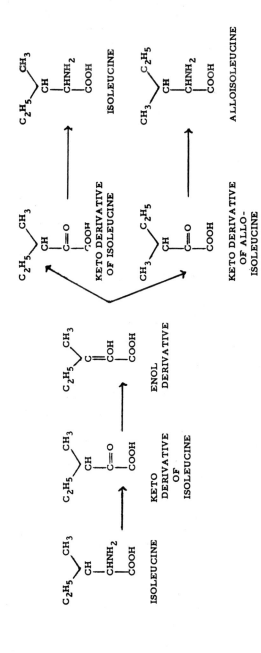

Figure 3.2. The formation of alloisoleucine from isoleucine

usually coincides with the elevation of the branched chain amino acids. Hypoglycaemia has also been observed, especially when the leucine concentration is abnormally high.

Pathology

The length of survival seems to influence the findings observed on postmortem examination[13]. There may be no abnormalities except for sponginess of the white matter in the brain if death occurs in the first few days of life. Deficient myelination and astrocytosis occur if the survival period is greater. The decreased myelin content seems to be the result of deficient synthesis rather than of increased destruction since products of myelin degradation have not been observed[14]. The diminished content of myelin lipids, cerebrosides and proteolipid protein also suggest deficient myelin formation[15].

The manner in which the metabolic block produces the extreme degree of central nervous system dysfunction is not at present known. A deleterious effect on brain metabolism by either the branched chain amino acids or their keto acid derivatives is a distinct possibility. Tashian[16] has shown that α-ketoisocaproic and α-methylvaleric acid inhibit the activity of L-glutamic acid decarboxylase in rat brain homogenates: Howell and Lee[17] have demonstrated that the keto acid derivatives of both the branched chain amino acids and of phenyl-alanine depress the oxygen utilisation of rat brain slices. Inhibition of the oxidation of pyruvate in rat brain homogenates by concentrations of α-ketoisocaproate of the order of magnitude present in the plasma of patients has also been observed[18]. Another possibility is that the elevated concentrations of branched chain amino acids may inhibit the transport of other essential amino acids across cell membranes. Aberrations in normal synaptic function may also account for the symptoms. Sustained alterations in both amino acid transport and in amino acid activating systems which result in impaired protein synthesis in the brain when either the levels of the branched chain amino acids or their keto acid derivates are elevated has been demonstrated by Appel[19]. He suggests that this may 'compromise newly forming synapses and intracellular communications being established in the developing brain'.

Diagnosis

The rapidity with which irreversible damage to the central nervous system can occur makes early diagnosis of this disease imperative. There should not be any problem in those families in whom the disease has previously occurred; however, it is frequently diagnosed too late when it is a first occurrence in a family. Often valuable time is lost in obtaining such procedures as electroencephalograms and pneumoencephalograms instead of pursuing possible metabolic causes for the central nervous system symptoms.

A clinical awareness as well as the use of a number of diagnostic tests, some of which are quite simple, should aid in establishing a diagnosis. The odour of these patients and their urine is quite remarkable. The 'nose test' should be part of the routine screening of all urine. Abnormal excretion of the keto acid derivatives of the branched chain amino acids can be detected by the use of 2,4-dinitrophenylhydrazine. This test has proved quite reliable if fresh urine is tested, and the reagent is reasonably fresh. In interpreting the results, one must remember that the newborn infant often has a slightly positive test and that a false positive may be obtained when ampicillin or one of its related compounds is being administered. A colour reaction is obtained with the ferric chloride test, a greyish-green colour results. More precise indication of elevation of keto acids may be obtained using thin-layer chromatography[20], and gas chromatographic techniques[21] are presently being developed. The concentration of branched chain amino acids in the plasma is usually sufficiently abnormal to be detected by one-dimensional paper chromatographic techniques. This can be confirmed by quantitative determination by ion-exchange column chromatography. Short column techniques will permit confirmation of this abnormality within one hour.

Final confirmation of the diagnosis can be made by determination of the enzyme activity of peripheral leukocytes[22]. Enzyme activity of the skin fibroblasts can also be determined, but the time required for cell culture reduces its utility as a diagnostic tool in the acute phase of the classical disease. However, it may prove to be quite useful in differentiating the several variants of the disease[23].

TREATMENT

Principles
In view of the rapidity of the downhill course in these infants, the institution of therapy must be considered to be a true medical emergency. It is quite possible that a delay even of hours may have an effect

77

on the eventual clinical state of the child. It might be considered expedient whenever the diagnosis is suspected, to immediately curtail the protein intake to the required level rather than continuing one of the usual infant formulas which contain a surfeit of protein.

Therapy is based on a limitation of intake of the 3 branched chain amino acids. The principle is similar to that of the therapy of a number of other disturbances of amino acid metabolism, to supply the requirement but not to allow any excess which the patient cannot catabolise because of the existence of the metabolic error. The difficulty in the nutritional management of maple syrup disease is the fact that the catabolism of 3 amino acids, all of which are essential, is impaired. In addition, the requirement of each, when expressed in terms of body weight, is different[24-26]: this then means that the intake of each must be adjusted individually. One cannot overemphasise the importance of the laboratory in monitoring therapy: good care of these children is impossible without accurate and rapid determination of the plasma amino acid concentrations. At present, the only method sufficiently precise is ion-exchange column chromatography.

There is no evidence that any of the compounds formed on the distal side of the block have any special nutritive function, hence supplementation with these would not seem to be necessary. Therapy is further complicated by the fact that the requirement in terms of body weight alters rapidly during the first months of life, and the fact that biochemical control is easily disturbed by a number of intercurrent events. Another factor is the inhibition of transamination that occurs as a result of keto acid accumulation; thus accumulated α-ketoisocaproic acid may not only inhibit leucine transamination, but that of isoleucine and valine as well. This has led us to try, whenever possible, to alter the intake of only one amino acid at a time (the one whose plasma concentration is most abnormal); of course, if all 3 are greatly elevated, then there must be readjustment of the intake of all.

Practical management

Dietary therapy is initiated as the sole therapy whenever treatment can be instituted before profound central nervous system disease is apparent. If convulsions, coma or respiratory depression have occurred, then some other form of emergency therapy (see next section) must also be employed. Since it is impossible to supply the protein requirement of the infant by any natural source without exceeding the requirement of the branched chain amino acids, it is necessary to supply the greater portion of the nitrogen moiety of the diet as a mixture of amino acids. The components of the diet with which we have had most experience are listed in Table 3.2. These components are mixed in our laboratory. Two other amino acid mixtures are available commercially in the United States. They have not yet been approved by the FDA, and are hence considered investigational. The other components of the diet may also be supplied by currently available products. (The carbohydrate, fat, vitamin, mineral portion of Lofenalac is available for such use.) Caloric requirement of infants on amino acid diets seem to be higher than those on diets of whole protein and we have tried to provide a caloric intake 10% above that usually recommended.

We have usually initiated the diet by providing it completely free of the branched chain amino acids while monitoring their plasma levels at intervals of 24–48 hours. As the plasma concentration of each of the branched chain amino acids approaches normal, individual supplementation is begun. Although the time to return to normal depends on the original degree of elevation, it has been our usual experience that isoleucine becomes normal first, usually within 2 or 3 days. This is followed in a day or two by normalisation of the valine level. Not only is the leucine level invariably the most abnormal, but it also takes the longest period of time to fall to normal levels; it usually takes a week to 10 days to do so. Pure solutions of L-leucine, L-isoleucine, and L-valine are utilised for this initial supplementation; this allows varying the intake of each individually which is not possible when natural foods with fixed ratio are utilised. Solutions containing 10 mg/ml are convenient for this purpose. The first weeks of therapy are usually characterised by great variations in plasma levels, thus frequent plasma monitoring (2–3 times weekly) and subsequent dietary readjustment are necessary. As soon as the plasma levels become fairly stationary, a carefully measured quantity of milk is substituted for part or all of the solutions. This is, of course dependent on the ratios of the pure solutions in use at the time. We have usually been successful in doing this between 2–3 months of age. This is important to avoid 'unidentified factor deficiency' which manifests itself as a failure to gain after 2–6 months on a completely synthetic diet that contains all the known nutritional factors[27]. This suggests the existence of still unknown dietary requirements for growth in the young infant. Other low protein natural foods such as fruits, certain vegetables and rice cereal are begun as soon as the levels have become stable on the milk supplement. It is

Table 3.2. Composition of the synthetic diet

Component	Amount (g)	Percentage of total calories
L-Amino acid mixture	100·00	12
L-Alanine	2·67	
L-Arginine	4·58	
L-Aspartic acid	8·78	
L-Cystine	2·14	
L-Glutamic acid	17·56	
Glycine	2·06	
L-Histidine	1·76	
L-Isoleucine	varied	
L-Leucine	varied	
L-Lysine hydrochloride	7·10	
L-Methionine	1·68	
L-Phenylalanine	4·89	
L-Proline	6·11	
L-Serine	5·34	
L-Threonine	4·58	
L-Tyrosine	4·58	
L-Tryptophan	1·68	
L-Valine	varied	
Corn oil	160·00	43
Dextrimaltose	375·00	45
Mineral mixture	22·30	
B vitamin mixture	10 ml/day	
Vitamins A, C, and D supplied at Tri Visol	0·6 ml/day	

The amino acid mixture, corn oil, dextrimaltose and mineral mixture are mixed with 176 g water, the caloric concentration of the diet is 4 calories/g and 125 calories/kg body weight are fed daily. The vitamins are administered separately.

The composition of the mineral mixture is as follows: NaCl 18·9 g; $CaHPO_4$ (anhydrous) 25·4 g; $MgSO_4$ (anhydrous) 6·8 g; $KHCO_3$ 44·4 g; KCl 2·88 g; Fe_3 citrate 2·21 g; $CuSO_4$ (anhydrous) 0·24 g; $MnSO_4$ (anhydrous) 0·15 g; KI 0·015 g; NaF 0·03 g.

The B vitamin mixture provides the following intake (mg/day): thiamine 0·38; riboflavin 2·0; nicotinamide 0·85; calcium pantothenate 3·5; pyridoxine 0·67; hexahydroxycylohexane 180; para-amino-benzoic acid 0·5; choline chloride 147; biotin 0·03; folic acid 0·05; cyanocobalamine 0·015.

usually possible, at this time, to reduce the frequency of monitoring to 1–2 times weekly.

Shortly after this, it is possible to make use of a mixture of gelatine and amino acids to supply the dietary nitrogen (Table 3.3). This has the advantage of reducing the cost of therapy since some of the amino acids contained in the gelatine are the most expensive, and it also reduces the number of individual components that must be weighed when the diet is being prepared locally. Occasionally an infant seems

Table 3.3. Gelatin-amino acid mixtures used in treatment of maple syrup urine disease (g/kg body weight)

Gelatin	2·0	1·75	1·25	0·86
L-Tryptophan	0·063	0·063	0·063	0·063
L-Threonine	0·134	0·139	0·148	0·156
L-Lysine	0·174	0·195	0·215	0·232
L-Methionine	0·048	0·051	0·055	0·057
L-Cystine	0·080	0·080	0·080	0·080
L-Tyrosine	0·163	0·164	0·166	0·168
L-Phenylalanine	0·143	0·148	0·158	0·166
L-Histidine	0·051	0·053	0·056	0·062
Provides in mg/kg				
Leucine	59·0	51·0	36·5	25·2
Isoleucine	27·0	23·8	17·0	11·7
Valine	48·0	42·5	30·0	20·8
Equivalent to				
g protein/kg	2·56	2·20	1·89	1·73

to prefer the taste of the gelatine mixture. The most important disadvantage of the gelatine is its appreciable content of branched chain amino acids. This greatly limits the intake of natural foods. It also makes it difficult to substantially reduce or completely omit the branched chain amino acids whenever biochemical control is lost.

At present, there is no way of determining just how rigid control should be to obtain the best therapeutic results. We have made efforts to maintain the plasma amino acids within the normal range, especially during the first years of treatment. This has been usually possible, except that small amounts of alloisoleucine do persist in the plasma in spite of normal concentrations of isoleucine.

Intercurrent infections or other untoward events, such as fractures, which cause a negative nitrogen balance, may result in a precipitous rise in the plasma branched chain amino acids and the excretion of appreciable amounts of their keto acid derivatives. Such episodes may be compared to feeding an unrestricted diet since all tissues contain the normal complement of these amino acids. We have frequently noted that these metabolic consequences of an infection may precede the clinical evidences by a period of 1–2 days. At such times, the supplement of branched chain amino acids should be omitted until the plasma concentrations once again approach normal. These episodes are also frequently associated with a severe acidosis which must be treated with the appropriate intravenous therapy. Any degree of dehydration should also be treated vigorously by intravenous therapy to prevent any concentration of toxic metabolites.

It has been our experience that the leucine concentration is that most closely associated with the onset of clinical symptoms. Irritability and ataxia are the two earliest clinical symptoms of chemical relapse. This ataxia is most often manifest as an unsteady gait, and several parents have described it as 'tipsy'. These symptoms may also persist for a day or two after biochemical control is restored. These neurological signs frequently seem to occur when plasma leucine exceeds 10 mg/100 ml. We have not been able to relate the appearance of neurological manifestations to the plasma concentrations of either isoleucine or valine: however, elevated isoleucine is usually accompanied by a return of the characteristic odour.

Another deficiency in our knowledge of the therapy of these children is how long therapy must be continued. It is the author's opinion that some degree of dietary control will have to be continued for life. The oldest child to be treated, now 14·5 years of age, still manifests clinical symptoms whenever biochemical control is lost. We have, however, been more liberal in our control of these older children and have been satisfied if the plasma concentrations of the branched chain amino acids are maintained at 3–4 times the normal values.

Results of therapy

There can be little doubt as to the benefit of therapy when one considers that without treatment, the disease was almost invariably fatal. Although there are still relatively few cases treated for really prolonged

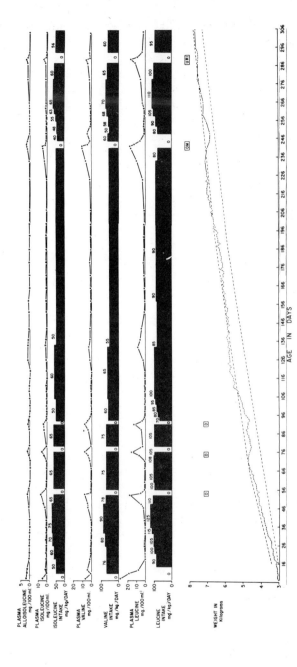

Figure 3.3. The protocol of an infant treated from the age of 6 days; the first 10 months

83

periods, the end results seem to be directly related to the age at which treatment is initiated, the condition of the infant at the time the diagnosis is established, and the number and severity of relapses[28-31]. Normal neurological and mental development has been observed in infants treated during the first week of life before the onset of the severe neurological manifestations of intractable convulsions and interference with respiration. Figures 3.3 and 3.4 illustrate the course of such a child.

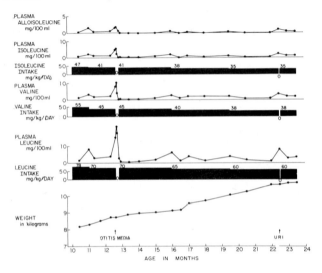

Figure 3.4. Further treatment course of patient illustrated in Figure 3.3. This child is physically, mentally and neurologically normal at 2·5 years of age

However, we have observed considerable improvement even if therapy is started later. Reinstitution of spontaneous respiration, return of swallowing and sucking, cessation of convulsive seizures, loss of rigidity, return of tendon reflexes, and reappearance of spontaneous activity have all been observed following the fall in plasma amino acid concentrations to normal. We have also observed normalisation of the electroencephalogram after 6 weeks to 3 months of dietary control. However, late initiation of therapy is invariably accompanied by mental retardation and neurological sequelae. Such children seem to have a certain degree of spasticity. We have 3 children under our care who are clinically indistinguishable from any other patients classified as having 'cerebral palsy', all were diagnosed after the first month of life.

Treatment during acute episodes

The condition of most of these infants, when first diagnosed, is so precarious that one cannot wait for the biochemical improvement to occur as a result of dietary therapy alone. Dramatic clinical and biochemical improvement can be achieved by a series of exchange transfusions or a prolonged course of peritoneal dialysis or a combination of both[32]. We do not know which of these two forms of acute therapy is more beneficial. It has been our experience, as well as that of others[33], that a single exchange transfusion is not sufficient; this results in only temporary improvement with both clinical and chemical relapse in a matter of hours. The condition of these infants is usually so desperate that both of these forms of therapy should be immediately employed (Figure 3.5).

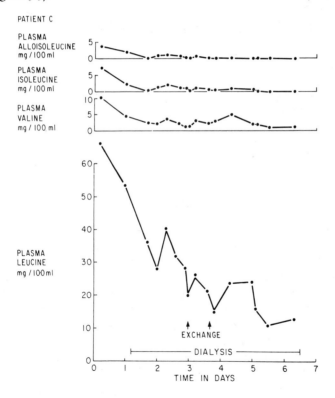

Figure 3.5. The effect of peritoneal dialysis and exchange transfusions on the plasma amino acids of a comatose infant

Although, as noted previously, mild relapse can usually be controlled by removal of the branched chain amino acids from the diet for a short period of time, we have also observed relapses that required much more vigorous therapy. In addition to the appropriate intravenous therapy for the occurrence of dehydration and acidosis, we have also employed peritoneal dialysis for periods of 1–3 days with very encouraging results. Supplying sufficient calories and an amino acid mixture free of the branched chain amino acids to prevent tissue breakdown is a very important, although less dramatic, part of the therapy during these acute episodes. Calories can be supplied intravenously by the use of carbohydrate and fat solutions, but at present no appropriate amino acid solution is available for intravenous use. We have had good results from administering the amino acid mixture by nasogastric tube when it was suspended in a small volume of fluid and fed at 4-hour intervals. This has been tolerated even in the presence of some form of assisted respiration. Careful monitoring of the plasma amino acids and of the urinary keto acids is necessary to determine how long this course of treatment must be carried out.

VARIANT FORMS

Two well-defined variant forms of branched chain keto aciduria have been described, a third possible variant has only been observed on one occasion. The first variant is episodic[34-37], the second has many of the same features at the classical disease, but the clinical manifestations are milder and the distinguishing feature of the third variety is the apparent therapeutic effectiveness of large doses of thiamine.

Episodic or intercurrent maple syrup urine disease, as the name implies, manifests clinical symptoms and abnormal plasma amino acid levels only with the advent of some special stress. The stress may be an infection, or any untoward occurrence that results in a negative nitrogen balance, or an unusually great protein intake. Several instances have been reported of apparently normal children who manifested convulsions, coma and death after a relatively mild infection. Between episodes, these children are perfectly well. The metabolic block is at the same site as in the classical form and there is apparently enough residual enzyme activity to maintain biochemical homeostasis on a normal diet, except when some untoward event occurs. No treatment is required except at the time of stress when therapy may have to be exactly the same as for the classical form with elimination of the branched chain amino acids and intravenous fluid therapy. Extremely high protein intakes should be avoided.

Mental retardation has been the presenting symptom of most of the children suffering from the second variant; acute episodes with the full-blown clinical picture occur frequently, usually in response to some stress[38-40]. Unlike the intermittent variety, some degree of biochemical derangement is always present when a normal diet is provided. The degree of impairment of enzyme activity is greater than in the intermittent variant, and lies between it and the classical variety. The two brothers we have observed are in complete biochemical control when their protein intake is maintained at or just above requirement. Since this has been provided as natural protein, this does exceed the requirement for the branched chain amino acids. More stringent limitation of intake of these amino acids has not been necessary except during acute episodes. The older boy was already retarded

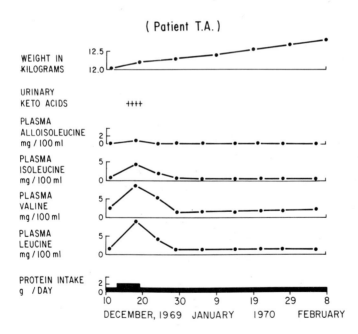

Figure 3.6. The response of the plasma amino acids to protein restriction in a child with a variant form of maple syrup urine disease

when he came under our observation, but has made considerable progress with this therapy. The younger sibling, who was put under surveillance immediately after birth, has had normal development with restricted protein intake. Calculation of the branched chain amino acid intake provided by the quantity of milk protein permitted, revealed that this child has been able to maintain his plasma amino acids in the normal range on an intake considerably above that tolerated by the child with classical maple syrup urine disease. In addition, his plasma is free of alloisoleucine, except during relapse. The clinical course of this child is illustrated in Figure 3.6.

The third variant, a form of the disease responsive to the administration of thiamine, has only been observed on one occasion[41]. This therapy has been tried a number of times in both the classical and variant forms of the disease, but without any therapeutic effect[42,43].

References

1. Menkes, J. H., Hurst, P. L. and Craig, J. M. (1954). A new syndrome: progressive familial infantile cerebral dysfunction associated with an unusual urinary substance. *Pediatrics*, **14**, 462
2. Lonsdale, D., Mercer, R. D. and Faulkner, W. R. (1963). Maple syrup urine disease. *Am. J. Dis. Child.*, **106**, 258
3. Linneweh, F. and Ehrlich, M. (1963). Heterozygoten-test für die ahornsirup-Krankheit. *Klin. Wchnschr.*, **41**, 255
4. Snyderman, S. E., Sansaricq, C. and Norton, P. (Unpublished data)
5. Dancis, J., Hutzler, J. and Levitz, M. (1965). Detection of the heterozygote in maple syrup urine disease. *J. Pediat.*, **66**, 595
6. Westall, R. G., Dancis, J. and Miller, S. (1957). Maple syrup urine disease—a new molecular disease. *Am. J. Dis. Child.*, **94**, 571
7. Mackenzie, D. Y. and Woolf, L. I. (1959). Maple syrup urine disease—an inborn error in the metabolism of valine, leucine, and isoleucine associated with gross mental deficiency. *Brit. Med. J.*, **i**, 90
8. Menkes, J. H. (1959). Maple syrup urine disease: isolation and identification of organic acids in the urine. *Pediatrics*, **23**, 348
9. Dancis, J., Levitz, M., Miller, S. and Westall, R. G. (1959). Maple syrup urine disease. *Brit. Med. J.*, **i**, 91
10. Bowden, J. A. and Connelly, J. L. (1968). Branched chain α-keto acid metabolism. II; Evidence for the common identity of α ketoisocaproic and α keto-β-methyl valeric acid dehydrogenases. *J. biol. Chem.*, **243**, 3526
11. Connelly, J. L., Danner, D. J. and Bowden, J. A. (1968). Branched chain α-keto acid metabolism. I; Isolation, purification, and partial character-

88

ization of bovine liver α-ketoisocaproic: α keto-β-methylvaleric acid dehydrogenase. *J. biol. chem.*, **243**, 1198

12. Norton, P. M., Roitman, E., Snyderman, S. E. and Holt, L. E. Jr. (1962). A new finding in maple syrup urine disease. *Lancet*, **i**, 26
13. Sander, C., Clotten, R., Noetzel, H. and Wehinger, H. (1968). The clinical aspects and the morbid anatomy of maple syrup urine disease. *Dtsch. Med. Wschr.*, **93**, 895
14. Prensky, A. L., Carr, S. and Moser, H. W. (1968). Development of myelin in inherited disorders of amino acid metabolism. *Arch. Neurol.*, **19**, 552
15. Prensky, A. L. and Moser, H. W. (1966). Brain lipids, proteolipids, and free amino acids in maple syrup urine disease. *J. Neurochem.*, **13**, 863
16. Tashian, R. E. (1961). Inhibition of brain glutamic decarboxylase by phenylalanine, leucine and valine derivatives: a suggestion concerning the neurologic defect in phenylketonuria and branched chain ketoaciduria. *Metabolism*, **10**, 393
17. Howell, R. K. and Lee, M. (1963). Influence of alpha-keto acids on the respiration of brain in vitro. *Proc. Soc. Exper. Biol. and Med.*, **113**, 660
18. Bowder, J. A., McArthur, C. L. III. and Fried, M. (1971). The inhibition of pyruvate decarboxylation in rat brain by α ketoisocaproic acid. *Biochem. Med.*, **5**, 101
19. Appel, S. H. (1966). Inhibition of brain protein synthesis: an approach to the biochemical basis of neurological dysfunction in the aminoacidurias. *Trans. N.Y. Acad. Scien.*, **29**, 63
20. Dancis, J., Hutzler, J. and Levitz, M. (1963). Thin layer chromatography and spectrophotometry of α-ketoacid hydrazones. *Biochem. Biophys. Acta*, **78**, 85
21. Greer, M. and Williams, C. M. (1967). Diagnosis of branched-chain ketonuria (maple syrup urine disease) by gas chromatography. *Biochem. Med.*, **1**, 87
22. Wendel, U., Wohler, W., Goedde, H. W., Langenbeck, U., Passarge, E. and Rudiger, H. W. (1973). Rapid diagnosis of maple syrup urine disease (branched chain ketoaciduria) by micro-enzyme assay in leukocytes and fibroblasts. *Clin. Chim. Acta*, **45**, 433
23. Dancis, J., Hutzler, J., Snyderman, S. E. and Cox, R. P. (1972). Enzyme activity in classical and variant forms of maple syrup urine disease. *J. Pediat.*, **81**, 312
24. Snyderman, S. E., Roitman, E., Boyer, A. and Holt, L. E. Jr. (1961). Essential amino acid requirements of infants: Leucine. *Am. J. Dis. Child.*, **102**, 157
25. Snyderman, S. E., Boyer, A., Norton, P. M., Roitman, E. and Holt, L. E. Jr. (1964). The essential amino acid requirements of infants. IX. Isoleucine. *J. Clin. Nutr.*, **15**, 313

26. Snyderman, S. E., Holt, L. E. Jr., Smellie, F., Boyer, A. and Westall, R. G. (1959). The essential amino acid requirements of infants: Valine. *Am. J. Dis. Child.*, **97**, 186

27. Snyderman, S. E., Holt, L. E. Jr., Nemir, R. L., Guy, L. P., Carretero, R. and Ketron, K. C. (1950). Observations on an unknown dietary factor essential for human growth. *J. Nutr.*, **42**, 31

28. Snyderman, S. E., Norton, P. M., Roitman, E. and Holt, L. E. Jr. (1964). Maple syrup urine disease with particular reference to dieto-therapy. *Pediatrics*, **34**, 454

29. Snyderman, S. E. (1967). The therapy of Maple Syrup Urine Disease. *Am. J. Dis. Child.*, **113**, 68

30. Westall, R. G. (1963). Dietary treatment of a child with maple syrup urine disease. *Arch. Dis. Child.*, **38**, 485

31. Goodman, S. I., Pollak, S., Miles, B. and O'Brien, D. (1968). The treatment of Maple Syrup Urine Disease. *J. Pediat.*, **75**, 485

32. Snyderman, S. E., Sansaricq, C. and Schacht, R. (Unpublished observations)

33. Schuchmann, L., Witt, I., Schulz, P., Schumacher, H. and Rudiger, H. (1972). Multiple exchange transfusion as treatment during the acute period in Maple Syrup Urine Disease. *Helv. Paediat. Acta*, **27**, 449

34. Morris, M. D., Lewis, B. D., Doolan, P. D. and Harper, H. A. (1961). Clinical and Biochemical observations on an apparently non-fatal variant of branched-chain ketoaciduria. *Pediatrics*, **28**, 918

35. Kiil, R. and Rokkones, T. (1964). Late manifesting variant of branched-chain ketoaciduria. *Acta Paediatrica*, **53**, 356

36. Van Der Horst, J. L. and Wadman, S. K. (1971). A variant form of branched chain ketoaciduria. *Act. Paediat. Scand.*, **60**, 594

37. Goedde, H. W., Langenbeck, U., Brackertz, D., Keller, W., Rokkones, T., Halvarsen, S., Kiil, R. and Merton, B. (1970). Clinical and biochemical-genetic aspects of intermittent branched chain ketoaciduria. *Acta. Paediat. Scand.*, **59**, 83

38. Schulman, J. D., Lustberg, T. J., Kennedy, J. L., Museles, M. and Seegmiller, J. E. (1970). A new variant of maple syrup urine disease (branched chain ketoaciduria). *Am. J. Med.*, **49**, 118

39. Fischer, M. H. and Gerritsen, T. (1971). Biochemical studies on a variant of branched chain ketoaciduria in a 19-year-old female. *Pediatrics*, **48**, 795

40. Snyderman, S. E., Sansaricq, C. and Garg, S. (Unpublished observations)

41. Scriver, C. R., Clow, C. L., Mackenzie, S. and Delvin, E. (1971). Thiamine-responsive maple syrup urine disease. *Lancet*, **i**, 310

42. Wong, P. W. K., Justice, P., Smith, G. F. and Hsia, D. Y. Y. (1972). A case of classical maple syrup urine disease 'thiamine non-responsive'. *Clin. Genetics*, **3**, 27

43. Snyderman, S. E., Sansaricq, C. and Norton, P. M. (Unpublished observations)

CHAPTER 4

The Galactosaemias

G. N. Donnell and W. R. Bergren

From the Genetics Research and the Biochemistry Laboratories, Childrens Hospital of Los Angeles, and the Departments of Pediatrics and of Biochemistry, School of Medicine, University of Southern California.

Galactose metabolism
Galactose is a constituent of many foodstuffs of both animal and plant origin. This sugar primarily occurs in complex compounds which are not readily digestible by man, and consequently not a source of free galactose. In most animal milks, however, galactose is found in the form of the disaccharide lactose, a major source of calories for the infant. Lactose is hydrolysed in the intestine to the monosaccharides galactose and glucose (Figure 4.1). Following absorption, these sugars are used for energy and for the synthesis of a number of cell components such as glycolipids, mucopolysaccharides and glycoproteins.

Galactose enters the mainstream of energy-producing metabolism via conversion to glucose-1-phosphate. The pathway in man is the same as that demonstrated in yeast by Leloir and co-workers[1-3]. Three enzymatic reactions are involved (Figure 4.2). A functional impairment of any one blocks effective galactose utilisation.

The first reaction in the Leloir pathway results in phosphorylation of galactose to galactose-1-phosphate (Gal-1-P), mediated by galactokinase in the presence of ATP and magnesium ion. Galactose-1-phosphate uridyl transferase (transferase) is the enzyme for the second step. There is an exchange of galactose-1-phosphate for the glucose-1-phosphate moiety of uridine diphosphate glucose (UDPG), resulting in release of glucose-1-phosphate and the formation of uridine diphosphate galactose (UDPGal). In the third step, UDPGal is transformed to UDPG: the enzyme UDPGal-4-epimerase (epimerase) catalyses the change in position of the hydroxyl group at carbon 4 of the galactose

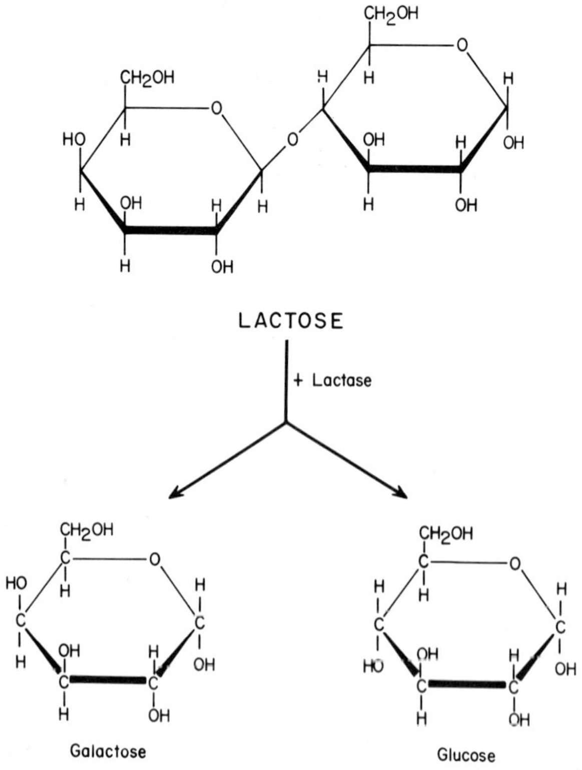

Figure 4.1. Hydrolysis of lactose

unit in UDPGal. This is the step that converts galactose to glucose. As the process continues, galatose is moved through the UDPG pool to give glucose-1-phosphate. The epimerase reaction has an important bearing on dietary treatment of galactosaemia. Because the reaction is reversible, galactose is not an essential nutrient. UDPGal, the starting point for synthesis of necessary galactose-containing compounds, can be derived from UDPG.

Well-defined deficiency states are known for 2 of the 3 enzymes in the pathway, each with recognised clinical manifestations. The defect in transferase has been the most studied, and it is to this condition that the term 'galactosaemia' has been applied. More recently, individuals with a galactokinase defect have been reported. Since this entity also is characterised by galactosaemia, it would be preferable to identify the

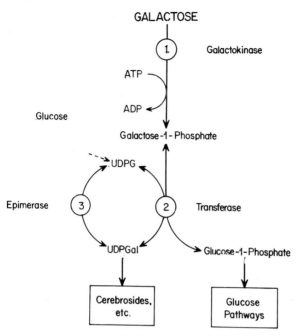

Figure 4.2. Major pathway of galactose metabolism

2 entities as transferase defect and galactokinase defect respectively. An epimerase defect has been reported in one asymptomatic individual[4]. Despite normal transferase activity, a substantial amount of galactose-1-phosphate was found to accumulate in erythrocytes upon feeding galactose to the child.

In addition to the main metabolic route for galactose, subsidiary pathways have been described. One involves reduction of free galactose by the enzyme aldose reductase to the sugar alcohol galactitol. Galactitol is not further metabolised. In normal individuals, this pathway does not represent an important route. However, in either the galactokinase defect or the transferase defect, galactitol accumulates and can be demonstrated in urine[5,6]. There is evidence to indicate that galactitol is directly or indirectly implicated in cataract formation[7]. Another known reaction for the disposal of galactose is oxidation to galactonic acid by a mechanism which has not been completely clarified[8-10]. Oral administration of galactose loads to transferase defect patients, or even to normal individuals, results in the appearance of galactonate in urine[11].

A reaction which at best has minor significance is the conversion of Gal-1-P to UDPGal by a pyrophosphorylase[12,13]. Another possibility is conversion of Gal-1-P to Gal-6-P by phosphoglucomutase, and subsequent oxidation by glucose-6-phosphate dehydrogenase[14]. No physiological significance for either of these routes has been established.

Although both galactokinase deficiency and transferase deficiency can be suspected on clinical grounds, laboratory confirmation is essential.

Laboratory diagnosis

Galactosuria, reflecting galactose intake, is common to untreated patients with either defect. A laboratory using only a glucose-specific method, based on glucose oxidase (Test Tape, Clinistix), will miss galactose. A non–specific test based on copper reduction (Benedict's test, Clinitest, etc.) will detect all reducing sugars. Comparison of the two can be indicative of the presence of galactose. Further identification of galactose can be made by chromatography or by specific enzymatic methods. It should be noted, however, that the presence of galactosuria is not by itself diagnostic, since measurable amounts of galactose can be found in urine of sick infants with a variety of problems[15].

Measurement of blood galactose can be a useful adjunct, since the concentration is substantially elevated in the untreated patient. At one time the oral galactose tolerance test was used for confirmation of diagnosis of galactosaemia. It is doubtful that this test now has any place in the diagnosis of galactosaemia. A prolonged tolerance curve is found, but the curve also may be abnormal whenever liver function is impaired. The galactose load may be harmful to some patients[16]. The test does not distinguish normal individuals from heterozygotes[17,18].

Testing for galactosaemia has been instituted in many places as an outgrowth of the screening of newborn infant populations for phenyl-ketonuria. Two major methods are in use. One, based on Guthrie's microbiological assay, is dependent upon the presence of galactose in the blood sample[19]. Consequently, both the transferase and the galactokinase defect may be recognised. The other, based on a pro-cedure developed by Beutler, detects a transferase deficiency but not a galactokinase defect[20]. Neither of the screening procedures provides a sufficient basis for diagnosis.

Definitive confirmation must be based on a specific enzyme assay. It is fortunate that the complete galactose pathway is present in the erythrocytes of normal individuals and that the defects are reflected in the red cells of affected patients. A number of satisfactory methods are available for assay of erythrocyte galactokinase and transferase[21-24]. The blood sample should be referred to a laboratory in which the methodology is regularly in use, since errors in diagnosis can occur as a result of laboratory inexperience.

Delays may occur in obtaining the results of laboratory tests. It is wise to initiate treatment as soon as galactosaemia is suspected on clinical grounds, rather than to await laboratory confirmation.

CLINICAL FEATURES

Galactokinase deficiency

Galactokinase deficiency was first reported by Gitzelmann in 1965[25]. The patient was a 42-year-old man of average intelligence who originally had been described as having galactose diabetes at 9 years of age by Fanconi[26]. Cataracts were present, and both galactose and galactitol were found in the urine. A deficiency was demonstrated in erythrocyte galactokinase activity. Later, an older sister also was shown to have the defect. Several additional patients now have been reported. The only major clinical manifestation in common is cataract. Hepatomegaly, jaundice and mental retardation have not been features of this disorder, in contrast to the transferase defect. In one patient, hyperbilirubinaemia was observed, in another, hepatosplenomegaly [27,28]. In neither of these patients did the condition persist, and any relationship of these findings to the basic disorder is unclear. In another reported case, cataracts were seen early; development was relatively normal until 17 years of age, at which time generalised seizures and mental deterioration began[29]. It was doubted that the neurological disease was related to the galactokinase defect, but this could not be established.

The defect is at the first step in the pathway. Therefore, galactose accumulates in the body but not galactose-1-phosphate. Both galactosuria and galactosaemia are present. The reduction of galactose to galactitol by aldose reductase in the lens is thought to account for the formation of cataracts[7].

Because the only clinical manifestation of the disorder is cataracts, the diagnosis can be missed early in life unless the infant is screened for abnormalities in galactose metabolism. A relatively simple approach, as a general measure for all infants seen, is to examine urine for reducing substance 1–2 hours after a milk feed. Early detection is important, since the development of cataracts can be prevented by exclusion of lactose from the diet. Preliminary information indicates that cataracts improve when treatment is begun quite early but that the results are not satisfactory if the cataracts have become more dense.

Treatment of the galactokinase defect is exclusion of lactose and other sources of galactose from the diet. Details of management are presented below in the section on the transferase defect.

It has been suggested by Monteleone[30] and by Beutler[31] that there is an increased risk of cataracts in carriers of the galactokinase deficiency. Beutler has advanced the view that consideration should be given to some degree of dietary restriction for carriers[32]. This could be of special importance in families at risk for producing an affected child. Galactokinase activity has been demonstrated in cultured amniotic cells, providing a basis for prenatal diagnosis[29,33].

Galactokinase deficiency appears to be transmitted as an autosomal trait. Both males and females have been found to be affected. Parents of affected children are carriers and have intermediate levels of erythrocyte galactokinase activity. Carrier frequency was found to be approximately one in a hundred by Mayes and Guthrie[34], corresponding to an estimated incidence of between 1 : 40 000 to 1 : 50 000.

Transferase deficiency
Galactosaemia as we know it today probably was first described in 1908 by von Reuss[35], but the first clear statement that galactosaemia is an inborn error of metabolism was made by Gorter in 1951[36]. Kalckar and his associates[37] established that the defect is in the activity of the enzyme galactose-1-phosphate uridyltransferase (Figure 4.2).

Most untreated patients with the transferase defect show distinctive clinical manifestations early in life. The affected infant usually appears normal at birth, and symptoms develop only after feeds containing lactose are given. Food often is refused, vomiting is common and diarrhoea is seen occasionally. The early manifestations include lethargy, hypotonia, jaundice, hepatomegaly, and susceptability to infection. Later, cataracts become evident, and physical and mental retardation occur in surviving, untreated patients. The frequency of signs and symptoms among symptomatic cases of galactosaemia seen at the Children's Hospital of Los Angeles is indicated in Table 4.1. Excluded from the table are affected children treated at birth because of a known family history.

Jaundice usually develops within 3–4 days after institution of milk feeding and may persist for a number of weeks. Mild haemolysis often

Table 4.1. Signs and symptoms at the time of diagnosis among 39 symptomatic cases of galactosaemia

Major organ system	Signs and symptoms	Percentage of occurrence
General	Anorexia and weight loss	59
	Pallor	8
	Lethargy	18
	Cyanosis	8
	Retarded growth	5
Hepatic	Hepatomegaly	100
	Jaundice	85
	Ascites	15
	Peripheral oedema	3
	Haemorrhagic phenomena	5
Gastrointestinal	Vomiting	41
	Abdominal distension	23
	Diarrhoea	8
Ophthalmologic	Cataract	38
Spleen	Splenomegaly	15
Renal	Galactosuria	100
	Proteinuria	100
	Dark urine (bile pigments)	15
Central nervous system	Bulging anterior fontanel	10
	Mental retardation (DQ < 70)	5

is evident. The pathogenesis of the liver damage is unclear, but retention of bilirubin may result from injury to hepatic cells by metabolites of galactose. It is doubtful that free galactose or galactitol is responsible, since liver involvement is absent in galactokinase deficiency but present in the transferase deficiency. A recent publication by Kepler and Decker[38] suggests that galactosamine-1-phosphate may be the responsible metabolite.

The results of conventional liver function tests for hepatocellular damage are abnormal in the majority of untreated patients. The bilirubin levels are usually moderately elevated, with variable ratios of direct and indirect forms. Occasionally, indirect bilirubin rises above

20 mg/100 ml and some of these infants have had exchange transfusions. Liver enlargement is a consistent finding, but enlargement of the spleen is variable. Oedema and ascites are present in about 15% of the untreated children, due in part to malnutrition, in part to liver dysfunction. Further evidence for liver disease is hypoprothrombinaemia, a hazard in relation to liver biopsy.

The untreated infant with severe galactosaemia appears to be highly susceptible to bacterial infections which do not respond favourably to therapy unless there is a concomitant restriction of dietary galactose. Many deaths in early infancy are due to infection. No primary immunological defect has been demonstrated in these children, and the causes of the increased susceptibility are not yet clear. The diagnosis of galactosaemia should always be considered in an infant suspected of sepsis.

All patients appear to have some renal involvement. The galactosuria is often associated with proteinuria and a generalised aminoaciduria. The renal tubular acidosis which has been described in some untreated patients may result in a metabolic acidosis. These findings disappear on a restricted galactose diet.

In the untreated patients who survive beyond infancy, physical development is unsatisfactory and there is a high risk of mental retardation. Surveys in institutions for the retarded have not revealed very many galactosaemics, due undoubtedly to the high mortality rate. Reports of untreated patients with normal intelligence are rare[39].

Lenticular opacities are present in most untreated patients. They are difficult to detect in the infant and can be missed. Without treatment, the cataracts may become dense and interfere with vision.

Clinical manifestations in classical galactosaemia differ in severity over a wide range. In some cases, the course is fulminant, and death occurs early in life consequent to inanition, infection or hepatic failure. In a few individuals, signs and symptoms are sufficiently mild to escape early detection. The majority of patients, however, demand prompt recognition and treatment to ensure an optimal prognosis.

Patients with a milder clinical picture have been described in older publications. In some, actual occurrence of a transferase defect is uncertain because of insufficient biochemical evidence. Some may have had a galactokinase deficiency[25,40]. Cataract was the only pertinent clinical feature in patients reported by Ritter and Cannon[41], and by Durand and Semach[42]. Cataracts and hepatomegaly, but normal intelligence were noted in a 65-year-old galactosaemic by Hugh-

Jones et al.[43] Beutler[44] has speculated that this individual may not have been homozygous for the classical transferase defect, but instead heterozygous for transferase deficiency and another variant of transferase (the Duarte variant).

There are 2 genetic variants of transferase known which are not usually associated with clinical manifestations. The Duarte variant enzyme[44,45] differs from the normal one in electrophoretic mobility. In addition it has a lesser activity (Table 4.5). The Los Angeles variant[46] also has a different electrophoretic mobility, but activity is normal or increased. Both variants are common in the population and are important in relation to genetic counselling.

There has been one report of an 8-month-old male infant, thought to be a Duarte variant homozygote, who was jaundiced during the first 2 months of life[47]. His liver was enlarged, and on biopsy, 'marked fatty infiltration, bile retention, periportal fibrosis and pseudoacinar changes' were noted. Urine analysis was normal. The child improved without treatment. It is not possible at this time to say whether or not the clinical manifestations were due to the presence of the variant enzyme.

Gitzelmann has described an infant, identified as having an elevated blood galactose concentration (10 mg/100 ml) by a screening procedure at 5 days of age[48]. The infant did well on breast feeding. Upon study at 1 month of age, the infant was found to be heterozygous for the Duarte variant and galactosaemia. In this particular case, with less than one quarter normal transferase activity, one would have expected to find symptoms if indeed the Duarte homozygote, with half normal value, exhibits manifestations. On the contrary, this patient was completely asymptomatic.

Most of the patients with clinical galactosaemia are thought to have a mutant transferase in which an alteration in protein structure has resulted in loss of activity[49]. Other transferase variants in symptomatic individuals are known. In two siblings, an electrophoretically different transferase was found[50], and in another patient an unstable transferase has been demonstrated[51]. In addition, there are individuals who exhibit the clinical manifestations of galactosaemia, but in whom the biochemical problem appears to be different. These individuals have virtually absent erythrocyte transferase activity but, at the same time, a demonstrable capacity to oxidise galactose in vivo[52]. These particular patients have been Negroes; liver and intestinal biopsies were found to have 10% of normal transferase activity[53,54].

The variants among symptomatic individuals with galactosaemia are of special interest from the genetic and biochemical standpoints, but the modes of treatment have been the same as for the classical type of transferase defect.

TREATMENT

Therapy must be initiated at once. Galactose or lactose must be eliminated from the diet. The frequently fulminant secondary manifestations rarely yield to treatment unless galactose intake has been minimised.

Symptomatic treatment

Vomiting, diarrhoea, dehydration and acidosis are common in the severely ill galactosaemic infant, and correction of fluid and electrolyte disturbances is paramount. The indications for parenteral fluid therapy are the same as in other disorders in which similar symptoms are present.

Septicaemia, pyelonephritis, and bronchial pneumonia are common. Since Gram-negative organisms predominate, it is recommended that treatment with broad spectrum antibiotics be instituted until bacteriological reports are available. The jaundice usually does not require specific therapy beyond restriction of galactose intake. In an occasional patient, the bilirubin level may be markedly elevated, and consideration must be given to phototherapy or to exchange transfusion. The indications are the same as for acute elevation of bilirubin from other causes.

The oedema and ascites usually do not interfere with physiological function. If specific therapy is required, albumin may be administered to correct the hypoproteinaemia, and diuretics may be used to mobilise some of the fluid. Abdominal paracentesis may be required to remove excess fluid.

A bleeding tendency due to hypoprothrombinaemia usually will respond to vitamin K.

Dietary restriction of galactose

The purpose of minimising galactose intake is to avoid the accumulation of galactose metabolites in tissues. At present, there is no known way of providing the body with a substitute functional enzyme.

Dietary management in galactosaemia is relatively simple, since galactose is not an essential nutrient. Galactose is an important constituent of a number of compounds in the body, but the donor molecule for galactose in biosynthesis of these substances (UDPGal) can be made from UDPG (Figure 4.2).

Restriction of galactose is accomplished primarily by avoidance of milk and milk products. Galactose in free form is rare in natural foodstuffs, and the principal dietary source is the disaccharide lactose. Human milk contains about 7% lactose (3·5% galactose). That of the cow and proprietary preparations, contain 5% lactose. Various commercial milk substitutes, essentially free of lactose, are available. Some are casein hydrolysates from which lactose has been removed. Others are based on lactose-free soya bean preparations.

As the infant grows older, cereals, vegetables, fruits and meats can be given safely. Particular care must be taken to avoid using commercial food products containing lactose as a sweetener. Foods which may be included in, or must be excluded from a galactose-restricted diet have been described[55]. Foods used in our own clinic are given in Table 4.2. The milk substitutes listed are those available in the United States. Recommendations in Britain for dietary treatment have been published by Francis and Dixon[56]. If lactose-free milk substitutes are not available, a meat-based formula can be prepared, including needed carbohydrate, lipids, vitamins and minerals.

In selecting foods, labels should be examined carefully. Any product which contains milk lactose, casein, whey, dry milk solids, or curds should be omitted. The terms lactic acid, lactalbumin or calcium lactate may be confusing to parents, and they should be assured that these do not refer to lactose. Food products which may contain lactose are:

(1) Creamed foods, breaded foods, gravies, cream soups, chowders.
(2) Frozen breaded meats and fish.
(3) Prepared meat products, such as sausages or cold cuts.
(4) Commercial mixes for muffins, biscuits, waffles, cakes, cookies or breads.
(5) Sweets, such as milk chocolate and caramels.

Margarines made without addition of milk or milk products are available. Bakeries should be contacted in each geographic area and a

Table 4.2. Foods which may be included in and excluded from the galactose-restricted diet

Type of food	Foods included	Foods excluded
Milk and milk products	Isomil (soya bean product)* Nutramigen (casein hydrolysate)† Prosobee (soya bean product)† Meat base formula Cream substitutes free of milk or milk derivatives	Breast milk Cow's milk or goat's milk or any other milk from an animal source in any form: whole, nonfat, evaporated, condensed: whey, casein, dry milk solids, curds, lactose Cream, butter, all cheeses, yogurt, ice cream, ice milk, sherbert, chocolate milk
Legumes	All may be included if laboratory facilities are available for periodic testing of blood (erythrocyte galactose-1-phosphate)	
Meat	Plain meats, fish, poultry, eggs	Liver, pancreas, brain or any organ meats Creamed, breaded, processed meats, fish, poultry which may contain lactose
Bread and cereal foods	Cooked and dry cereals without milk or lactose added Bread or crackers without milk or lactose added; saltines, graham crackers Macaroni, spaghetti, noodles, rice	Cereals, breads, crackers which have milk, milk products or lactose added

Fats	Vegetable oils, such as soy bean, corn, cottonseed, safflower, olive, peanut oils Shortening, lard, margarines which do not contain milk or milk products Olives, nuts, bacon	Butter, cream Margarine containing milk products
Fruits and vegetables	Any fresh, frozen, canned or dried fruits, unless processed with lactose Any vegetable unless excluded, or if processed with lactose White potatoes, sweet potatoes, yams	Fruits processed with lactose Peas; vegetables processed with lactose Most brands of instant mashed potatoes
Soups	Clear soups; vegetable soups which do not contain peas; cream soups made with milk substitutes listed	Cream soups, chowders, commercially prepared soups containing lactose
Desserts	Water and fruit ices; gelatin, angel food cake, home-made cakes, pies and cookies made from acceptable ingredients; fruit-flavoured corn-starch pudding made with water	Ice cream, ice milk, sherbert, custard Most commercial mixes for cakes and cookies
Miscellaneous	Unbuttered popcorn, marshmallows, sugar, corn syrup, molasses, honey, carbonated beverages, colas, root beer, instant coffee, unsweetened cocoa, unsweetened cooking chocholate Pure spices, punch base without lactose	Caramels, toffee Milk chocolate Pre-sweetened punch base with lactose

* Ross Laboratories.
† Mead–Johnson Laboratories.

103

list of acceptable products prepared. In case of doubt about any product, the manufacturer should be consulted.

The advisability of feeding peas, beans and other legumes containing galactose in the form of oligosaccharides was questioned at one time. However, these complex sugars are not digested to free galactose, and their intake in limited quantities should not result in any problem.

Nutritional adequacy must not be overlooked in providing for maximum restriction of galactose intake. Calcium supplementation may be necessary, and adequacy of mineral and vitamin contents must be assured. We have found that having a nutritionist or dietitian involved in management is very helpful.

As the child grows older, the diet can become more varied. The parents will need advice in the selection of new foods. Meat, poultry, fish and eggs are excellent protein sources, but processed meats containing fillers should be carefully scrutinised to make sure that no milk products are included.

Monitoring the diet

For dietary monitoring, the most important criteria are the clinical state of the child, a careful dietary history, and evaluation of the attitudes of the parents. One objective measure is determination of erythrocyte galactose-1-phosphate concentration[57]. In the infant, it is useful in observing the initial response to treatment (Figure 4.3). In older children, each patient tends to stay in a range particular to

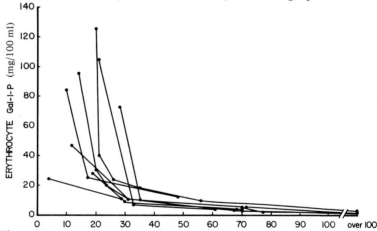

Figure 4.3 Time course of erythrocyte galactose-1-phosphate concentration after initiation of dietary treatment

himself (Figure 4.4). The erythrocyte galactose-1-phosphate concentration increases after a single galactose intake of any consequence, but it returns to the individual's baseline value within 24 hours. Such a single dietary violation may be missed, but the test does have value for detecting a systematic deviation from the prescribed diet.

The measurement of urinary galactitol for dietary monitoring has not been successful in our hands[58]. A large amount of galactose must be ingested before it is reflected in galactitol excretion, and the response to ingestion is delayed.

There is no question that rigid exclusion of galactose during the first year of life is essential. There is some difference of opinion on how restricted the dietary regime must remain thereafter. It has been our policy to restrict intake of milk throughout life. At the time the children enter school, they are allowed to eat breads, sauces and other prepared foods which may contain small amounts of milk products.

It has been proposed that relaxation of dietary restriction is possible on the assumption that there is adaptation to galactose with age through development of an alternate pathway. None of those described have been shown to have the capacity of substituting for the conventional pathway. A practical consideration is the difference in lactose intake in relation to size between the infant and the adult. Galactose makes a large contribution to the infant's total energy intake (up to

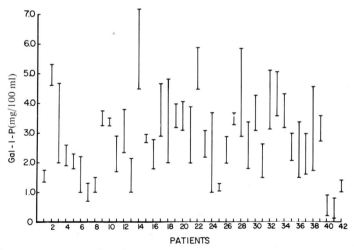

Figure 4.4 Range of erythrocyte galactose-1-phosphate values in individual treated patients

40% comes from the lactose in mother's milk). A reasonable estimate for the adult, with the usual intake of milk products, is that only 3–4% of calories come from lactose. In these terms, the ability to tolerate a more nearly normal diet cannot be considered as adaptation to galactose.

Results of treatment

By now there has been more than 20 years of experience with dietary management of transferase-defect galactosaemia. The immediate effects usually are dramatic. The patient becomes more alert, takes feeds well and gains weight. The jaundice disappears in a few days, and the liver diminishes in size. The severely ill patient generally responds well to antibiotics and other supportive measures. Some patients have been described as being slow to respond, but this has not been our experience.

Over the longer term, galactose restriction provides for good general health. While there have been a number of isolated reports on various aspects of treatment, surveys of long-term outcome in large patient groups have been published from only 3 centres[59-61]. These cover both physical and intellectual progress.

It is generally accepted that growth and development is poor in the untreated patient. It has been stated by workers in 2 studies that, as a group, even the treated galactosaemic may exhibit some growth retardation. The data are difficult to evaluate. Many factors influence growth, including those of genetic origin, nutrition, time of starting therapy, degree of dietary restriction and time of dietary relaxation. It has been the experience of our group that adequate treatment is compatible with achieving average stature.

In the infant, development of cataract is arrested under dietary treatment, and there usually is improvement. If the lenses have become opaque before treatment is begun, as in children diagnosed late, very little improvement can be expected. In these cases recourse to surgery may be necessary.

Based on the 3 major reports published, it can be concluded that treated patients, as a group, can achieve at least a low normal intelligence score (Table 4.3). The spread of values among individuals is large, and there is no good explanation as yet why some children develop better than others. There is an impression that outcome is better with earlier treatment, but the information available is still too meagre for a conclusion to be reached. Neither is it known whether or not the developing homozygote foetus can be adversely affected *in utero* from accumulation of galactose metabolites. Some few infants have been known to have had symptoms at birth. In most, accumulation of galactose-1-phosphate can be demonstrated in erythrocytes. Because of the uncertainty involved, it has been our practice to restrict galactose intake by the pregnant woman at risk.

It has not been possible to conduct studies on patients to compare treatment and non-treatment. The closest approach to the use of controls has been comparison of mean IQ values for affected children to those of their parents and unaffected siblings (Table 4.4). The spread of values in any one group is too large to permit individual judgment. The mean for the treated affected children, while lower than that for their parents and unaffected siblings, is not dramatically different.

Visual motor problems, which are common in treated galactosaemic children, may be responsible for learning difficulties. There is no

Table 4.3. Intelligence score of treated patients by age groups

Age group	Number	Mean IQ	Range of IQ
18–23 y	6	90	80–104
12–17 y	12	88	48–121
6–11 y	20	88	50–118
0– 5 y*	9	107	100–125
Total	47	92	48–125

* Values represent primarily Developmental Quotient (DQ)

Table 4.4. Comparison of IQ scores between affected children and family members

Group	Number	Mean IQ	Range of IQ
Parents	60	109	70–138
Heterozygous siblings	22	104	86–125
Normal siblings	12	99	82–116
Affected children	51	92	48–125

clearly-defined correlation between the intelligence quotient and the degree of visual perceptual deviation, although in one study[62], the patients with severest degree of visual perceptual handicap had IQ's of 48, 51 and 52. Children under treatment for galactosaemia require special assistance in school. Early evaluation and therapy has proved to be very helpful in making necessary adjustments.

Most children with galactosaemia manifest some psychological problems[62]. The younger patients tend to be shy, sensitive and sometimes withdrawn. In their psychological tests, feelings of hostility and defiance of authority figures emerge. In later life, there is excessive dependence upon parents. It is not possible to implicate any single factor as being of particular importance in the social adjustment of children with galactosaemia. The many variables include parental attitudes, the burden of dietary restriction, the effects of being subject to continuing study and evaluation, and the attitudes of other children. The scholastic difficulty adds to problems that may already exist.

Genetic counselling
Counselling of families of affected children may involve questions concerning not only direct management and prognosis but also the genetic implications of the disease. Galactosaemia is transmitted as an autosomal recessive condition, and thus the parents of an affected child are heterozygotes. For such a mating, the risk of having an affected child is one in four for each pregnancy, two in four of having a child who is a carrier and one in four of a child who is completely normal with respect to transferase. Once the disease is known to be present in a kindred, relatives of the immediate family group may become concerned. Since there are methods for determining the carrier state, information can be provided to family members about the presence and continued transmission of the gene.

Specific assays are available for determination of activity of galactose-1-phosphate uridyltransferase. Erythrocytes from affected individuals have little or no transferase activity, erythrocytes from known carriers have about half that of normal individuals (Table 4.5). It must be noted that the finding of half-normal transferase activity does not identify the individual as being heterozygous for galactosaemia. At least one low-activity genetic variant of transferase, the Duarte variant, has been described[44]. Homozygotes for the Duarte variant have half normal erythrocyte transferase activity, and in this respect they are indistinguishable from galactosaemia carriers. How-

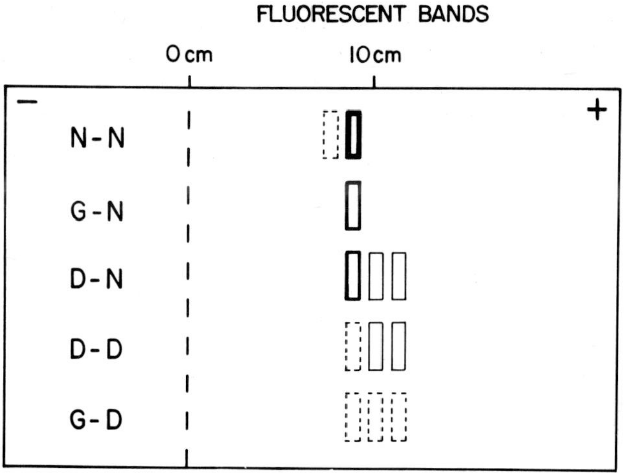

FLUORESCENT BANDS

Figure 4.5. Starch gel electrophoretic patterns of erythrocyte galactose-1-phosphate uridyl transferase. Normal, galactosaemic, and Duarte genes are denoted by N, G and D

ever, the Duarte variant transferase and normal transferase can be distinguished from each other by gel electrophoresis (Figure 4.5). A combination of transferase assay and electrophoresis is necessary for definitive genetic study[63].

The Duarte variant homozygote is asymptomatic, and transmission

Table 4.5. Erythrocyte galactose-1-phosphate uridyl transferase activity

Genotype		Transferase activity*	
		Mean	SD
Normal homozygote	(N–N)	23·7	3·00
Galactosaemia/normal heterozygote	(G–N)	10·9	2·04
Galactosaemia homozygote	(G–G)	0·1	–
Duarte/normal heterozygote	(D–N)	17·6	2·24
Duarte homozygote	(D–D)	10·4	–
Duarte/galactosaemia heterozygote	(D–G)	5·1	1·48

* Transferase activity is expressed as μ mol UDPGalactose formed/g Hb

of the gene for this variant cannot result in a galactosaemic child even in a mating with a galactosaemia carrier. Duarte variant carriers are relatively common in the population, with an incidence of 12–13%.

Most of the published figures on the incidence of galactosaemia have been based on work done before the effect of the Duarte variant could be evaluated. Consequently the calculations based on hetero-zygote incidence have resulted in too high an occurrence figure for affected individuals. Estimates available vary greatly, but the true incidence of galactosaemia appear to be less than 1 : 60 000.

A frequent question raised by families at risk is the feasibility of prenatal diagnosis. It has been established that the presence or absence of transferase activity can be determined in cultured amniotic cells. It is possible to make a diagnosis *in utero* of an affected foetus, but this is not the sole criterion of whether or not amniocentesis should be performed. Since galactosaemia is treatable, the issues involved are more complex than for a number of other diseases in which there are definitive indications for the termination of pregnancy. In our own clinic, amniocentesis is considered to have value in decisions on dietary restriction of the mother during pregnancy, but at the present time termination of pregnancy is not encouraged.

Early diagnosis and successful treatment have provided for the survival of galactosaemia homozygotes to child-bearing age. This has been of concern, since it is known that many non-phenylketonuric offspring of phenylketonuric mothers are mentally retarded. One of our patients has had two clinically normal heterozygous children at term after uneventful pregnancies[64]. Dietary restriction was carefully maintained throughout.

This work was supported by Grants AM-04135 and AM-04837 of the United States Public Health Service.

REFERENCES

1. Leloir, L. F. (1951). The enzymatic transformation of uridine diphosphate glucose into a galactose derivative. *Arch. Biochem.*, **33**, 186
2. Trucco, R. E., Caputto, R., Leloir, L. F. and Mittelman, N. (1948). Galactokinase. *Arch. Biochem.*, **18**, 137
3. Leloir, L. F. (1971). Two decades of research on the biosynthesis of saccharides. *Science*, **172**, 1299
4. Gitzelmann, R. (1972). Deficiency of uridine diphosphate galactose-4-

epimerase in blood cells of an apparently healthy infant. *Helv. Paediat. Acta*, **27**, 125

5. Wells, W. W., Pittman, T. A. and Egan, T. J. (1964). The isolation and identification of galactitol from the urine of patients with galactosemia. *J. biol. Chem.*, **239**, 3192

6. Gitzelmann, R., Curtius, H. C. and Muller, M. (1966). Galactitol excretion in the urine of a galactokinase-deficient man. *Biochem. Biophys. Res. Comm.*, **22**, 437

7. Van Heyningen, R. (1959). Formation of polyols by the lens of the rat with sugar cataract. *Nature (London)*, **184**, 194

8. Cuatrecasas, P. and Segal, S. (1966). Mammalian galactose dehydrogenase. I; Identification and purification in rat liver. *J. biol. Chem.*, **241**, 5904

9. Cuatrecasas, P. and Segal, S. (1966). Mammalian galactose dehydrogenase. II; Properties, substrate specificity and developmental changes. *J. biol. Chem.*, **241**, 5910

10. Srivastava, S. K. and Beutler, E. (1969). Auxiliary pathways of galactose metabolism. *J. biol. Chem.*, **244**, 6377

11. Bergren, W. R., Ng, W. G., Donnell, G. N. and Markey, S. P. (1972). Galactonic acid in galactosemia: identification in the urine. *Science*, **176**, 683

12. Isselbacher, K. J. (1957). Evidence for an accessory pathway of galactose metabolism in mammalian livers. *Science*, **126**, 652

13. Chacko, C., McCrone, L. and Nadler, H. (1972). Uridine diphosphoglucose pyrophosphorylase and uridine diphosphogalactose pyrophosphorylase in human skin fibroblasts derived from normal and galactosemic individuals. *Biochem. Biophys. Acta*, **268**, 113

14. Inouye, T., Schneider, J. and Hsia, D. (1964). Enzymatic oxidation of galactose-6-phosphate. *Nature, (London)*, **204**, 1304

15. Tengstrom, B. (1969). The discriminatory ability of a galactose tolerance test and some other tests in the diagnosis of cirrhosis of the liver, hepatitis and biliary obstruction. *Scand. J. Clin. Lab. Invest.*, **23**, 159

16. Holzel, A. (1959). Some aspects of galactosemia. *Mod. Prob. Pediat.*, Vol. 4, p. 388. (E. Rossi, *et al.*, editors) (Basel: S. Karger)

17. Holzel, A. and Komrower, G. M. (1955). A study of the genetics of galactosemia. *Arch. Dis. Childh.*, **30**, 155

18. Donnell, G. N., Bergren, W. R. and Roldan, M. (1959). Genetic studies in galactosemia. I; The oral galactose tolerance test and the heterozygous state. *Pediat.*, **24**, 418

19. Guthrie, R. G. (1968). Screening for 'Inborn Errors of Metabolism' in the Newborn Infant—A Multiple Test Program. *Birth Defects Original Article Series*, Vol. 4, No. 6, p. 92. (D. Bergsma, editor) (New York: The National Foundation)

20. Beutler, E. and Baluda, M. C. (1966). A simple spot screening test for galactosemia. *J. Lab. Clin. Med.*, **68**, 137

21. Ng, W. G., Donnell, G. N. and Bergren, W. R. (1965). Galactokinase activity in human erythrocytes of individuals at different ages. *J. Lab. Clin. Med.*, **66**, 115

22. Ng, W. G., Bergren, W. R. and Donnell, G. N. (1967). An improved procedure for the assay of hemolysate galactose-1-phosphate uridyl transferase activity by the use of ¹⁴C-labeled galactose-1-phosphate. *Clin. Chim. Acta*, **15**, 489

23. Beutler, E. and Baluda, M. C. (1966). Improved method for measuring galactose-1-phosphate uridyltransferase activity of erythrocytes. *Clin. Chim. Acta*, **13**, 369

24. Mellman, W. J. and Tedesco, T. A. (1965). An improved assay of erythrocyte and leucocyte galactose-1-phosphate uridyl transferase, stabilization of the enzyme by a thiol protective reagent. *J. Lab. Clin. Med.*, **66**, 980

25. Gitzelmann, R. (1965). Deficiency of erythrocyte galactokinase in a patient with galactose diabetes. *Lancet*, **ii**, 670

26. Fanconi, G. (1933). Hochgradige Galaktose-intoleranz (Galaktose-diabetes) bei einem Kinde mit Neurofibromatosis Recklinghausen. *Jb. Kinderheilk*, **138**, 1

27. Cook, J. G. H., Don, N. A. and Mann, T. P. (1971). Hereditary galactokinase deficiency. *Arch. Dis. Childh.*, **46**, 465

28. Thalhammer, O., Gitzelmann, R. and Pantlitischko, M. (1968). Hypergalactosemia and galactosuria due to galactokinase deficiency in a newborn. *Pediat.*, **42**, 441

29. Pickering, W. R. and Howell, R. R. (1972). Galactokinase deficiency: clinical and biochemical findings in a new kindred. *J. Pediat.*, **81**, 50

30. Monteleone, J. A., Beutler, E., Monteleone, P. L., Utz, C. L. and Casey, E. C. (1971). Cataracts, galactosemia and hypergalactosemia due to galactokinase deficiency in a child. *Am. J. Med.*, **50**, 403

31. Beutler, E., Matsumoto, F., Kuhl, W., Krill, A., Levy, N., Sparkes, R. and Degnan, M. (1973). Galactokinase deficiency as a cause of cataracts. *New Eng. J. Med.*, **288**, 1203

32. Beutler, E. (1972). Cataracts and galactokinase deficiency. *New Eng. J. Med.*, **287**, 202

33. Olambiwonnu, N. O., McVie, R., Ng, W. G., Frasier, S. D. and Donnell, G. N. (1974) Galactokinase deficiency in twins: clinical and biochemical studies. *Pediatrics*, **53**, 314

34. Mayes, J. S. and Guthrie, R. (1969). Detection of heterozygotes for galactokinase deficiency in a human population. *Biochem. Genetics*, **2**, 219

35. Von Reuss, A. (1908). Zuckerausscheidung in Sauglingsalter. *Wien. Med. Wochshr.*, **58**, 799

36. Gorter, E. (1951). Familial galactosuria. *Arch. Dis. Childh.*, **26**, 271

37. Kalckar, H. M., Anderson, E. P. and Isselbacher, K. J. (1956). Galactosemia,

a congenital defect in a nucleotide transferase: a preliminary report. *Proc. Nat. Acad. Sci.*, **42**, 49

38. Keppler, D. and Decker, K. (1969). Studies on the mechanism of galactosamine hepatitis: accumulation of galactosamine-1-phosphate and its inhibition of UDPGlucose pyrophosphorylase. *Europ. J. Biochem.*, **10**, 219

39. Hsia, D. Y.-Y. and Walker, F. A. (1961). Variability in the clinical manifestations of galactosemia. *J. Pediat.*, **59**, 872

40. Gitzelmann, R. (1967). Hereditary galactokinase deficiency, a newly recognized cause of juvenile cataracts. *Ped. Res.*, **1**, 14

41. Ritter, J. A. and Cannon, E. J. (1955). Galactosemia with cataracts. *New Eng. J. Med.*, **252**, 747

42. Durand, P. and Semach, F. (1955). Formes tardives, atténuées de galactosémie chez deux fréres. Interprétation clinique et classement génétique de la maladie. *Arch. Franc. Pédiat.*, **12**, 958

43. Hugh-Jones, K., Newcomb, A. J. and Hsia, D. Y.-Y. (1960). The genetic mechanism of galactosaemia. *Arch. Dis. Childh.*, **35**, 521

44. Beutler, E., Baluda, M. C., Sturgeon, P. and Day, R. W. (1966). The genetics of galactose-1-phosphate uridyl transferase. *J. Lab. Clin. Med.*, **68**, 646

45. Beutler, E., Baluda, M. C., Sturgeon, P. and Day, R. (1965). A new genetic abnormality resulting in galactose-1-phosphate uridyltransferase deficiency. *Lancet*, **i**, 353

46. Ng, W. G., Bergren, W. R. and Donnell, G. N. (1973). A new variant of galactose-1-phosphate uridyltransferase in man: the Los Angeles variant. *Ann. hum. Genet. (London)*, **37**, 1

47. Kelly, S., Desjardins, L. and Ali Khera, S. (1972). A Duarte variant with clinical signs. *J. med. Genet.*, **9**, 129

48. Gitzelmann, R., Poley, J. R. and Prader, A. (1967). Partial galactose-1-phosphate uridyltransferase deficiency due to a variant enzyme. *Helvet. Paediat. Acta*, **22**, 252

49. Tedesco, T. A. and Mellman, W. J. (1971). Galactosemia: evidence for a structural gene mutation. *Science*, **172**, 727

50. Schapira, F. and Kaplan, J. C. (1969). Electrophoretic abnormality of galactose-1-phosphate uridyl transferase in galactosemia. *Biochem. Biophys. Res. Commun.*, **35**, 451

51. Chacko, C. M., Christian, J. C. and Nadler, H. L. (1971). Unstable galactose-1-phosphate uridyl transferase: a new variant of galactosemia. *J. Pediat.*, **78**, 454

52. Segal, S., Blair, A. and Topper, Y. J. (1962). Oxidation of carbon-14 labeled galactose by subjects with congenital galactosemia. *Science*, **136**, 150

53. Segal, S., Rogers, S. and Holtzapple, P. G. (1971). Liver galactose-1-phosphate uridyl transferase: activity in normal and galactosemic subjects. *J. Clin. Invest.*, **50**, 500

54. Rogers, S., Holtzapple, P. G., Mellman, W. J. and Segal, S. (1970). Characteristics of galactose-1-phosphate uridyl transferase in intestinal mucosa of normal and galactosemic humans. *Metabolism*, **19**, 701

55. Koch, R., Acosta, P., Ragsdale, N. and Donnell, G. N. (1963). Nutrition in the treatment of galactosemia. *J. Am. Diet. Assoc.*, **43**, 216

56. Francis, D. E. M. and Dixon, D. J. W. (1970). *Diets for Sick Children*, p. 165. (Oxford: Blackwell) (New edn. in press, 1974)

57. Donnell, G. N., Bergren, W. R., Perry, G. and Koch, R. (1963). Galactose-1-phosphate in galactosemia. *Pediat.*, **31**, 802

58. Roe, T. F., Ng, W. G., Bergren, W. R. and Donnell, G. N. (1973). Urinary galactitol in galactosemic patients. *Biochem. Med.*, **7**, 266

59. Nadler, H. L., Inouye, T. and Hsia, D. Y.-Y. (1969). Classical galactosemia. *Galactosemia*, p. 127. (D. Y.-Y. Hsia, editor) (Springfield, Illinois: C. C. Thomas)

60. Donnell, G. N., Koch, R. and Bergren, W. R. (1969). Observations on Results of Management of Galactosemic Patients. *Galactosemia*, p. 247. (D. Y.-Y. Hsia, editor) (Springfield, Illinois: C. C. Thomas)

61. Komrower, G. M. and Lee, D. H. (1970). Long-term follow-up of galactosemia. *Arch. Dis. Childh.*, **45**, 367

62. Fishler, K., Donnell, G. N., Bergren, W. R. and Koch, R. (1972). Intellectual and personality development in children with galactosemia. *Pediat.*, **50**, 412

63. Ng, W. G., Bergren, W. R., Fields, M. and Donnell, G. N. (1969). An improved electrophoretic procedure for galactose-1-phosphate uridyl transferase: demonstration of multiple activity bands with the Duarte variant. *Biochem. Biophys. Res. Commun.*, **37**, 354

64. Roe, T. F., Hallatt, J. G., Donnell, G. N. and Ng, W. G. (1971). Childbearing by a galactosemic woman. *J. Pediat.*, **78**, 1026

CHAPTER 5

Hepatic Glycogen Storage Diseases

J. Fernandes

The study of glycogen storage disease of the liver (GSD) dates from 1928 when Van Creveld[1] described a patient with hepatomegaly and an hitherto unrecognised disturbance of carbohydrate metabolism. The symptoms were interpreted as being due to an accumulation of glycogen which could be mobilised only with great difficulty. Further understanding of the biochemical and clinical features of GSD was provided by the Cori's[2] who in 1952 for the first time described a patient with glucose-6-phosphatase deficiency. Later other enzyme deficiencies related to impaired glycogenolysis were detected, and it soon became clear that in the great majority of patients with GSD, the underlying enzyme defect could be established. This is important because the symptoms caused by each separate GSD enzyme deficiency vary greatly in severity and some are limited to a single enzyme deficiency. Thus treatment aimed at the alleviation or prevention of the metabolic disturbances is not the same for all types of GSD and some aspects may even be related to one enzyme deficiency only.

Table 5.1. Distribution of enzyme deficiencies in children with glycogen storage disease of the liver

Enzyme deficiency	Number of patients
Glucose-6-phosphatase	14
Lysosomal 1,4-glucosidase	7
Debranching enzyme	10
Branching enzyme	2
Phosphorylase system	43
Total	76

The main questions are therefore:

(1) Which enzyme deficiencies are most frequent
(2) Which diagnostic procedures are suitable for detection
(3) Which metabolic disturbances are most marked
(4) What treatment is most appropriate

Relative frequency of different enzyme deficiencies

The enzyme deficiencies occurring in our 73 patients with GSD are given in Table 5.1 (for comparison see the Tables of Illingworth[3], and Van Hoof et al.[4]). Thus deficiencies of glucose-6-phosphatase, the debranching enzyme system, and the phosphorylase system are those most frequently diagnosed.

Of the remainder, lysosomal α-glucosidase deficiency is an untreatable generalised enzyme defect which usually causes death in early infancy: less severe variants are very rare. Treatment until now has been symptomatic, except for the few unsuccessful trials with enzyme substitution[4][6]. Antenatal diagnosis by biochemical analysis of cultured amnion cells[7,8], and abortion of a diseased foetus is the most appropriate preventive measure at the moment, and this enzyme deficiency will not be discussed further.

Branching enzyme deficiency is another very rare untreatable glycogenosis which will not be further discussed. Here too antenatal diagnosis and abortion of an affected foetus seems feasible[9].

Thus, in the following sections, only the most frequent types of GSD, deficiencies of glucose-6-phosphatase, the debranching enzyme system and the phosphorylase system, will be discussed.

Diagnosis

Diagnosis of GSD and the further differentiation of the 3 most frequent enzyme deficiencies can be made by the following procedure.

First a patient with hepatomegaly and a tendency to hypoglycaemia should be shown to have normal liver function tests, with exception of serum transaminases which are often elevated in GSD patients. Malabsorption and hormone imbalances as primary causes of hypoglycaemia should also be excluded, but such abnormalities are rarely associated with marked hepatomegaly.

Having made a tentative diagnosis of GSD, the 3 enzyme deficiencies can be distinguished as follows[10] (Figure 5.1). First, the patient in the fasting state is subjected to an oral glucose load and glucose and

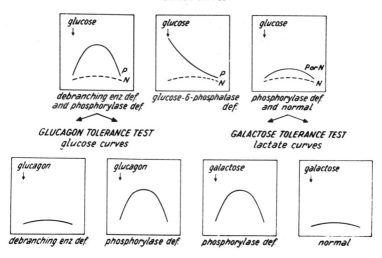

Figure 5.1. Screening procedure for differentiating patients (P) with a deficiency of glucose-6-phosphatase, the debranching enzyme system, the phosphorylase system, and normal children (N). (From: Fernandes *et al. Archives of Disease of Childhood*, **44**, 311, 1969, with permission of the Editor)

lactate determined in the blood every 30 minutes for 3 hours. The lactate curves are of greatest importance for diagnosis and only these curves are shown in the 3 diagrams at the top of Figure 5.1. There are 3 possible results of this test.

(1) The fasting lactate concentration is abnormally high and decreases steadily after glucose ingestion (Figure 5.1, upper centre). In this case glucose-6-phosphatase deficiency is very probable and should be confirmed by assay of this enzyme in a liver biopsy.

(2) The fasting lactate concentration is normal and increases markedly after glucose ingestion (Figure 5.1, upper left). If this abnormal increase of lactate is observed unequivocally and if a similar lactate curve is obtained following an oral galactose load (Figure 5.1, lower half, curve 3) a deficiency of debranching enzyme or of the phosphorylase system is very probable.

(3) The lactate curve is in the upper normal range (Figure 5.1, upper right). This type of lactate curve does not exclude debranching enzyme or phosphorylase deficiency and an oral galactose curve is

needed to differentiate these deficiencies from liver disease due to other causes (Figure 5.1, lower right).

For the differentiation of debranching enzyme deficiency from that of the phosphorylase system a glucagon test in the fasting state is required (Figure 5.1, lower left). In this case the glucose curves are the most important and lactate determination may be omitted. If a normal glucose curve is observed deficiency of phosphorylase kinase is probable (Figure 5.1, lower half, curve 2) and this has to be confirmed by assay of this enzyme in leucocytes. If a flat glucose curve is observed deficiency of debranching enzyme is probable (Figure 5.1, lower left) and this, too, has to be confirmed by assay of the enzyme in leucocytes. The only exceptions to this test leading to a correct preliminary diagnosis were two brothers with a flat glucagon tolerance test, who did not have debranching enzyme deficiency as anticipated, but deficiency of phosphorylase enzyme proper (as distinct from its activating kinase) with a concomitant normal activity of phosphorylase kinase. These two cases could, in retrospect, be recognised by a second glucagon test, performed postprandially. Their glucose curves remained flat, whereas a postprandial glucagon test in a patient with debranching enzyme deficiency would have given a normal result[11].

In summary, this screening procedure allows a tentative diagnosis of patients with deficiency of either debranching enzyme or the phosphorylase system after 2 or 3 tolerance tests, and of glucose-6-phosphatase deficiency after only one test. It should be stressed, however, that such a scheme of investigation can only yield a tentative diagnosis which should be confirmed by enzyme assay using leucocytes or liver. However, it does allow selection of the patients in whom an enzyme assay should be carried out and indicates the tissue (leucocytes or liver) in which the enzyme assay has to be performed. Puzzling cases of hepatomegaly with tolerance tests which cannot be interpreted in accordance with the scheme described should be examined for one of the rarer enzyme deficiencies.

Main metabolic disturbances

The main metabolic disturbances observed in our patients are summarised in Table 5.2. Specific symptoms, though common to all 3 enzyme deficiencies, can be of different severity in the 3 diseases, and some symptoms are limited to one enzyme deficiency. It is important to look for these metabolic deviations in every patient with GSD because, until now, only these symptoms can be treated or prevented. This is especially so for infants and young children, because often the younger the patient, the more severe are the symptoms. If the patient is adequately treated in his first years of life symptoms, at first life-threatening, may later become less serious. In the pre-adolescent and adolescent period some abnormalities may diminish or disappear completely, but others will remain. This age-dependent adaptation or gradual change of symptoms has been mentioned by several authors[12-14]. An adequate explanation for this phenomenon has not been found.

Table 5.2. Main metabolic disturbances in children with glycogen storage disease of the liver

Metabolic characteristics	Enzyme deficiency		
	Glucose-6-phosphatase	Debranching enzyme system	Phosphorylase system
Hypoglycaemia	++	+	±
Acidosis	+	−	−
Ketosis	−	+	±
Hyperlipidaemia	++	+	±
Hyperuricaemia	+	±	−

GLUCOSE-6-PHOSPHATASE DEFICIENCY

Glucose-6-phosphatase deficiency is the most severe of all hepatic glycogenoses for the following reasons. The tendency to hypogly-caemia is most outstanding (Table 5.2) and can be life-threatening, especially during infections. Hyperlactacidaemia is almost always present and can rapidly increase during prolonged fasting and during infections. A bleeding tendency has been observed by many authors[14]. In a patient of Kelsch and Oliver[15] this complication even required blood transfusions and we have observed severe bleeding in two sisters after tonsillectomy. It was recently demonstrated by Czapek et al.[16] that decreased platelet adhesiveness is the cause of the haemorrhagic tendency and that the degree of this platelet dysfunction is correlated

with the patients' general clinical condition. In the light of these findings the utmost care should be taken during the performance of dental
and surgical procedures and tonsillectomy and adenectomy are almost
absolutely contra-indicated. Hypoglycaemia, lactic acidosis and severe
post-tonsillectomy bleeding were the causes of death in 6 of 14 of
our glucose-6-phosphatase-deficient patients. This demonstrates the
severity of the illness of these patients and it indicates the need for
supervising them as closely as possible.

Treatment of metabolic disturbances

Hypoglycaemia

Glucose is the only carbohydrate, which can be directly utilised by
all tissues. Repeated and timely ingestion of glucose and its polymers,
such as starch and maltose, is essential for blood glucose homeostasis,
because the formation of glucose from endogenous sources is very
small. The absence of glucose-6-phosphatase in the liver prevents
glucose production by gluconcogenesis since glucose-6-phosphate
cannot be hydrolysed. Glucose from glycogen can be liberated only
to the extent that hydrolytic cleavage of branching points by the
action of debranching enzyme can occur—approximately 8% of the
total glycogen store[17].

It is therefore essential to ensure that patients with this enzyme
deficiency have sufficient glucose both day and night. The omission

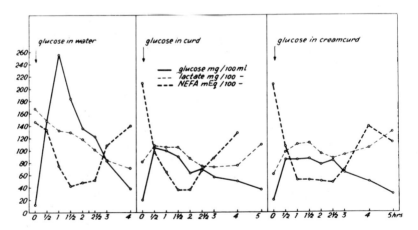

Figure 5.2. The effect of oral glucose in water, curd, or creamcurd, in a child
with a glucose-6-phosphatase deficiency

of night feeding is seldom warranted and perhaps only feasible for adults who can tolerate longer fasting periods. As sources of exogenous glucose a mixture of glucose and starch, with a prevalence of the latter should be given with every meal, because the more protracted release of glucose from starch maintains normoglycaemia for a longer period. Not only the source of exogenous glucose but also the vehicle in which it is administered is of importance. Figure 5.2 shows that glucose in curd or creamcurd is more slowly absorbed, and hence available for longer, than an equal amount of glucose in water. This can be deduced from the slower increase and decrease of glucose concentration, and from the slope of the curve of the blood free fatty acids (NEFA). NEFA increased later and more gradually from its minimum after a glucose-curd mixture than after glucose in water.

As regards fructose and galactose, it is clear that the conversion of these hexoses into glucose is not possible and the same is true for the fructose and galactose components of the disaccharides sucrose and lactose. These sugars should be omitted from the diet, because they increase lactic acidaemia. This lactate overproduction from these sugars is further discussed below.

Hyperlactic acidaemia
It is well known that the blood lactate concentration in these patients increases during fasting and during infections. During fasting the liver is unable to sustain normoglycaemia and a variety of secondary effects ensue, such as the release of epinephrine, glucagon, growth hormone and later also glucocorticoid, if hypoglycaemia persists[17]. Phosphorylase is activated, hepatic glycogenolysis is increased and the resultant metabolite is lactate rather than glucose which, for the reasons already given, is only liberated from glycogen to a small extent. Thus the liver produces lactate and the muscles utilise this substrate[18,19] which is the reverse of the normal pattern. Lactate may also be utilised by the brain, but this has not been established. Lactate utilisation by the brain might explain the fact that patients with very high lactate and very low glucose levels may stay free from cerebral symptoms or electro-encephalographic abnormalities[20]. The reverse phenomenon, i.e. a decrease of hyperlactacidaemia by oral glucose administration is shown in Figure 5.3. It follows that the frequent and timely supply of glucose or starch over the 24 hours is of equal importance for the prevention of both lactic acidosis and of hypoglycaemia.

As regards other carbohydrates, the effects of alternate ingestion of

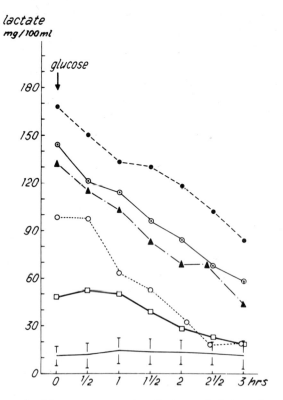

Figure 5.3. Blood lactate concentrations during oral glucose tolerance tests in 5 children with glucose-6-phosphatase deficiency. The control curve is the average $\pm$ 2 S.D. from 12 normal children. (From: Fernandes *et al. Archives of Disease of Childhood*, **44**, 311, 1969, with permission of the Editor)

glucose and fructose and of glucose and galactose are shown in Figure 5.4. This shows that both fructose and galactose cause lactate and glucose concentrations to change reciprocally and in an unfavourable direction. The administration of sucrose or lactose is not followed by hypoglycaemia, but we have found that blood lactate increases rapidly and markedly. Sucrose and lactose should therefore be restricted in the diets of these children. Sucrose should be replaced by glucose; lactose as a constituent of cow's milk should be restricted by supplying other cow's milk products with a low lactose content, such as butter-milk and curd, or by the replacement of cow's milk by soy milk.

In this context the dietary experiments of Kelsch and Oliver[15] are of interest. They performed short-term and long-term experiments in one patient, in whom a low-frequency home diet, which contained sucrose, was replaced by a high-frequency diet containing glucose instead of sucrose. During the short-term experiment the lactic acidaemia and lactic aciduria decreased considerably (Figure 5.5) and therefore the blood pH increased. At the same time the negative calcium balance became positive (Figure 5.6), blood urate fell sharply and urate excretion increased temporarily. During the long-term experiment, a similar diet of frequent meals every 3 hours around the clock was continued for 9 months at home. Growth rate and bone calcification improved markedly and serum lipids remained at almost normal levels, but serum lactate and urate increased again, and the patient became much more susceptible to symptomatic hypoglycaemia than he had been before.

Not only dietary factors influence hepatic lactate production, this is even more markedly enhanced by infections. The cause of this is probably multifactorial. Anorexia and vomiting may interfere with

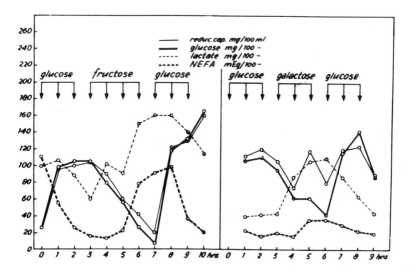

Figure 5.4. The effect of oral glucose, fructose, glucose, respectively (left) and of glucose, galactose, glucose, respectively (right), in a child with glucose-6-phosphatase deficiency. (From: Fernandes and Van de Kamer, *Pediatrics*, **35**, 470, 1965, with permission of the Editor)

adequate supply of calories and glucose and the further need for these created by the hypermetabolism associated with fever may further aggravate the already increased lactate production. An example of a lactic acidosis provoked by a febrile viral infection in a one-year-old child with glucose-6-phosphatase deficiency is shown in Table 5.3. The hyperlactic acidaemia in this case may be a consequence of increased hepatic production, decreased hepatic utilisation or decreased renal excretion of lactate. The striking hyperlactic aciduria, however, strongly

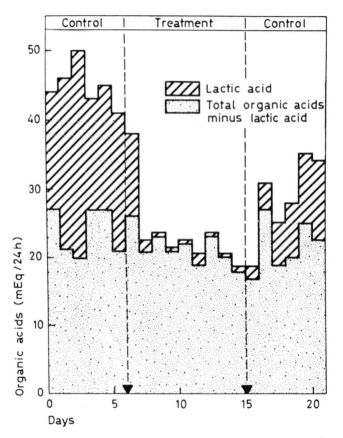

Figure 5.5. The effect of frequent carbohydrate feeding on urinary excretion of organic acids in a child with glucose-6-phosphatase deficiency. (From: Kelsch and Oliver, *Pediatric Research*, **3**, 160, 1969, with permission of the Editor)

points to hepatic lactate over-production. In the light of these data the need for supplementary sodium bicarbonate administration is evident. A daily oral dose of 1–2 mmol/kg/day, which could be adequate for steady-state conditions, has to be rapidly increased to approximately 2–4 mmol/kg/day intravenously during infections. If higher doses of sodium bicarbonate are needed, THAM might be supplemented instead in order to avoid sodium overloading.

In summary the hyperlactic acidaemia of glucose-6-phosphatase-deficient children should be suppressed by regular feedings around the

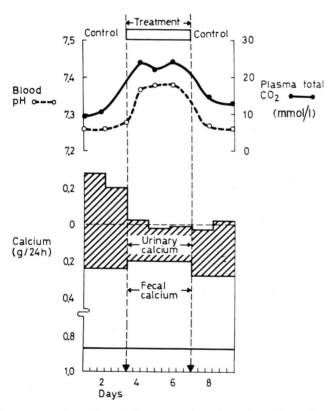

Figure 5.6. The effect of frequent carbohydrate feeding on the external calcium balance in a child with glucose-6-phosphatase deficiency. Calcium intake is plotted from the base line downward; excretion is plotted from the intake line upward. (From: Kelsch and Oliver, *Pediatric Research*, **3**, 160, 1969, with permission of the Editor)

clock (older children and adults excepted), the administration of starch and glucose, the restriction of sucrose and lactose, and the extra supplementation of sodium bicarbonate. These measures should be particularly stringent during infections.

Hyperlipidaemia

Hyperlipidaemia is observed in many children with GSD, but is most pronounced in glucose-6-phosphatase-deficient patients. Their serum may be milky because of the particularly high blood levels of tri-glycerides (Figure 5.7), resulting in hyper-β and hyper-pre-β-lipo-proteinaemia[21] (own observations). Xanthomata and lipaemia retinalis may be noted[17]. Hyperlipidaemia and xanthomata may increase during infections[18].

The aetiology of the hyperlipidaemia associated with glucose-6-phosphatase deficiency is complex. Two factors probably play a causative role: increased liponeogenesis in the liver, and decreased fatty acid elimination from the blood.

Several observations are in favour of increased liponeogenesis. The

Table 5.3. Effect of a febrile viral infection on blood and urine lactate in a one-year-old child with glucose-6-phosphatase deficiency

		Urine			Blood
Day	Volume (ml/day)	Creatinine (mmol/l)	Lactate (mmol/l)	Lactate/ Creatinine	lactate (mmol/l)
1	125	8·50	4·94	0·58	9·49
6	140	6·97	31·60	4·53	13·99
7	130	4·12	64·50	15·65	12·88
9	110	5·86	22·90	3·91	–
13	225	3·27	5·81	1·78	–
14	145	3·54	1·10	0·31	–
15	140	3·22	2·01	0·62	7·45
20	190	4·24	1·45	0·32	8·41
Normal range n = 10	50–450	1·11–12·12	0·09–0·93	0·01–0·17	0·5–2·2

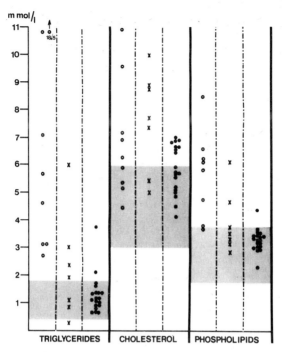

Figure 5.7. Serum lipids in children with deficiencies of glucose-6-phospha-tase, the debranching enzyme system and the phosphorylase system. The shaded areas represent the range of the serum lipids in normal children. o = glucose-6-phosphate deficiency; x = branching enzyme deficiency; • = phosphorylase deficiency

augmented production of NADPH, NADH, glycerol-1-phosphate, and pyruvate, derived from increased glycogenolysis might promote fatty acid synthesis in the liver[22]. Increased activity of fatty acid synthetase in the liver of glucose-6-phosphatase-deficient children has indeed been found[23]. The increased palmitate concentration of the serum fatty acids in these patients is also in favour of increased liponeo-genesis[24]. Increased splanchnic triglyceride production has been found[25].

Concerning the second possible cause of hyperlipidaemia, a decreased activity of post-heparin lipoprotein lipase was found[25,26], and these patients also showed a decreased triglyceride elimination rate[26]. According to Havel et al.[25] the decreased lipoprotein lipase activity is a consequence of low insulin levels, which have been demonstrated by several authors[25-28]. It might therefore be concluded that the hyper-lipidaemia is caused by both increased liponeogenesis and decreased fatty acid elimination.

The hyperlipidaemia might influence the life expectancy unfavourably as in other diseases with secondary hyperlipidaemia. Mason et al.[18] found atheromatous plaques of the left coronary artery and the aorta in a 10-year-old glucose-6-phosphatase-deficient girl. It therefore seems important to control the serum lipids of these patients and to aim at a reduction of the serum lipids by dietary measures. The influence of dietary fats on serum lipids has been investigated by Cuttino et al.[29] and by us[24]. The former authors found a striking reduction of serum triglycerides and a concomitant disappearance of xanthomata with a diet containing 40% MCT (medium-chain triglycerides). When a normal diet without MCT, but with the same fat content (type of fat not specified) was resumed the serum triglycerides again increased, but these decreased again after reinstitution of MCT. We, however, observed an increase of the serum lipids when MCT was substituted for corn oil in an isocaloric diet with a constant fat, carbohydrate and protein composition. The value of MCT therefore seems unresolved as yet.

The ratio of fat to carbohydrate in the diet may also affect the level of serum triglycerides. Diets high in fat, whatever the type, should only be administered with caution, because the high fat intake can further overload the low fat clearing capacity and the concomitant low carbohydrate intake will entail a risk of hypoglycaemia, increased lactate production and increased liponeogenesis.

The effect of different types of carbohydrate on serum lipids has been examined by Kelsch and Oliver[15], who compared a sucrose-containing home diet with an isocaloric glucose-containing diet, which was administered with a higher frequency every 2 or 3 hours around the clock. Serum triglycerides and cholesterol decreased considerably during the latter diet, but this effect probably is due to the high frequency of the diet rather than to its carbohydrate composition.

It might be concluded, that a high-carbohydrate, low-fat diet with a prevalence of polyunsaturated fat, administered around the clock at regular intervals, is the most appropriate diet to decrease the serum lipids of glucose-6-phosphatase-deficient children.

In the context of abnormal lipid metabolism there is much confusion concerning the existence of hyperketonaemia and ketonuria in patients with glucose-6-phosphatase deficiency. Though ketonuria has been found by many authors, only very few state the degree of elevated ketones in the blood[19,30] whereas others reported normal ketone concentrations[18,31-33].

Havel et al.[25] found normal or even decreased splanchnic production rates for 3-ketobutyrate and 3-hydroxybutyrate. We never found a fasting ketosis in our glucose-6-phosphatase-deficient patients, even under circumstances of severe hypoglycaemia and lactic acidosis, whereas a marked ketosis was a common finding in our patients with debranching enzyme deficiency or deficiency of the phosphorylase system[34] and these are discussed further below. It has to be stressed that the acidosis often found in glucose-6-phosphatase-deficient children is not a ketoacidosis but a lactic acidosis.

Hyperuricaemia, gout

Hyperuricaemia is a metabolic abnormality often found in young children with glucose-6-phosphatase deficiency. The sequelae of hyperuricaemia, i.e. acute gouty arthritis, gouty nephropathy and tophi may become a major problem in adolescent or adult patients[32]. Hyperuricaemia appears to be the result of both increased uric acid production[35] and decreased uric acid elimination[19]. The mechanism by which a deficiency of glucose-6-phosphatase causes uric acid over-production is not known. It has been suggested that as one of the major pathways of glucose-6-phosphate conversion is blocked, a greater fraction of this substrate is converted to ribose, which may lead to an increased *de novo* purine synthesis[14].

Decreased uric acid elimination can result from competitive inhibition of renal tubular secretion by lactate. Thus, the hyperlactaciduria of these patients may negatively affect renal uric acid elimination[15] (own observations). Early treatment of hyperuricaemia is essential to prevent or postpone the later sequelae of urate accumulation.

Zangeneh et al.[36] treated their patient, who had gout at the age of 12, with colchicine, Probenecid and Allopurinol. We compared the results of Probenecid and Allopurinol in 2 patients. Probenecid inhibits the tubular urate reabsorption. Allopurinol, a xanthine oxidase inhibitor, promotes the excretion of the uric acid precursors hypoxanthine and xanthine, which are highly soluble in the urine, whereas the excretion of uric acid, which is less soluble, decreases. It appeared that Allopurinol was much more effective in decreasing serum uric acid levels and alleviating gouty symptoms than Probenecid (Figures 5.8, 5.9).

In summary, treatment with Allopurinol is indicated in most

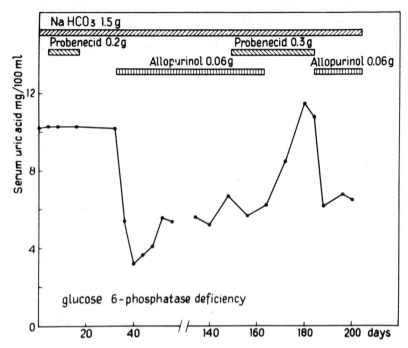

Figure 5.8. Effect of Probenecid and Allopurinol on serum uric acid concentration in a one year old child with glucose-6-phosphatase deficiency during a short-term study

glucose-6-phosphatase-deficient children as soon as serum urate concentration has been found to be repeatedly elevated. It is recommended that this treatment should be started in early childhood in order to prevent the pathology of urate accumulation at a later age.

Treatment of non-metabolic complications
It is probable, though not proven, that the number of liver malignancies which has been reported in glucose-6-phosphatase-deficient children is higher than expected by chance. Hepatomata of the liver have been reported in a 10-year-old girl[18], carcinoma of the liver with metastasis to the lymph nodes of the hepatic pedicle in a 14-year-old boy[36], and a stemmed liver tumour consisting of nodules with a tendency to hepatoma formation in a 23-year-old woman[37]. The first 2 patients died, the last patient in whom the stemmed tumour could be

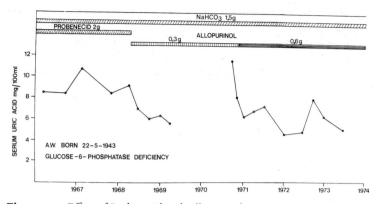

Figure 5.9. Effect of Probenecid and Allopurinol on serum uric acid concentration in an adult with glucose-6-phosphatase deficiency during long-term treatment

removed *in toto*, survived. It is therefore very important to be on the alert for these malignancies of the liver. A regular careful examination of the liver, a liver scan if the surface of the liver is not smooth, and timely laparoscopy or surgical exploration are all indicated.

Surgical treatment

A surgical approach to the management of GSD was first conceived of by Field[38] who postulated that creating a portocaval shunt might maintain a relatively constant and high blood glucose concentration. Further interest was created by Sexton *et al.*[39] who found a reduction of hepatic glycogen content following portocaval transposition in dogs. Based upon this experimental observation and the concept that a diversion of portal blood from the liver to the vena cava would make glucose more available for peripheral utilisation, 4 patients with a glucose-6-phosphatase deficiency have so far been operated upon. Two techniques have been used: portocaval transposition[40,41] and end-to-side portocaval shunt[42,43]. The portocaval shunt is the least complicated operation and therefore the most recommended procedure[41,43]. One patient had a temporary ascites but the subsequent course was very satisfactory[40], one patient died within 2 days, apparently because the portal system was overloaded with the caval inflow from the portocaval transposition[41], one patient had severe hypocalcaemia with apnoea and repeated convulsions[42].

The effect on the metabolic abnormalities of the 3 surviving patients, was that the hypoglycaemia, hyperlactacidaemia, hyperlipidaemia, and hyperuricaemia disappeared almost completely, growth progressed very satisfactorily but reduction of hepatomegaly is recorded in only 1 patient. As the long-term effects on liver function and the possible development of encephalopathy are not yet known, it is too early to evaluate the ultimate value of such surgical treatment. Patients with severe metabolic abnormalities such as repeated hypoglycaemic convulsions, life-threatening attacks of lactic acidosis or even gouty arthritis, might be candidates for a portocaval shunt.

Treatment with hormones or related agents
Lowe *et al.*[22] treated some patients with intravenous infusions of glucagon and observed shrinking of the liver within a few hours in 1 patient, but this has not been observed in other patients. The same investigators administered glucagon postprandially in order to impair glycogen synthesis in the liver and thus spare glucose for peripheral utilisation. This resulted in a favourable effect on the levels of glucose, lactate, and lipids.

The long-term effect with a long-acting zinc-glucagon complex was favourable too. This treatment has not been repeated by other investigators and so awaits confirmation. Zangeneh *et al.*[36] treated a patient with cortisone, DOCA and anabolic steroids without success. Rennert and Mukhopadhyay[44] treated two brothers with Diazoxide, and noted an improved glucose and lactic acid homeostasis, and a reduction in the hepatomegaly of 1 patient.

No definite conclusions can be drawn from these observations and it is the opinion of the author that hormonal treatment of glucose-6-phosphatase-deficient children is seldom justified.

DEFICIENCY OF THE DEBRANCHING ENZYME SYSTEM

The clinical symptoms associated with debranching enzyme deficiency are less severe than those seen in glucose-6-phosphatase deficiency. This is easy to understand if the site of the enzyme defect in the glycogenolytic pathway is considered. Glycogenolysis, unimpaired for the outer chains of the glycogen molecule, comes to a stop at the primary branch points. This means that approximately 12% of glycogen can still be degraded in a debranching enzyme-deficient liver compared with the 25–41% that occurs in a normal liver[13].

However, after a short fast hypoglycaemia will ensue unless gluconeogenesis can rapidly and adequately compensate for the deficient glycogenolysis. It is therefore surprising that hypoglycaemia is reported to play a minor role in this particular type of GSD[13,17]. Among our 10 patients with debranching enzyme deficiency, severe hypoglycaemia occurred in 4. Two of them are mentally retarded, probably as a consequence of repeated hypoglycaemic convulsions. We therefore consider hypoglycaemia as a main metabolic disturbance in early infancy (Table 5.2).

Other metabolic abnormalities such as hyperlipidaemia, are not acute dangers, but may have long-term consequences. It is therefore important to treat them (see below), the more so, because the life expectancy of patients with this enzyme defect appears to be good. The first GSD patients, described by Van Creveld[1,45] when reinvestigated[12] appear to have a debranching enzyme deficiency. These now adult patients are in good health and have normal children. The hepato-megaly has disappeared, and only some tolerance tests are still abnormal.

Periportal fibrosis has been reported in some patients[21,46] and we have seen it in one patient and even liver cirrhosis with portal hypertension has been found[47]. Attacks of icterus were noted by Roget et al.[46] and by us in the patient with fibrosis mentioned above. Markedly elevated levels of serum transaminases are common findings in these patients. Considering these clinical, histological and chemical signs of liver dysfunction, the ultimate favourable prognosis of most patients indicated by the literature and in our own experience is remarkable.

Extensive investigation of this enzyme defect[48,49] has led to the suggestion that there are 3 or 4 subgroups depending on the deficiency of one or both enzymes of the debranching enzyme complex, i.e. amylo-1,6-glucosidase and maltotriosyl transferase and depending on the localisation of the enzyme defect in both liver and muscle or in the liver alone. Much work has also been done on parallel measurements of enzyme activity in leucocytes and liver[50,51].

It is the opinion of the author that the differentiation of the enzymes of the debranching enzyme complex and the localisation of the enzyme defect in different organs probably has no relevance to the treatment of the patients. The only procedure essential for diagnosis is the measurement in leucocytes of the overall activity of the debranching

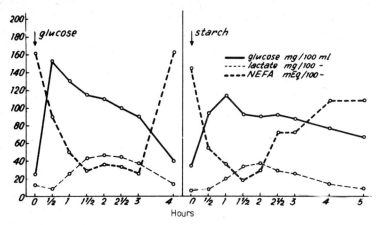

Figure 5.10. The effect of oral glucose (left) and starch (right), in a child with a deficiency of the debranching enzyme system. (From: Fernandes and Van de Kamer, *Pediatrics*, **41**, 935, 1968, with permission of the Editor)

enzyme system by determining glucose production from phosphorylase limit-dextrin: this assay reflects enzyme deficiencies of all subtypes.

Prevention of the disease is feasible since antenatal diagnosis of debranching enzyme deficiency has been demonstrated[52]. However, this procedure has, in the opinion of the author, little point, because prevention by abortion of a debranching enzyme-deficient foetus would not be justified when the disease is easy to treat and has a good prognosis.

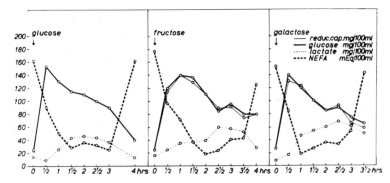

Figure 5.11. The effect of oral glucose, fructose and galactose in a child with a deficiency of the debranching enzyme system

Treatment of metabolic disturbances

Hypoglycaemia

Glucose homeostasis in debranching enzyme-deficient patients depends on the utilisation of glucose and starch, the conversion of fructose and galactose into glucose, and gluconeogenesis from non-glucose substrates. Oral administration of starch boiled in water is compared with the effect of glucose, administered in the same dose of 2 g/kg body weight in Figure 5.10. It is apparent that normoglycaemia is maintained longer after starch than after glucose. Oral administration of glucose, fructose and galactose in doses of 2 g/kg body weight are compared in one patient in Figure 5.11. Fructose and galactose were so rapidly converted into glucose, that non-glucose reducing substances could not be detected after fructose or galactose ingestion (specific fructose and galactose determinations were not available at the time of this study). The conversion of these sugars into glucose after intravenous administration had been demonstrated earlier[53-55]. The rapid conversion of these hexoses into glucose in patients deficient in debranching enzyme, allows fructose, galactose, sucrose and lactose to be included in their diet in complete contrast to the situation in patients deficient in glucose-6-phosphatase. This does not mean that carbohydrates may be given in unrestricted quantities, because a carbohydrate-induced hyperlipidaemia would then ensue (see below).

The most important aspect of glucose homeostasis, gluconeogenesis, was investigated more closely by the oral administration of different proteins and amino acid mixtures[56]. These were all administered in a dose of 1·5 g protein or amino acid mixture/kg body weight, and Figure 5.12 shows that they caused a rapid and sustained increase in the concentration of blood glucose. The tolerance tests indicate that in debranching enzyme deficiency, gluconeogenesis is a very active process. The sustained effect of protein on blood glucose levels explains the value of a high-protein diet in general and a high-protein meal at night, in particular, as already suggested by Van Creveld[57].

In summary, high-protein feeding, containing sufficient carbohydrate of any nature, and an extra feed at night, is appropriate for debranching enzyme-deficient children. It is wise to administer an extra night feed in early infancy and during infections.

Hyperlipidaemia

Hyperlipidaemia is a metabolic abnormality, which has often been observed in debranching enzyme-deficient children[12,21,22,24,58]. The

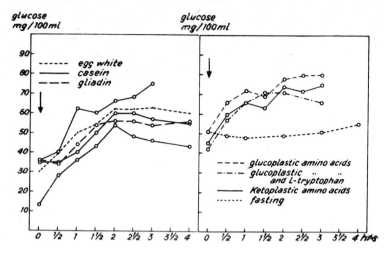

Figure 5.12. The effect of oral proteins (left) and amino acid mixtures (right) in a child with a deficiency of the debranching enzyme system. (From: Fernandes and Van de Kamer, *Pediatrics*, **41**, 935, 1968, with permission of the Editor)

hyperlipidaemia can be so severe that xanthomata result[46]. We found in our patients a combined elevation of triglycerides, cholesterol, and phosphatides (Figure 5.7), which resulted in a hyper β-lipoprotein-aemia[21]. The aetiology of the hyperlipidaemia associated with debranching enzyme deficiency is probably different from that in glucose-6-phosphatase deficiency. The latter has been shown to be due to both increased liponeogenesis and decreased fatty acid elimination, whereas the former appears to be caused by increased liponeogenesis[24], fatty acid elimination being in the low normal range[26].

As it is important to aim at a reduction of the serum lipid concentration by dietary means, the influence of the ratio of carbohydrate to fat and the type of fat in the diet on the serum lipids have been investigated. Substitution of dietary fat for carbohydrates lowered the serum lipids concentration in most patients, but not in all. The type of fat is important: corn oil and olive oil have a favourable effect and coconut oil and medium-chain triglycerides (MCT) an unfavourable effect on the hyperlipidaemia[24]. It was concluded that the hyperlipidaemia is mainly carbohydrate-induced, and the type of fat can influence the level of serum lipids.

The hyperlipidaemia of patients with a deficiency of debranching enzyme is thus amenable to reduction by restriction of the carbohydrate intake. This should not be attempted during the first year of life because of the tendency to hypoglycaemia in very young infants. This tendency gradually subsides, because gluconeogenesis from protein increasingly meets the glucose need and so, during the second year the proportion of carbohydrates in the diet may be gradually reduced in favour of an increased proportion of fat which should preferably be polyunsaturated.

Ketosis
Ketosis has generally been considered to be a characteristic feature of GSD[1,6,15,19,22], but pertinent data on ketone body levels in the blood,

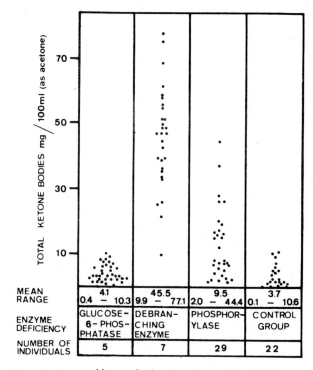

Figure 5.13. Fasting total ketone bodies in patients with a deficiency of glucose-6-phosphatase, the debranching enzyme system, the phosphorylase system, and normal children. (From: Fernandes and Pikaar, *Archives of Disease of Childhood*, **47**, 41, 1972. With permission of the Editor)

which more reliably reflect the existence of ketosis than the finding of ketonuria, are scanty. Figure 5.13 represents the fasting blood concentrations of total ketone bodies in our GSD patients. A marked ketosis was found in most children with a debranching enzyme deficiency. Figure 5.14 shows how rapidly ketosis developed in a debranching enzyme-deficient child during a 12-hour fast. We reasoned that these patients, like diabetics, compensate for a deficient glucose supply to peripheral tissues by both increased gluconeogenesis from protein and increased ketone body formation from fatty acid oxidation. As exogenous carbohydrates (and protein) suppress fatty acid oxidation and promote fatty acid re-esterification, it follows that a pathological ketosis can be prevented or suppressed by the same measures as are indicated for the prevention of hypoglycaemia. Therefore, a high-carbohydrate, high-protein meal at night and a relatively short fasting

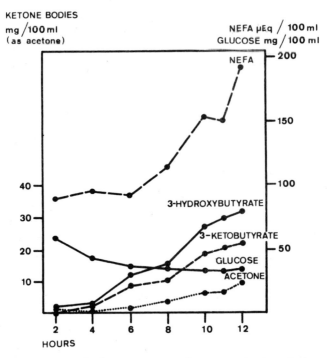

Figure 5.14. Ketone body concentrations during a twelve-hour fasting period in a child with debranching enzyme deficiency. (From: Fernandes and Pikaar, *Archives of Disease of Childhood*, **47**, 41, 1972. With permission of the Editor)

period during the night are both essential to prevent fasting ketosis and fasting hypoglycaemia.

Hyperuricaemia

Hyperuricaemia has only incidentally been reported in debranching enzyme-deficient children[58-60]; there have been no complications arising from it and no treatment of hyperuricaemia has been recommended. The aetiology of hyperuricaemia in debranching enzyme-deficient children is not known. Overproduction and reduced elimination of uric acid might both be involved. Increased glycolysis after carbohydrate ingestion[61] might enhance ribose and purine formation and lead to excessive urate formation. Elimination of urate could be reduced by competitive inhibition of tubular excretion of urate by ketone bodies[19] which are often elevated in the fasting state.

Hyperuricaemia in debranching enzyme deficiency may prove to be more common than appears from the few reports in the literature, if serum urate was determined routinely in all GSD patients. Treatment with Allopurinol may be started, if serum urate levels are repeatedly elevated, though gouty arthritis in patients deficient in debranching enzyme has not yet been reported.

Other complications

Liver malignancies have not been reported in patients with a debranching enzyme deficiency, although periportal fibrosis has already been mentioned. A portocaval transposition has been performed in an 8-year-old girl with hepatosplenomegaly[47]. At the operation liver cirrhosis and portal hypertension were found. A catching-up of growth and a decrease in the hepatosplenomegaly were observed 8 months after operation. As the ultimate prognosis as regards both growth and the normalisation of the metabolic abnormalities is very good[12], a surgical approach is seldom if ever indicated.

DEFICIENCY OF THE PHOSPHORYLASE SYSTEM

The clinical symptoms of GSD due to a deficiency of one of the enzymes of the phosphorylase system are usually mild or may even escape attention until hepatomegaly is found at a routine examination. Hepatomegaly, usually very marked in infancy, may diminish gradually and disappear before or at puberty[57,62] (own observations).

Symptoms of hypoglycaemia are absent or mild, or develop only after prolonged fasting. There may be a slight muscular weakness, which may cause the child to stand up, walk and climb at a later age than normal. Growth, though slightly retarded during the first 3 or 4 years, catches up gradually into the normal range.

Involvement of the liver is indicated by the fact that serum trans-aminases are often elevated, especially in early childhood, whereas other liver function tests are normal. Liver cell architecture is usually normal, except for the glycogen accumulation. Periportal fibrosis[62] and a malignant hepatoma with renal metastasis[63] have been reported, however. Except for these observations, the prognosis as regards development and life expectancy is good.

Deficiency of the phosphorylase system is the most frequent type of GSD[4,64] (own observations, see Table 5.1), but diagnostic criteria differ. Van Hoof[4] states that 'the diagnosis of type VI glycogenosis is made by exclusion: all the patients with hepatomegalic glycogenosis who could not be classified as types I, III or IV, are included in this group which is obviously heterogeneous'. It is the opinion of the author, that the deficiencies of the phosphorylase system are indeed heterogeneous, but only deficiencies of phosphorylase or its activating system should be included in this group, and glycogenoses of unknown origin excluded.

It is mainly due to the investigations of Hug and Huying that insight into the mechanism of the activation of phosphorylase has increased. Figure 5.15 illustrates the phosphorylase cascade. It has been pointed out by Huying[65] that at least in the leucocytes, the phosphory-lase assay has to be performed both in the absence and presence of AMP in order to differentiate a phosphorylase from a phosphorylase b kinase deficiency. Patients with phosphorylase deficiency show a low activity which cannot be stimulated by the addition of AMP[66]. Patients with a phosphorylase b kinase deficiency show a low activity of phosphorylase which can be restored to almost normal values by the addition of AMP[67]. It follows that the diagnosis of phosphorylase b kinase deficiency can be missed, if the enzyme assay is only performed in the presence of AMP. When a deficient activity of phosphorylase has been found, phosphorylase b kinase should be assayed in leucocytes in order to confirm the tentative diagnosis, obtained by the first 'overall assay'.

Differentiation between phosphorylase and phosphorylase b kinase deficiency is important, because the first type of glycogenosis is probably characterised by an autosomal recessive mode of inheritance[68],

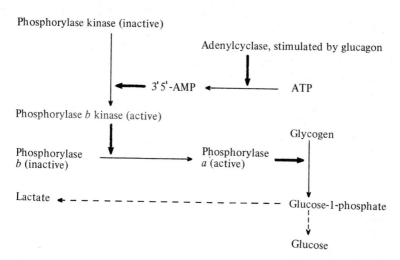

Figure 5.15. The phosphorylase activating system (activation is indicated by broad arrows)

and the latter by an x–chromosomal inheritance[69]. Although the subtyping of the enzyme deficiencies of the phosphorylase system is important from a genetic point of view, the clinical symptoms of both glycogenoses appear to be similar. The metabolic disturbances of both glycogenoses will therefore be discussed together.

Treatment of metabolic disturbances
Hypoglycaemia
The glycogenolysis of patients deficient in phosphorylase or phosphorylase b kinase is not seriously impaired by the enzyme defect, possibly because zero activity of the deficient enzyme has not been demonstrated except by Koster *et al.*[66]. The extent of glycogenolysis is more or less substantiated by the glucagon test. This test is usually characterised by a normal glucose increase in phosphorylase b kinase-deficient children[10,70], whereas the glucagon test in phosphorylase-deficient children is usually characterised by a slow and small increase of the glucose levels[66,71,72]. Theoretically, patients with a phosphorylase deficiency should be more prone to hypoglycaemia than those with phosphorylase b kinase deficiency. It appears that glucose homeostasis is only moderately disturbed in patients with either enzyme

deficiency, although glycogen accumulation in the liver can be considerable (15% in one of the patients of Huying and Fernandes[69]).

The factors affecting glucose homeostasis resemble those discussed under debranching enzyme deficiency. Fructose and galactose are rapidly converted into glucose although the concomitant pathological increase in blood lactate indicates that these hexoses are utilised less efficiently than normal. Gluconeogenesis from non-glucose substrates is adequate (own observations). The conclusion should therefore be that no dietary measures are indicated to maintain normoglycaemia, except an extra feed at night in infants and during infections.

Hyperlipidaemia

A moderate hyperlipidaemia is often present in children deficient in one of the enzymes of the phosphorylase system, although a severe hyperlipidaemia has been reported[73]. This 5-year-old child even had small xanthomatous eruptions. We found in our patients that serum cholesterol was moderately increased, whereas serum triglycerides and phosphatides were only slightly increased or normal (Figure 5.7). In some patients a dense β-lipoprotein band was present on the electropherogram. The hyperlipidaemia, if present, is caused by increased liponeogenesis only[24], not by decreased fatty acid elimination[26]. The increased liponeogenesis appears to be carbohydrate-induced. Figure 5.16 shows, that the total fatty acid concentration was high and cholesterol moderately elevated during a high-carbohydrate diet. After substitution of an isocaloric amount of corn oil for carbohydrate the total fatty acid concentration fell precipitously and the cholesterol decreased moderately. Reintroduction of the high-carbohydrate diet resulted in a prompt rise of total fatty acids and cholesterol to the original levels. The influence of the nature of dietary fat on serum lipids has not been separately studied, but the use of a polyunsaturated fat seems indicated in order to keep the serum cholesterol as low as possible.

In summary, a gradual reduction of carbohydrates and increase of dietary fat, preferably polyunsaturated fat, is appropriate for the treatment of the carbohydrate-induced hyperlipidaemia of these children.

Ketosis

A marked ketosis was present in most children deficient in one of the enzymes of the phosphorylase system as can be seen from Figure 5.13. The tendency to ketosis, which is most marked in the youngest

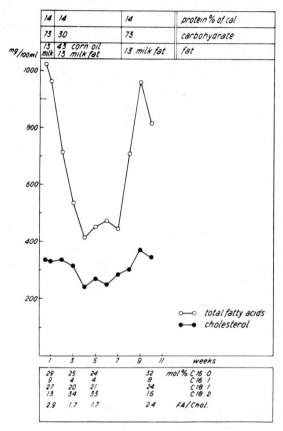

14	14		14		protein % of cal
73	30		73		carbohydrate
13 milk	43 corn oil	13 milk fat	13 milk fat		fat

29	25	24		32	mol % C 16 : 0
9	4	4		8	C 16 : 1
27	20	21		24	C 18 : 1
13	34	33		16	C 18 : 2
2.9	1.7	1.7		2.4	FA/Chol.

Figure 5.16. Effect of high- and low-carbohydrate diets, in which carbo-hydrates were replaced by corn oil, on serum total fatty acid (open circles) and cholesterol (closed circles) in a child with a deficiency of phosphorylase b kinase. (From: Fernandes and Pikaar, *Amer. J. Clin. Nutrition*, **22**, 617, 1969. With permission of the Editor)

patients, decreases with age. The origin of the ketosis related to defici-encies of the phosphorylase system is probably identical with that of the debranching enzyme deficiency-related ketosis. Therefore similar treatment may be applied, consisting of a high-carbohydrate, high-protein meal at night and an adaptation of the length of the fasting period during the night to the fasting concentrations of ketone bodies and glucose in blood.

Table 5.4. Schematic presentation of the treatment of children with glycogen storage disease of the liver

Enzyme deficiency	Glucose-6-phosphatase	Debranching enzyme system	Phosphorylase system
Carbohydrate			
Requirement	70–75% of calories	50% of calories	
Preference	Starch, dextromaltose, glucose	Starch, dextromaltose, glucose	
Restriction	Sucrose, lactose Instead: curd, bag cheese, soymilk	—	
Protein			
Requirement	10% of calories Combine with carbohydrate	15–20% of calories Combine with carbohydrate	
Fat			
Requirement	15–20% of calories Polyunsaturated fat: corn oil, sunflower oil, safflower oil	30–35% of calories Polyunsaturated fat: corn oil, sunflower oil, safflower oil	
Remarks	Frequent meals, night feeds; divide all nutrients, especially, carbohydrates equally over all meals $NaHCO_3$: maintenance 2 mmol/kg/24 h, increase during infections Allopurinol: 8 mg/kg/24 h	High-protein, high-carbohydrate supper recommended Night feeding in infancy and during infections	Dietary measures not very stringent Extra supper during infections

Other complications
Periportal fibrosis has been reported by Sokal *et al.*[62] in a patient at ages of 15 and 23, and in a boy at 2 years of age (low phosphorylase activity in the liver was found in both patients, phosphorylase b kinase activity was not measured). A hepatoma with a very low activity of phosphorylase b kinase, renal metastasis, and death of the infant at the age of 7 months, has been reported by Christiansen *et al.*[63], but this hepatoma was located in an otherwise normal liver. This complication could therefore be coincidental. Other abnormalities such as hyperuricaemia, have not been found. The control of patients with a deficiency of one of the enzymes of the phosphorylase system, can therefore be focused on the treatment of a mild tendency towards hypoglycaemia and hyperlipidaemia.

Summary

Table 5.4 presents an outline of our treatment of patients with glycogen storage disease of the liver, as based upon the suppression or prevention of the main metabolic disturbances related to the 3 most frequently occurring enzyme deficiencies. The stringency of the treatment of any patient should depend on the severity of the metabolic disturbances which is often age-dependent.

REFERENCES

1. Van Creveld, S. (1928). Over een bijzondere stoornis in de koolhydraat-stofwisseling in de kinderleeftijd. *Ned. Maandschr. Geneeskd.*, **75**, 349
2. Cori, G. T. and Cori, C. F. (1952). Glucose-6-phosphatase of the liver in glycogen storage disease. *J. biol. Chem.*, **199**, 661
3. Illingworth, B. (1961). Glycogen storage disease. *Am. J. Clin. Nutr.*, **9**, 683
4. Van Hoof, F., Hue, L., de Barsy, T., Jacquemint, P., Devos, P. and Hers, H. G. (1972). Glycogen storage diseases. *Biochimie*, **54**, 745
5. Baudhuin, P., Hers, H. G. and Loeb, H. (1964). An electron microscopic and biochemical study of type II glycogenosis. *Lab. Invest.*, **13**, 1139
6. Hug, G. and Schubert, W. K. (1967). Lysosomes in type II glycogenosis; changes during administration of extract from *Aspergillus Niger*. *J. Cell Biol.*, **35**, C1
7. Nadler, H. L., Bigley, R. H. and Hug, G. (1970). Prenatal diagnosis of Pompe's disease. *Lancet*, **ii**, 369
8. Galjaard, H., Fernandes, J., Jahodova, M., Koster, J. F. and Niermeyer, M. F. (1972). Prenatal diagnosis of genetic disease. *Bull. Europ. Soc. Hum. Genetics*, p. 79

9. Howell, R. R., Kaback, M. M. and Brown, B. I. (1971). Type IV glycogen storage disease: branching enzyme deficiency in skin fibroblasts and possible heterozygote detection. *J. Pediatr.*, **78**, 638

10. Fernandes, J., Huijing, F. and Van de Kamer, J. H. (1969). A screening method for liver glycogen diseases. *Arch. Dis. Childh.*, **44**, 311

11. Hug, G. (1962). Glucagon tolerance test in glycogen storage disease. *J. Pediatr.*, **60**, 545

12. Van Creveld, S. and Huijing, F. (1964). Differential diagnosis of the type of glycogen disease in two adult patients with long history of glycogenosis. *Metabolism*, **13**, 191

13. Hsia, D. Y.-Y. (1968). The diagnosis and management of the glycogen storage diseases. *Am. J. Clin. Pathol.*, **50**, 44

14. Howell, R. R. (1972, 3rd edn.). The glycogen storage diseases. *The Metabolic Basis of Inherited Disease*, p. 149. (J. B. Stanbury, J. B. Wyngaarden, and D. S. Fredrickson, editors) (New York: McGraw-Hill)

15. Kelsch, R. C. and Oliver, W. J. (1969). Studies on dietary correction of metabolic abnormalities in hepatorenal glycogenosis. *Pediatr. Res.*, **3**, 160

16. Czapek, E. E., Deykin, D. and Salzman, E. W. (1973). Platelet dysfunction in glycogen storage disease, type I. *Blood*, **41**, 235

17. Cornblath, M. and Schwartz, R. (1967). Disorders of carbohydrate metabolism in infancy. *Major Problems in Clinical Pediatrics*, **3**, 131. (Philadelphia and London: Saunders)

18. Mason, H. H. and Andersen, D. H. (1955). Glycogen disease of the liver (Von Gierke's disease) with hepatomata: case report with metabolic studies. *Pediatrics*, **16**, 785

19. Howell, R. R., Ashton, D. M. and Wyngaarden, J. B. (1962). Glucose-6-phosphatase deficiency glycogen storage disease: studies on the interrelationships of carbohydrate, lipid, and purine abnormalities. *Pediatrics*, **29**, 553

20. Schulman, J. L. and Saturen, P. (1954). Glycogen storage disease of the liver. I. Clinical studies during the early neonatal period. *Pediatrics*, **14**, 632

21. Jakovcic, S., Khachadurian, A. K. and Hsia, D. Y.-Y. (1966). The hyperlipidaemia in glycogen storage disease. *J. Lab. Clin. Med.*, **68**, 769

22. Lowe, C. U., Sokal, J. E., Mosovich, L. L., Sarcione, E. J. and Doray, B. H. (1962). Studies in liver glycogen disease; effects of glucagon and other agents on metabolic pattern and clinical status. *Am. J. Med.*, **33**, 4

23. Hülsmann, W. C., Eijkenboom, W. H. M., Koster, J. F. and Fernandes, J. (1970). Glucose-6-phosphatase deficiency and hyperlipaemia. *Clin. Chim. Acta*, **30**, 775

24. Fernandes, J. and Pikaar, N. A. (1969). Hyperlipaemia in children with liver glycogen disease. *Am. J. Clin. Nutr.*, **22**, 617

25. Havel, R. J., Balasse, E. O., Williams, H. E., Kane, J. P. and Segel, N.

(1969). Splanchnic metabolism in Von Gierke's disease (glycogenosis type I). *Trans. Assoc. Am. Physicians*, **82**, 305

26. Forget, P. P., Fernandes, J. and Haverkamp Begemann, P. (1974). Triglyceride clearing in glycogen storage disease. *Pediatr. Res.*, **8**, 114

27. Hug, G., Schubert, W. K. and Howell, R. R. (1967). Serum insulin in type I glycogenosis; effect of galactose or fructose administration. *Diabetes*, **16**, 791

28. Lockwood, D. H., Merimee, T. J., Edgar, P. J., Greene, M. L., Fujimoto, W. Y. and Seegmiller, J. E. (1969). Insulin secretion in type I glycogen storage disease. *Diabetes*, **18**, 755

29. Cuttino, J. T., Summer, G. K., Hill, H. D. and Mitchell, B. J. (1970). Response to medium chain triglycerides in Von Gierke's disease. *Pediatrics*, **46**, 925

30. Brante, G., Kaijser, K. and Öckerman, P. A. (1964). Glycogenosis type I (lack of glucose-6-phosphatase) in four siblings. *Acta Paediatr. Scand.*, **53**, Suppl. 157

31. Matschke, I., Neubaur, J., Willms, B. and Wolf, H. (1969). Stoffwechsel Untersuchungen bei Kindern und jungen Erwachsenen mit Glykogenosen. *Monatschr. Kinderheilkd.*, **117**, 259

32. Neubaur, J., Willms, B., Söling, H. D. and Creutzfeldt, W. (1969). Gicht als Komplikation der Glykogenspeicherkrankheit beim Erwachsenen. *Arch. Klin. Med.*, **216**, 148

33. Binkiewicz, A., Sadeghi-Nejad, A. and Senior, B. (1972). Hypoketonemia in Von Gierke's disease (Glucose-6-phosphatase deficiency) glycogen storage disease (GSD) type I. (Abstract). *Pediatr. Res.*, **6**, 396

34. Fernandes, J. and Pikaar, N. A. (1972). Ketosis in hepatic glycogenosis. *Arch. Dis. Childh.*, **47**, 41

35. Kelley, W. N., Rosenbloom, F. M., Seegmiller, J. E. and Howell, R. R. (1968). Excessive production of uric acid in type I glycogen storage disease. *J. Pediatr.*, **72**, 488

36. Zangeneh, F., Limbeck, G. A., Brown, B. I., Emch, J. R., Arcasoy, M. M., Goldenberg, V. E. and Kelley, V. C. (1969). Hepatorenal glycogenosis (type I glycogenosis) and carcinoma of the liver. *J. Pediatr.*, **74**, 73

37. Spycher, M. A. and Gitzelmann, R. (1971). Glycogenosis type I (glucose-6-phosphatase deficiency): ultrastructural alterations of hepatocytes in a tumor bearing liver. *Virchows Arch. (Zellpathol.)*, **8**, 133

38. Field, R. A. (1960). Glycogen deposition diseases. *The Metabolic Basis of Inherited Disease*, p. 156. (J. B. Stanbury, J. B. Wyngaarden, and D. S. Fredrickson, editors) (New York: McGraw-Hill)

39. Sexton, A. W., Waddell, W. R. and Starzl, T. E. (1964). Liver deglycogenation after portocaval transposition. *Surg. Forum*, **15**, 120

40. Riddell, A. G., Davies, R. P. and Clark, A. D. (1966). Portocaval transposition in the treatment of glycogen storage disease. *Lancet*, **ii**, 1146

The Treatment of Inherited Metabolic Disease

41. Starzl, T. E., Brown, B. I., Blanchard, H. and Brettschneider, L. (1969). Portal diversion in glycogen storage disease. *Surgery* **65**, 504
42. Hermann, R. E. and Mercer, R. D. (1969). Portocaval shunt in the treatment of glycogen storage disease; report of a case. *Surgery*, **65**, 499
43. Boley, S. J., Cohen, M. I. and Gliedman, M. L. (1970). Surgical therapy of glycogen storage disease. *Pediatrics*, **46**, 929
44. Rennert, O. M. and Mukhopadhyay, D. (1968). Diazoxide in Von Gierke's disease, *Arch. Dis. Childh.*, **43**, 358
45. Van Creveld, S. (1932). Chronische hepatogene Hypoglykämie im Kindesalter. *Z. Kinderheilkd.*, **52**, 299
46. Roget, J., Beaudoing, A., Tizzani, R. and Gilbert, Y. (1959). Polycorie glycogénique du foie chex deux frères, par absence d'enzyme débranchant ou amylo-1,6-glucosidase. *Pediatrie*, **14**, 197
47. Starzl, T. E., Marchioro, T. L., Sexton, A. W., Illingworth, B., Waddell, W. R., Faris, T. D. and Hermann, T. J. (1965). The effect of portocaval transposition on carbohydrate metabolism; experimental and clinical observations. *Surgery*, **57**, 687
48. Manners, D. J. and Wright, A. (1961). A case of limit dextrinosis. *Biochem. J.*, **79**, 18P
49. Van Hoof, F. and Hers, H. G. (1967). The subgroups of type III glycogenosis. *Eur. J. Biochem.*, **2**, 265
50. Huijing, F. (1964). Amylo-1, 6-glucosidase activity in normal leucocytes and in leucocytes of patients with glycogen storage disease. *Clin. Chim. Acta*, **9**, 269
51. Chayoth, R., Moses, S. W. and Steinitz, K. (1967). Debrancher enzyme activity in blood cells of families with type III glycogen storage disease. *Isr. J. Med. Sci.*, **3**, 422
52. Justice, P., Ryan, C., Hsia, D. Y.-Y. and Krompotik, E. (1970). Amylo-1, 6-glucosidase in human fibroblasts; studies in type III glycogen storage disease. *Biochem. Biophys. Res. Commun.*, **39**, 301
53. Schwartz, R., Ashmore, J. and Renold, A. E. (1957). Galactose tolerance in glycogen storage disease. *Pediatrics*, **19**, 585
54. Hers, H. G. and Malbrain, H. (1959). Etude biochimique d'un cas de maladie glycogénique. *Probl. Actuels Pediatrie*, **4**, 203
55. Moses, S. W., Levin, S., Chayoth, R. and Steinitz, K. (1966). Enzyme induction in a case of glycogen storage disease. *Pediatrics*, **38**, 111
56. Fernandes, J. and Van de Kamer, J. H. (1968). Hexose and protein tolerance tests in children with liver glycogenosis caused by a deficiency of the debranching enzyme system. *Pediatrics*, **41**, 935
57. Van Creveld, S. (1963). The clinical course of glycogen disease. *Can. Med. Assoc. J.*, **88**, 1
58. Neimann, N., Piesson, M. and Gentin, G. (1960). Quatre observations de polycorie glycogénique avec étude enzymologique. *Sem. Hop. Paris*, **36**, 2617

148

59. Brombacher, P. J., Van Creveld, S., Damme, J. P., Huijing, F. and Ploem, J. E. (1964). A report on two adult patients with glycogen storage disease. *Acta Med. Scand.*, **176**, 269
60. Orsini, A., Pierron, H., Vo Van, L. and Perrimond, H. (1968). Glycogénose hépato-musculaire par déficit en amylo-1, 6-glucosidase (type IIIA) associé à une hyper-lactacidémie. *Arch. Fr. Pediatr.*, **25**, 845
61. Fernandes, J. and Van de Kamer, J. H. (1965). Studies on the utilization of hexoses in liver glycogen disease. *Pediatrics*, **35**, 470
62. Sokal, J. E., Lowe, C. U., Saks, G. L., Leahy, M. and Stowens, D. (1964). Liver glycogen disease in two generations of a family; clinical studies and tissue analyses during overt disease and after apparent recovery. *Am. J. Med.*, **36**, 847
63. Christiansen, R. O., Page, L. A. and Greenberg, R. E. (1968). Glycogen storage in a hepatoma; dephosphophosphorylase kinase defect. *Pediatrics*, **42**, 694
64. Hers, H. G. (1964). Glycogen storage disease. *Advances in Metabolic Disorders*, Vol. I, p. 1. (R. Levine, and R. Luft, editors) (New York: Academic Press)
65. Huijing, F. (1967). Phosphorylase kinase in leucocytes of normal subjects and of patients with glycogen storage disease. *Biochim. Biophys. Acta*, **148**, 601
66. Koster, J. F., Fernandes, J., Slee, R. G., Van Berkel, Th. J. C. and Hülsmann, W. C. (1973). Hepatic phosphorylase deficiency; a biochemical study. *Biochem. Biophys. Res. Commun.*, **53**, 282
67. Huijing, F. (1970). Phosphorylase kinase deficiency. *Biochem. Genet.*, **4**, 187
68. Schwartz, D., Savin, M., Drash, A. and Field, J. (1970). Studies in glycogen storage disease IV. Leucocyte phosphorylase in a family with type VI GSD. *Metabolism*, **19**, 238
69. Huijing, F. and Fernandes, J. (1969). X-Chromosomal inheritance of liver glycogenosis with phosphorylase kinase deficiency. *Am. J. Hum. Genet.*, **21**, 275
70. Ludwig, M., Wolfson, S. and Rennert, O. (1972). Glycogen storage disease type VIII. *Arch. Dis. Childh.*, **47**, 830
71. Drummond, G. I., Hardwick, D. F. and Israels, S. (1970). Liver glycogen phosphorylase deficiency. *Can. Med. Assoc. J.*, **102**, 740
72. Guibaud, P. and Mathieu, M. (1972). Hétérogénéité de la glycogenose type VI. Etude de l'activité de la phosphorylase leucocytaire dans deux familles. *Arch. Fr. Pediatr.*, **29**, 1043
73. Öckerman, P. A., Jelke, H. and Kaijser, K. (1966). Glycogenosis type VI (liver phosphorylase deficiency); a case followed for ten years with normal phosphorylase activity in white blood cells and jejunal mucosa. *Acta Paediatr. Scand.*, **55**, 10

CHAPTER 6

Hereditary Fructose Intolerance and Fructose-1,6-Diphosphatase Deficiency

E. R. Froesch

Hereditary fructose intolerance (HFI) is an inborn error of fructose metabolism characterised by a primary deficiency of hepatic aldolase (aldolase B)[1-3]. Normal hepatic aldolase splits fructose-1-phosphate and fructose-1,6-diphosphate at saturation concentrations of each substrate with approximately equal velocity[4]. In patients with HFI the activity of fructose-1,6-diphosphate aldolase is reduced to anywhere between 10 and 50% of normal, whereas the fructose-1-phosphate splitting activity is 1–10% of normal[5-8]. At substrate saturation concentrations the hepatic aldolase of patients with HFI splits fructose-1,6-diphosphate at least 5 times as fast as fructose-1-phosphate[7]. Even though the activity of hepatic aldolase towards fructose-1,6-diphosphate is also considerably reduced the remaining enzyme activity appears to be sufficient not to become limiting either for glycolysis or gluconeogenesis.

Biochemical consequences of fructose-1-phosphate aldolase deficiency

Symptoms occur in HFI only when sucrose (saccharose) or fructose are ingested[9,10]. Most of the symptoms can be explained by the accumulation of fructose-1-phosphate in those tissues which metabolise fructose by the following specific pathway. In the liver, in the proximal renal tubule and in the mucosa of the small bowel fructose is first phosphorylated to fructose-1-phosphate by the enzyme fructokinase[11]. Fructose-1-phosphate is then split by hepatic aldolase to glyceraldehyde and dihydroxyacetone-phosphate[12,13]. There is a triose kinase in liver which can phosphorylate glyceraldehyde directly to glyceraldehyde-phosphate[14,15], thereby funnelling fructose into the regular glycolytic pathway.

HFI is characterised by a lack of the fructose-1-phosphate splitting activity of hepatic aldolase. Therefore, fructose-1-phosphate accumulates. The biochemical consequences of fructose-1-phosphate accumulation are numerous. First the intracellular concentration of ATP and inorganic phosphorus decrease rapidly as reflected in the serum by a sharp and prolonged drop of the level of inorganic phosphorus[9,16]. Fructose-1-phosphate then leads to a secondary inhibition of several enzymes such as fructokinase, phosphorylase and the remaining activity of hepatic fructose-1,6-diphosphate aldolase. The block of fructokinase renders further phosphorylation of fructose impossible so that the fructose concentration in the blood rises to high levels. Between 10 and 20% of administered fructose is excreted in the urine.

This secondary block of fructokinase leads to fructosuria, which is the only chemical sign of essential fructosuria, a harmless anomaly

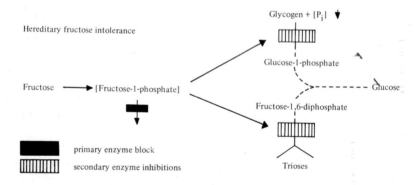

primary enzyme block
secondary enzyme inhibitions

Figure 6.1. Mechanisms of fructose-induced hypoglycaemia in HFI. Other signs and symptoms of HFI such as vomiting, renal tubular defects, and liver cell damage also result from the accumulation of fructose-1-phosphate which must be removed by as yet unknown mechanisms (possibly lysosomal enzymes). In all likelihood other biochemical consequences such as changes in the redox potential, a fall of the concentration of inorganic phosphorus and ATP and resulting alterations of energy metabolism play a major role in the 'toxicity' of fructose-1-phosphate. All these acute and chronic biochemical and clinical alterations are fully reversible when a fructose-free diet is administered

characterised by a primary deficiency of fructokinase. The other 2 enzyme inhibitions are much more serious since they lead to hypoglycaemia. Fructose-1-phosphate is an effective competitive inhibitor of phosphorylase at fructose-1-phosphate concentrations of 10^{-2} molar[17]. Low inorganic phosphorus levels in the cells accentuate phosphorylase inhibition by fructose-1-phosphate, so that glycogen breakdown by phosphorylase may be reduced to a few percent of normal. Glucagon and adrenaline are completely ineffective in stimulating glycogenolysis in patients with HFI during fructose induced hypoglycaemia. Whereas fructose-1-phosphate stimulates the condensation of trioses to fructose-1,6-diphosphate by normal hepatic aldolase[18], the reverse is true for muscle aldolase[5]. In this respect hepatic aldolase of patients with HFI reacts in the same manner as muscle aldolase and is also inhibited by fructose-1-phosphate[18].

Other substrates of fructokinase, such as L-sorbose cause only one secondary enzyme inhibition, namely that of further phosphorylation of L-sorbose by fructokinase[5]. The reason for this is that fructokinase has a much smaller affinity for L-sorbose than for D-fructose[19]. Therefore, the accumulation of a small amount of L-sorbose-1-phosphate leads to a block of further L-sorbose phosphorylation by fructokinase. However, when fructose is subsequently administered to such a patient, fructose is phosphorylated normally and fructose-1-phosphate leads to all the other secondary enzyme inhibitions which L-sorbose-1-phosphate failed to produce.

Serum insulin has been measured many times in patients with HFI and insulin has been excluded as the cause of the hypoglycaemia in this condition[1]. A block in hepatic glucose production during fructose induced hypoglycaemia has been directly demonstrated by the administration of labelled glucose which was no longer diluted by unlabelled glucose from the liver during fructose induced hypoglycaemia[20]. After small doses of fructose, patients recover spontaneously from hypoglycaemia in a few hours. It is not known how fructose-1-phosphate is metabolised by these patients. In the electron-microscope one can observe lysosomal activation shortly after the administration of fructose, indicating that lysosomal phosphatases may break down some of the fructose-1-phosphate[21]. Fructose-1-phosphate accumulation has also been demonstrated in the mucosa of the small bowel[22] and in the proximal tubules of the kidney[23].

Hypoglycaemia is only one of many symptoms caused by fructose ingestion by patients with HFI. The most prominent symptoms after an acute load of fructose are nausea and vomiting. Chronic fructose poisoning of patients with HFI cannot be fully explained by what we know about the biochemistry of HFI and the symptoms of this will be described in a later section.

Genetics of HFI

HFI is transmitted by an autosomal recessive gene[1]. One of the very early cases of HFI was from a family with many consanguineous marriages[9]. However, this is the exception. Therefore, HFI is likely to be a relatively uncommon disorder. There are 3 reports of children with HFI whose fathers also had HFI. It is very unlikely that this means true dominant inheritance[1,30,31]. In all likelihood a homozygous father married a heterozygous mother, resulting in offsprings with HFI. It is not yet possible to detect heterozygous carriers of HFI either by fructose tolerance tests or by biochemical or immunological detection of an abnormal hepatic aldolase[32].

Recognition of HFI in adults

It may be of interest how we discovered some patients with HFI. A lady who had dinner with her friends, one of whom was a geneticist who had just heard about this new disorder, refused any dessert. The geneticist asked her whether she didn't like any sweets or whether she didn't feel well. She told him that she had never been able to take anything sweet because of nausea and vomiting. She was referred to us and the diagnosis of HFI was established.

A dental technician who, in contrast to his family, had exceptionally healthy teeth, read about the disorder in a dental journal and spontaneously visited me to ask whether he had hereditary fructose intolerance. Sure enough, he did. A brother of his who had the same disorder was afraid to visit us because he thought he, a state employee, might lose his job if his disease was diagnosed.

While in military service I once sat at the same table with a surgeon who did not take any dessert. I asked him why and he gave me the most beautiful description of the acute fructose induced symptomatology of HFI. He was the only adult with HFI who had a few dental cavities[24,25], and I asked him therefore, whether he had taken any sweets when he was young. He said that his father, a country physician, had forced him to eat cookies and cake because he would not make any exceptions in the education of his children.

These examples show that patients with HFI may reach adulthood without diagnosis and without any serious disadvantage. Formerly, when babies were nursed, the most important endowment of fate in the life of such patients was the common sense or intelligence of their mother. Now it is the intelligence of the doctor which is more important since babies have contact with sucrose or other fructose containing foodstuffs much earlier in life. Not uncommonly the oldest child with HFI may die or become severely ill from fructose ingestion until the mother or the doctor discovers what is wrong, whereafter the following children do perfectly well because those responsible suspect or are aware of HFI. Although HFI is one of the more common inborn errors of metabolism and although it has been described many times in the English literature[2,5,26-29], unbelievable mishaps may still occur to such patients. Thus, I know of a tragic recent incident which happened to an 8-year-old boy who had to undergo surgery. His mother told the surgeon and the anaesthetist that her boy had hereditary fructose intolerance. They both assured her that they knew quite well what this meant and went ahead with the operation. The boy died within 3 days because the medical staff infused him with invert sugar, obviously unaware of the fact that this is a hydrolysate of sucrose.

Nowadays small babies and newborns are in great danger because many milk products contain sucrose. In our opinion, foodstuffs containing fructose or sucrose should not be used within the first 3 months of life. In this way babies with HFI have a good start in life, and gain 1 kg or more before the diagnosis of HFI is established. The child is then in much less danger if exposed to fructose for the first time after having grown and thrived well for the first 3 months of life.

Diagnosis of HFI

The diagnosis of HFI in the adult is very easy. Patients report that they do not tolerate anything sweet, that they have nausea and vomiting for several hours after eating sweet things. They give an exact list of all the foodstuffs which contain fructose, and when administered fructose orally, experience acute hypoglycaemia, nausea and vomiting.

Since intravenous administration of fructose does not lead to vomiting, we prefer it for diagnostic purposes. The diagnosis can be made by giving 0·25 g fructose intravenously per kg of body weight. After this dose the blood sugar falls to between 20 and 30 mg/100 ml after 45–60 minutes, and then returns spontaneously but slowly to normal. If the patient experiences severe symptoms of hypoglycaemia, one may have to administer glucose. Hypophosphataemia develops

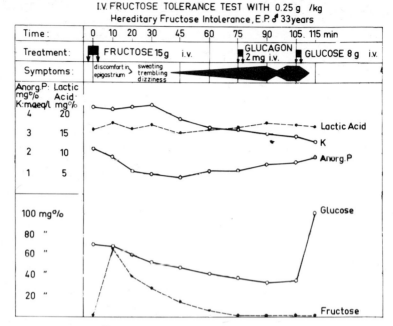

Figure 6.2. The IV fructose tolerance test is preferred for diagnostic purposes since it leads to the classical hypoglycaemia without causing nausea and vomiting. The failure of the blood glucose level to respond to glucagon proves the hepatic origin of hypoglycaemia. It is of interest, albeit unexplained, that glucagon somehow brings about a temporary relief of hypoglycaemic symptoms (from Froesch et al., Amer. J. Med., **34**, 151 (1963); with permission of the Editor)

more rapidly than hypoglycaemia and may also last for several hours. The normal blood phosphorus of around 3 mg/100 ml may fall below 1·5 mg/100 ml without any symptoms. Since hypoglycaemia and hypophosphataemia after fructose infusion are shared by patients with fructose-1,6-diphosphatase deficiency one may want to establish the diagnosis of HFI by a liver biopsy. In adults with HFI who have normal liver function, the fructose-1,6-diphosphate splitting aldolase activity is reduced to between 20 and 50%, whereas the fructose-1-phosphate aldolase activity is reduced to between 2 and 6% of normal[1].

In otherwise healthy older children the diagnosis of HFI may be just as easy. Our first patient with HFI was referred to the children's hospital at the age of 6 years. She was perfectly normal and healthy. Since she had not been taking any fructose for several years, the diagnosis was established by means of a fructose tolerance test.

However, it is much more difficult to establish the diagnosis of HFI in severely ill, chronically intoxicated newborns and small babies. One should think of HFI in the following situations: failure to thrive, vomiting, hepatosplenomegaly, ascites, oedema, dehydration, seizures and other neurologic symptoms, hyperbilirubinaemia[27,33]. All these symptoms may be caused by fructose intoxication in children with HFI and the right diagnostic steps must be taken immediately. One should investigate immediately whether the formula which the baby gets contains any sucrose or fructose. Secondly, fructose must be looked for in the urine and possibly also in the blood. Fructose is a reducing sugar and, in general, is excreted by such children in the urine for some hours after meals. If the 'Clinitest' or any other reducing test is positive and the glucose oxidase test ('Test Tape') negative, one should look for fructose.

The simplest way to do this is to use the hexokinase-glucose-6-phosphatase method. This method is very specific for glucose. In the absence of glucose or when no glucose is left in the reaction mixture, fructose is phosphorylated by hexokinase to fructose-6-phosphate[34]. If, at this point, the enzyme phosphohexose isomerase is added, which converts fructose-6-phosphate to glucose-6-phosphate, the reaction continues to proceed as with glucose[34]. Therefore, the difference between the measurement of NADH in the presence of hexokinase-glucose-6-phosphate-dehydrogenase plus phosphohexose isomerase minus the NADH which one gets with hexokinase and glucose-6-phosphate-dehydrogenase alone yields an accurate value of the fructose concentration in the urine. Fructose can be determined by a simple colour reaction with resorcinol[35]. However, this reaction is not entirely specific. To identify fructose one has to resort to paper chromatography[36]. In our view it is faster and just as specific to use the modified hexokinase-method with phosphohexose isomerase to determine whether the sugar excreted in the urine is fructose. This method can also be used for the quantitative determination of glucose and fructose in plasma and serum.

If large amounts of fructose are found in the urine of patients the diagnosis of HFI is not definitive but very likely. It is reasonable to let the patient recover on a fructose-free diet and to perform a fructose tolerance test later when the patient is in better general health. A liver biopsy may be dangerous in severely ill children with a prolonged clotting time. It should be carried out only if the clotting time can be restored to normal by intravenous injection of vitamin K. The interpretation of the result of aldolase determination is also relatively difficult in children with severe liver disease in a chronic stage of fructose intoxication, because all enzyme activities are decreased and aldolase activity so low that it may be difficult to determine.

Fructose tolerance tests should not be carried out in a severely ill, chronically intoxicated child with HFI. It is very harmful and may endanger the child's life. Furthermore, since the child is chronically intoxicated it has a low phosphorus to start with and may have relatively low blood sugar values at the beginning of the test, so that the results may be difficult to interpret. Larger doses of fructose may have to be used to be sure of the results of the test, but then, these large doses of fructose are even more harmful.

Symptoms of hereditary fructose intolerance

As mentioned earlier, there is an acute syndrome in HFI which occurs in subjects in good health after fructose ingestion. It consists of hypoglycaemia, nausea and vomiting. Children have a more rapid glucose turnover than adults and, therefore, hypoglycaemia develops sooner. Hypoglycaemic symptoms may occur in as little as 20–30 minutes and may be so severe that glucose must be administered. It is essential to give glucose intravenously, since these children experience nausea and may vomit when glucose is given orally. A large dose of fructose may produce hyperbilirubinaemia for a few days and a rapid increase in the serum levels of liver enzymes. The renal changes are classical; as soon as fructose is given, the kidney loses its capacity to acidify the urine[37]. Renal tubular acidosis has been described in chronically fructose intoxicated children with HFI. This syndrome is reversible. At the same time, amino acids are lost in the urine, and phosphate reabsorption is impaired[38]. All these changes point to the proximal tubule, the metabolism of which is impaired due to fructose-1-phosphate accumulation and severe alterations in energy metabolism.

It is very typical that children with HFI, and only these children, develop a strong distaste and aversion for all sweet foodstuffs and fruits[1]. The children cannot distinguish between glucose and fructose and, therefore, reject everything that has a sweet taste to it. Thus, they protect themselves from their disease. We realise again how important

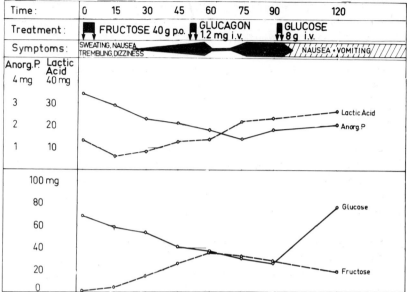

Figure 6.3. As demonstrated in this figure, fructose by mouth causes not only hypoglycaemia but prolonged nausea and vomiting in patients with HFI (from Froesch *et al., Amer. J. Med.,* **34,** 15 (1963); with permission of the Editor)

it is that these children have contact with fructose late in life when they can show their distaste and can protest. At the age of 3–4 months they can already show their own will and recognise that the sweet stuff in the food is harmful. In contrast, they are completely helpless as newborns or small babies.

The classical case history is that of a baby which has been nursed for 2 or 3 months and did perfectly well. Then, fruit juices or sucrose were added to the formula and suddenly the child starts to vomit, fails to thrive and is drowsy after meals. The mother gives a classical dietary history, from which the diagnosis can be made. In such children, who have been exposed to fructose for only a few days, a fructose-tolerance test is not harmful and can be used to establish the diagnosis.

Recognition of HFI in the newborn and infant

Because newborns are no longer breast-fed in many parts of the 'civilised' world and because sucrose is the cheapest carbohydrate, babies nowadays are exposed to this sugar very early in life. It goes without saying that this is deleterious for babies with HFI. Severely intoxicated small babies show the following syndrome which is by no means specific for HFI: failure to thrive and to gain weight, loss of adipose tissue despite a big belly with hepato– and maybe also spleno-megaly and sometimes ascites. Oedema may be present if anorexia, liver damage and hypoalbuminaemia are severe enough. Haemorrhages may be present because of liver damage. Renal function is impaired because of dehydration and because of the specific effect of fructose-1-phosphate on the proximal tubule leading to tubular acidosis, a defect in phosphate reabsorption and a defect in amino acid reabsorption resulting in aminoaciduria which, of course, is also of hepatic origin.

Table 6.1. Signs and symptoms of hereditary fructose intolerance

Acute signs and symptoms beginning 20 minutes after oral administration of fructose	Chronic syndrome after prolonged exposure to fructose, reversible by fructose-free diet
Sweating	Failure to thrive
Trembling	Jaundice
Dizziness	Hepatomegaly
Nausea	Vomiting
Vomiting	Dehydration
Various degrees of disturbed consciousness to deep coma	Oedema
	Ascites
Fructosuria	Seizures
Hypophosphataemia	Fructosuria
Fructosaemia (not excessive)	Fructosaemia
Amino aciduria	Hypophosphataemia
Hyperbilirubinaemia	Hyperbilirubinaemia
Rise of serum levels of hepatic enzymes	Rise of serum levels of hepatic enzymes
	Fibrosis or cirrhosis of liver
	Aversion towards sweet food
	Lack of dental caries

It is of interest in this respect, that severely intoxicated children with HFI have been confounded with patients with primary tyrosinosis[39,40]. HFI may lead to almost the same clinical picture and to the same biochemical findings as tyrosinosis. The neurologic and cerebral signs and symptoms of hypoglycaemia are manifold and by no means specific for HFI.

The procedures by which the diagnosis of HFI in such babies can be established are the following: (1) accurate dietary history, (2) search for fructose in the urine and (3) determination of phosphate and fructose in the blood after a meal. A fructose tolerance test and a liver biopsy should not be carried out in this situation.

TREATMENT OF HEREDITARY FRUCTOSE INTOLERANCE

Treatment of acute hypoglycaemia
As in any hypoglycaemia of hepatic origin it does not help to give glucagon or epinephrine, since phosphorylase is completely blocked. Patients with fructose-induced hypoglycaemia must be treated with intravenous glucose. Hypoglycaemia in HFI may be somewhat prolonged since fructose-1-phosphate remains in the liver for several hours. However, hypoglycaemia in HFI has a lesser tendency to recur than insulin hypoglycaemia or hypoglycaemia induced by tolbutamide. Therefore, it is usually sufficient to give an adequate amount of glucose in one intravenous injection, which may, if necessary, be repeated after a certain period of time. Usually it is not necessary to give glucose by continuous intravenous infusion because of hypoglycaemia but rather because of the poor nutritional state of the baby.

Treatment of the severely intoxicated newborn baby and infant
The first and most important step is to omit fructose from all foodstuffs. The baby may then be rehydrated carefully, starting with intravenous infusions of glucose and electrolytes. Since phosphorus has been lost in rather large amounts in the urine and since a lot of it is sequestered in the liver in the form of fructose-1-phosphate and also because the intravenous infusion of glucose will lead to a further decrease of inorganic phosphorus, one should carefully monitor the serum phosphorus and one may have to add inorganic phosphorus to

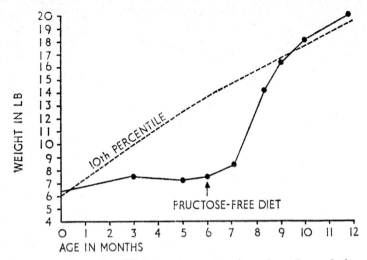

Case 3. Weight chart showing the effect of the introduction of a fructose-free diet.

Figure 6.4. Weight chart showing the effect of a fructose-free diet in a case of HFI (from Black, J. A. and Simpson, K., *Brit. Med. J.*, **iv**, 139 (1967); with permission of the Editor)

the infusion. Some children have a low serum potassium so that this may have to be supplemented.

Due to malnutrition and severe liver disease, the glucose infusion may lead to transient hyperglycaemia which may be prevented by small doses of insulin which will help to bring the baby more rapidly from a very catabolic and toxic state into one more anabolic. Amino acids should not be added at the beginning of treatment, since the liver function of these children is poor and since the plasma level of amino acids is elevated. The bleeding tendency may be partially corrected by vitamin K, if it is due to malnutrition and not solely to liver disease. The baby now has a chance to recover within a few days and is again able to retain food. As usual in such toxic children, feeds must at first be frequent and small.

Diet in hereditary fructose intolerance
In the adult and in children diet is absolutely no problem, since the patients protect themselves from everything that contains the noxious

agent fructose. Every time they take fructose, they feel sick and, therefore, soon learn to avoid sweets and all fructose containing food-stuffs. If medication is to be administered for any reason, one should make sure that it does not contain sucrose which is present in all syrups and is used for the coating of almost all drugs in pill form. The doctor is very likely to make mistakes. My last patient with HFI in the hospital complained of constipation. I told the nurse to give her a harmless laxative. Sure enough the patient received some fig syrup which made her vomit for several hours but did not help her constipation. The patient surely would not have taken any fig syrup at home because she was quite aware that it contains sucrose. Since I prescribed it in the hospital she was willing to take it in the firm belief that I know!

The smaller the baby, the more difficult is the prescription of a correct diet. First of all, any baby with HFI who has never experienced the effect of sucrose is likely to try to get at fruit, chocolate, etc. After all, his brothers and sisters take it, why shouldn't he also? Some such mistakes are perfectly harmless and cannot be prevented because every child will try a few times and will have to find out by himself. It is like smoking a cigar. One may try it once at the age of 5 to impress one's friends, but one will probably not repeat it until judgment and memory get worse at the age of 25 or so.

An important question which has not yet been resolved is whether or not one should use anything sweet at all in the diet of children with HFI. In my own opinion the patient should know that everything sweet is bad for him, because otherwise he will make one mistake after another and will anyway stop taking sweets. None of my patients, adult or children with HFI, showed any signs of psychological disturbance. Since these children can eat as much starch as they want, they certainly get enough carbohydrate in their food. One of my adult patients with HFI has carbohydrate induced hyperlipoproteinaemia. There were never any signs of any deficiency of nutrients or vitamins reported in any such patient.

One should also remember that sorbitol is metabolised via fructose and that it is just as toxic as fructose both in the diet and in the infusion. Before using any formula or any infusion solution in a patient with hereditary fructose intolerance one should check carefully and make sure that it does not contain fructose, sorbitol, invert sugar or laevulose which happens to be the same thing as fructose.

Last, but not least, I should mention that fructose is an endogenously formed carbohydrate. It was long believed to be produced from glucose via sorbitol in the prostate and seminal vesicles only[41]. Recent investigations make it likely that many tissues can make fructose from glucose particularly at high glucose concentrations[42]. It is possible that increased fructose production due to diabetes might get a patient with HFI into trouble. So far, we know of no patient in whom diabetes mellitus coincided with HFI.

FRUCTOSE-1,6-DIPHOSPHATASE DEFICIENCY

This rare inborn error of metabolism is characterised by a primary deficiency of hepatic fructose-1,6-diphosphatase[43–45]. This is a one-way enzyme in the gluconeogenic (glycolytic) pathway permitting the cleavage of fructose-1,6-diphosphate to fructose-6-phosphate. If the enzyme is lacking, hypoglycaemia must occur during prolonged fasting. Children with fructose-1,6-diphosphatase deficiency maintain a normal blood sugar for as long as 12–16 hours after the last meal, i.e. as long as they can mobilise hepatic glycogen stores. When the glycogen stores are depleted, they cannot turn to gluconeogenesis because of the lack of this essential gluconeogenetic enzyme and they then become hypoglycaemic. Therefore, fasting hypoglycaemia is one of the major symptoms of fructose-1,6-diphosphatase deficiency. However, since it occurs only after 12–16 hours of fasting, it is relatively rare.

The second, and more important spontaneously occurring abnormality is lactic acidosis. The primary enzyme deficiency in these children explains the lactic acidosis. Whereas the normal liver converts a large portion of amino acids and glycerol to glucose, the liver of these children can convert these substrates only to lactate or fat. The normal 'buffering' capacity of the liver which consists of taking up lactate and of making glucose from lactate during muscular exercise is completely deficient in these children. Therefore, they are prone to develop lactic acidosis, firstly during stress when glycerol release from adipose tissue is increased, and secondly during physical exercise. Infectious diseases precipitate first lactic acidosis and only later hypoglycaemia. The reason why fructose-1,6-diphosphatase deficiency is dealt with in this particular chapter is that these children do not only present fasting hypoglycaemia, but also fructose-induced hypoglycaemia. The mechanism by which fructose precipitates hypoglycaemia is the same as that in HFI. Fructose can be phosphorylated and fructose-1-phosphate is readily broken down. However the major fate of fructose in the normal organism is its conversion to glucose, a process which is blocked in these children. Therefore, fructose administration leads to excessive lactic acid accumulation and to a backward substrate inhibition of several enzymes ultimately leading to the accumulation of fructose-1-phosphate. The latter causes a block of phosphorylase and a block of glycogenolysis as in HFI.

Fructose-1,6-diphosphatase deficiency should be suspected when children show repeated attacks of acidosis with high serum lactate

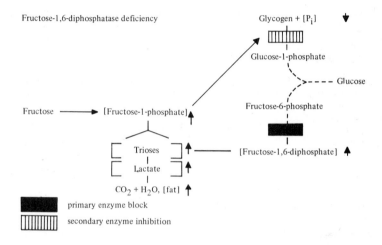

Fructose-1,6-diphosphatase deficiency

Glycogen + [P_i]

Glucose-1-phosphate

Glucose

Fructose ⟶ [Fructose-1-phosphate]

Fructose-6-phosphate

Trioses

[Fructose-1,6-diphosphate]

Lactate

CO_2 + H_2O, [fat]

primary enzyme block

secondary enzyme inhibition

Figure 6.5. This figure shows only the primary enzyme deficiency of fructose-1,6-diphosphatase deficiency and the biochemical consequences of fructose ingestion. The main symptomatology, i.e. fasting hypoglycaemia and fasting lactic acidosis is also explained by the primary fructose-1,6-diphosphatase deficiency. When the hepatic glycogen stores are exhausted no glucose can be produced from gluconeogenic precursors so that hypoglycaemia results. The major fate of glycerol and in part also of amino acids in the normal liver is their conversion to glucose which is blocked in patients with fructose-1,6-diphosphatase deficiency. Stress and catabolic situations increase the flux of glycerol and amino acids to the liver. The fastest way to deal with these substrates is to release them as lactate. This explains lactic acidosis in patients with fructose-1,6-diphosphatase deficiency. Hepatomegaly is likely to be caused by increased fat synthesis from these same substrates and by chronic fructose intoxication since these patients, in contrast to HFI, do not vomit after fructose intake and, therefore, do not develop an aversion to sweet foodstuffs

concentrations and spontaneous attacks of hypoglycaemia in the presence of hepatomegaly. The diagnosis can be established by prolonged fasting for 12–16 hours after which time the blood sugar must fall. An intravenous fructose tolerance test with 0·25 g/kg body weight shows typical short lasting hypoglycaemia with concomitant hypophosphataemia. Both are a little bit less severe in this condition than in HFI.

These children do not have nausea and do not vomit and, therefore, do not develop a distaste for sweet foodstuff. In contrast to HFI, they continue eating fructose containing foodstuffs, grow normally and have an ordinary incidence of dental caries. The signs of fructose intoxication are much less severe than in HFI, probably because the accumulation of fructose esters in the liver cells is much less pronounced and because there are regular ways of disposing of fructose-1-phosphate. The definitive diagnosis of fructose-1,6-diphosphatase deficiency must be established by means of a liver biopsy and the determination of fructose-1,6-diphosphatase in the tissue.

The treatment of fructose-1,6-diphosphatase deficiency consists of frequent feeds and prompt treatment of infections including, if necessary, intravenous glucose feeding. Fructose and sorbitol should be omitted from the diet if at all possible, since they always lead to acute, more or less severe lactic acidosis. Whereas the prognosis of HFI is very good, the same cannot be said for fructose-1,6-diphosphatase deficiency. This enzyme is essential for life, notwithstanding exogenous factors. It is possible to prevent somebody who detests fructose from taking fructose, but it is more difficult to impose upon someone the habit of eating regularly every 2–3 hours and impossible to prevent him from catching common infectious diseases which may lead to death in lactic acidosis and hypoglycaemia. It is essential that children with fructose-1,6-diphosphatase deficiency and their parents are accurately informed about their disease, that they always carry a note on themselves which tells the doctor who may find them in an acidotic or unconscious state exactly what he has to do.

The original work carried out in the laboratories of the Metabolic Unit, Department of Medicine, University of Zurich, was supported by a Grant (3.7180.72) from the Schweizerischer Nationalfonds.

REFERENCES

1. Froesch, E. R. (1972). *The Metabolic Basis of Inherited Disease*, 3rd edn. (J. B. Stanbury, J. B. Wyngaarden, and D. S. Fredrickson, editors) (New York: McGraw-Hill)

2. Levin, B., Snodgrass, G. J. A. I., Oberholzer, V. G., Burgess, E. A. and Dobbs, R. H. (1968). Fructosemia: observation on seven cases. *Amer. J. Med.*, **45**, 826

3. Royer, P., Lestradet, H., Habib, R., Lardinois, R. and Desbuquois, B. (1964). L'intolérance héréditaire au fructose. *Bull. Soc. Med. Hop. Paris.*, **115**, 805

4. Gürtler, B., Bally, C. and Leuthardt, F. (1971). Reindarstellung und Eigenschaften der menschlichen Leberaldolase. *Hoppe-Seyler's Z. Physiol. Chem.*, **352**, 1455

5. Froesch, E. R., Wolf, H. P., Baitsch, H., Prader, A. and Labhart, A. (1963). Hereditary fructose intolerance: an inborn defect of hepatic fructose-1-phosphate splitting aldolase. *Amer. J. Med.*, **34**, 151

6. Hers, H. G. and Joassin, G. (1961). Anomalie de l'aldolase héptique dans l'intolérance au fructose. *Enzym. Biol. Clin.*, **1**, 4

7. Wolf, H. P. and Froesch, E. R. (1963). Ueber Aldolasen. IV; Mitteilung. Enzymaktivitäten in der Leber bei hereditärer Fructoseintoleranz. *Biochem. Ztschr.*, **337**, 328

8. Nikkilä, E. A., Somersalo, O., Pitkänen, E. and Perheentupa, J. (1962). Hereditary fructose intolerance, an inborn deficiency of liver aldolase complex. *Metabolism*, **11**, 727

9. Froesch, E. R., Prader, A., Labhart, A., Stuber, H. W. and Wolf, H. P. (1957). Die hereditäre Fructoseintoleranz, eine bisher nicht bekannte kongenitale Stoffwechselstörung. *Schweiz. Med. Wschr.*, **87**, 1168

10. Perheentupa, J., Pitkänen, E., Nikkilä, E. A., Somersalo, O. and Hakosalo, J. (1962). Hereditary fructose intolerance, a clinical study of 4 cases. *Ann. Paediat. Fenn.*, **8**, 221

11. Hers, H. G. (1952). La fructokinase du foie. *Biochim. Biophys. Acta*, **8**, 416

12. Leuthardt, F., Testa, E. and Wolf, H. P. (1953). Der enzymatische Abbau des Fructose-1-phosphats in der Leber. III. Mitteilung über den Stoffwechsel der Fructose in der Leber. *Helv. Chim. Acta*, **36**, 227

13. Hers, H. G. and Kusaka, T. (1953). Le métabolisme du fructose-1-phosphate dans le foie. *Biochim. Biophys. Acta*, **11**, 427

14. Heinz, F. and Lamprecht, W. (1961). Anreicherung und Charakterisierung einer Triosekinase aus Leber. Zur Biochemie des Fruchtosestoffwechsels, III. *Z. Physiol. Chem.*, **324**, 88

15. Hers, H. G. (1955). The conversion of fructose-1-^{14}C and sorbitol-1-^{14}C to liver and muscle glycogen in the rat. *J. biol. Chem.*, **214**, 373

16. Froesch, E. R., Prader, A., Wolf, H. P. and Labhart, A. (1959). Die hereditäre Fructoseintoleranz. *Helv. Paediat. Acta*, **14**, 99

17. Kaufmann, U. and Froesch, E. R. (1973). Inhibition of phosphorylase-a by fructose-1-phosphate, a-glycerophosphate and fructose-1,6-diphosphate: explanation for fructose-induced hypoglycemia in hereditary fructose intolerance and fructose-1,6-diphosphatase deficiency. *Europ. J. clin. Invest.*, **3**, 407

18. Bally, C. and Leuthardt, F. Aldolase and hereditary fructose intolerance. (In preparation)

19. Kuyper, Ch. M. A. (1959). Studies on fructokinase. (1) Substrate specificity. *Koninkl. Nederl. Akad. Wetenschap. Proc. ser. B*, **62**, 137

20. Dubois, R., Loeb, H., Ooms, H. A., Gillet, P., Bartmann, J. and Champenois, A. (1961). Etude d'un cas d'hypoglycémie fonctionelle par intolérance au fructose. *Helv. Paediat. Acta*, **16**, 90

21. Phillips, M. J., Little, J. A. and Ptak, T. W. (1968). Subcellular pathology of hereditary fructose intolerance. *Amer. J. Med.*, **44**, 910

22. Milhaud, G. (1964). Téchnique nouvelle de mise en évidence d'erreurs congénitales du métabolisme chez l'homme. *Arq. Brasil Endocr.*, **13**, 49

23. Morris, R. C. Jr., Ueki, I., Loh, D., Eanes, R. Z. and McLin, P. (1967). Absence of renal fructose-1-phosphate aldolase activity in hereditary fructose intolerance. *Nature (London)*, **214**, 920

24. Marthaler, T. M. and Froesch, E. R. (1967). Hereditary fructose intolerance. Dental status of eight patients. *Brit. Dent. J.*, **123**, 597

25. Marthaler, T. M. and Froesch, E. R. (1967). Ist Weissbrot kariogen? *Schweiz. Mschr. Zahnheilk.*, **77**, 630

26. Swales, J. D. and Smith, A. D. M. (1966). Adult fructose intolerance. *Quart. J. Med.*, **35**, 455

27. Black, J. A. and Simpson, K. (1967). Fructose intolerance. *Brit. Med. J.*, **iv**, 138

28. Cornblath, M., Rosenthal, I. M., Reisner, S. H., Wybregt, S. H. and Crane, R. K. (1963). Hereditary fructose intolerance. *New Eng. J. Med.*, **269**, 1271

29. Levin, B., Oberholzer, V. G., Snodgrass, G. J. A. I., Stimmler, L. and Wilmers, M. J. (1963). Fructosaemia: an inborn error of fructose metabolism. *Arch. Dis. Childh.*, **38**, 220

30. Wolf, H., Zschokke, B., Wedemeyer, F. W. and Huebner, W. (1959). Angeborene hereditäre Fructoseintoleranz. *Klin. Wschr.*, **37**, 693

31. Auricchio, S. and Prader, A. (Personal communication)

32. Raivio, K., Perheentupa, J. and Nikkilä, E. A. (1967). Aldolase activities in the liver in parents of patients with hereditary fructose intolerance. *Clin. Chim. Acta*, **17**, 275

33. Sacrez, R., Juif, J.-G., Metais, P., Sofatzis, J. and Dourof, N. (1962). Un cas mortel d'intolérance héréditaire au fructose. Etude biochimique et enzymatique. *Pédiatrie*, **17**, 875

34. Bernt, E. and Bergmeyer, H. U. (1970). D-Fructose. Bergmeyer, H. U., *Methoden der Enzymatischen Analyse*. 2nd edn., Vol. II, p. 1266 (Weinheim: Verlag Chemie)

35. Roe, J. H., Epstein, J. H. and Goldstein, N. P. (1949). A photometric method for the determination of inulin in plasma and urine. *J. biol. Chem.*, **178**, 839

36. Lederle, E. and Lederle, M. (1957). *Chromatography: A review of Princples and Applications*. 2nd edn., p. 245. (Amsterdam: Elsevier)

37. Morris, R. C. Jr. (1968). An experimental renal acidification defect in patients with hereditary fructose intolerance. I; Its resemblance to renal tubular acidosis. *J. Clin. Invest.*, **47**, 1389

38. Morris, R. C. Jr. (1968). An experimental renal acidification defect in patients with hereditary fructose intolerance. II; Its distinction from classical renal tubular acidosis; its resemblance to the renal acidification defect associated with the Fanconi syndrome of children with cystinosis. *J. Clin. Invest.*, **47**, 1648

39. Lindemann, R., Gjessing, L. R., Merton, B. and Halvorsen, S. (1969). Fructosaemia/ 'acute tyrosinosis'. *Lancet*, **i**, 891

40. Lindemann, R., Gjessing, L. R., Merton, B., Löken, A. Ch. and Halvorsen, S. (1970). Amino acid metabolism in hereditary fructosemia. *Acta Paediat. Scand.*, **59**, 141

41. Hers, H. G. (1960). L'aldose-réductase. Le mécanisme de la formation du fructose séminal et du fructose foetal. *Biochim. Biophys. Acta*, **37**, 120, 127

42. Morrison, A. D., Clements, R. and Winegrad, A. I. (1972). Effects of elevated glucose concentration on the metabolism of the aortic wall. *J. Clin. Invest.*, **51**, 3114

43. Baker, L. and Winegrad, A. I. (1970). Fasting hypoglycaemia and metabolic acidosis associated with deficiency of hepatic fructose-1,6-diphosphatase activity. *Lancet*, **ii**, 13

44. Baerlocher, K., Gitzerlmann, R., Nüssli, R. and Dumermuth, G. (1971). Infantile acidosis due to hereditary fructose-1,6-diphosphatase deficiency. *Helv. Paediat. Acta*, **26**, 489

45. Hülsmann, W. C. and Fernandes, J. (1971). A child with lactacidemia and fructose diphosphatase deficiency in the liver. *Pediat. Res.*, **5**, 633

CHAPTER 7

Wilson's Disease (Hepatolenticular Degeneration)

J. M. Walshe

Time was when genetic disease was thought of as a visitation of divine justice, 'the sins of the parents shall be visited upon the children'; any attempt to modify the course of such an illness was clearly reprehensible. With the advancement of medicine came a clearer understanding of the laws of inheritance leading inevitably to therapeutic nihilism; what treatment, other than palliative, could be given to an individual whose very constitution had resulted in the development of a progressive and perhaps fatal illness. The introduction of biochemistry into medicine led to renewed hope that an understanding of the metabolic lesion in some genetic diseases might result in therapeutic advances which would arrest if not reverse the progress of the illness. One of the first so approached was hepatolenticular degeneration, Wilson's disease, and the therapeutic attack upon this devastating malady must, in its modest way, be considered as one of the success stories of modern medicine.

HISTORY

The story began in 1911 with the description by Kinnier Wilson[1] of a new syndrome, 'progressive lenticular degeneration: a familial nervous disease associated with cirrhosis of the liver'. The first clue pointing to the nature of the illness came only two years later when Rumpel[2] reported finding excess copper in the liver of a patient dying of this disease. Further support for the hypothesis that copper was involved in the pathogenesis came from the observation of Siemerling and

Oloff[3] that a patient with Wilson's disease had a 'sunflower cataract' which closely resembled the lens changes found in association with a copper containing intraocular foreign body. During the 1930s and 1940s further isolated case reports all pointed to an association between the disease and abnormal concentrations of copper in brain and liver[4].

Cumings[5] in 1948 confirmed this association beyond doubt and went on to suggest that the chelating agent 2,3-dimercaptopropanol (BAL) might be of value in mobilising these abnormal copper stores thereby halting the progression of the illness. Despite the strength of the copper–BAL bond this proved to be, for a variety of reasons and with a few notable exceptions[6], somewhat of a disappointment as a method of treatment.

Another powerful chelating agent, calcium disodium versenate, proved even more unrewarding[7] but the third such compound to be tried, penicillamine[8] (β,β-dimethyl cysteine) has completely revolutionised the prognosis of this hitherto invariably fatal disease[9]. Patients may now not only expect the disease process to be halted but actually reversed so that most can make a virtually complete recovery, return to a normal way of life and enter into gainful employment or, should they feel so inclined, proceed to propagate the species and hence the abnormal gene.

DIAGNOSIS

It is a truism to say that effective treatment of a disease cannot be initiated before the diagnosis has been made; nevertheless it is a painful fact that many patients with Wilson's disease undergo a long drawn-out series of investigations, provisional diagnosis and therapeutic trials all to no effect before the true nature of their malady is established. Unhappily such delays can have disastrous consequences as they may permit both the structural and the biochemical lesions to proceed to the point of no return. To those familiar with the clinical picture of Wilson's disease these diagnostic vicissitudes may seem hard to justify but, in practice, it is inevitably difficult to diagnose a rare disease on the first occasion it is met, particularly one as pleomorphic as Wilson's disease.

In order to attain to a reasonable degree of diagnostic competence there is but one golden rule that needs always to be remembered; namely that this disease can present not only with symptoms involving the liver and brain but also the blood, kidneys and skeleton; psychiatric disturbances are not uncommon and sometimes there is an apparently unexplained deterioration in performance of a previously bright school child. Even endocrinopathies are occasionally seen. Only the more important signs and symptoms will be considered here.

Any and every child with an attack of jaundice for which there is no cast-iron diagnosis, whether the jaundice be hepatic or haemolytic, should be considered as a possible case of Wilson's disease and investigated accordingly. Those with a mixed hepatic and haemolytic jaundice and cases of 'chronic active hepatitis', particularly those with a familial history must rate a very high index of suspicion. Before puberty this is the common way for Wilson's disease to present and it may do so occasionally even into the twenties; such cases will subsequently be referred to as 'hepatic Wilson's disease'.

Similarly any child, adolescent or young adult with choreiform movements, dystonia, parkinsonism or ataxia should be considered as a case of Wilson's disease until proven otherwise. The presenting symptoms may be a subtle personality change, unexplained falling off in performance at school, difficulty in writing, the development of a speech defect or, more rarely, a schizophrenia-like illness. In all such cases the eyes should be examined for the possible presence of a Kayser Fleischer ring (Figure 7.1a). Seen in the earliest stages this appears as a small, brown, granular pigmented crescent in Descemet's membrane of the cornea in the arc 10 o'clock to 2 o'clock, only later becoming a complete corneal ring (Figure 7.1b). In doubtful cases the aid should always be sought of an experienced observer using a slit lamp[10]. The undisputed finding of Kayser Fleischer corneal pigment confirms the diagnosis of Wilson's disease for this is one of the few truly diagnostic signs in clinical medicine. Pigment is probably always present once the nervous system has become involved but may be absent or only detected with difficulty in the early hepatic stages of the illness.

However the diagnosis must, ultimately, be confirmed by bio-chemical means; that is by the demonstration of a reduced concentration of copper and caeruloplasmin in the serum and of an excess of copper in the urine. Occasionally these tests remain equivocal; should they do so it is necessary to demonstrate a high concentration of copper in the liver (by biochemical rather than histochemical means) or a great reduction in the rate of incorporation of radiocopper into caeruloplasmin. In assessing both the clinical picture and the biochemical results it must be remembered that no two patients with Wilson's disease are ever the same, that perhaps 5% have a normal or near normal concentration of serum caeruloplasmin[11] and that a small number of patients with severe liver damage have reduced concentrations of this protein in the blood which will return to normal if and when the patient recovers[12].

It is not within the scope of this book to describe the technical details of biochemical determinations which are mentioned but as a general rule it is safe to say that the simpler the method used to determine copper in serum or urine the more accurate the result is likely to be; extreme care to avoid contamination of the specimen and all reagents must be taken not only during the determination but also during collection. This is particularly true of 24-hour urine specimens which are so vulnerable to interference from the nursing staff; on occasions it may be wise to collect for accurately timed short periods when full supervision can be given. The methods which have been used in this laboratory over the last 15 years are discussed in a recent review article, these have been found to be both reliable and very reproducible[13].

Normal values vary from one laboratory to another so that it is not possible to give absolute figures, furthermore the range of biological variation is so great that normal and abnormal results inevitably show overlap, thus no single test can ever be considered an absolute criterion for diagnosis. The figures given in Table 7.1 for copper values can therefore be taken as no more than a rough guide.

Figure 7.1. Kayser Fleischer Rings
(a) R.P., easily seen dense brown top crescent; stages of partial reabsorption of a previously complete ring
(b) B.M., ring viewed obliquely from above showing a brown fuzz across the pupil. The ring is not easily seen when viewed directly against a brown iris

Figure 7.2. The early liver lesion in Wilson's disease; presymptomatic stage
(a and b) P.K.S., aged 12; two different areas are from the same biopsy, one showing cellular infiltration in the portal tract, the other fatty vacuolation of hepatocytes
(c) R.M., aged 9; cellular infiltration of portal tract—more advanced fatty changes—prominent glycogen nuclei
(d) J.T., aged 19; cellular infiltration and early portal fibrosis. Marked fatty change and glycogen nuclei in hepatocytes

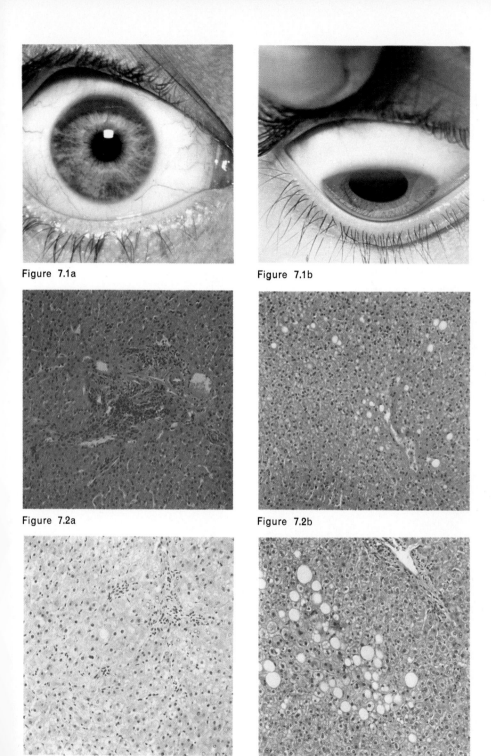

Figure 7.1a

Figure 7.1b

Figure 7.2a

Figure 7.2b

Figure 7.2c

Figure 7.2d

Table 7.1. Copper concentration in Wilson's disease and control groups

	Normal	Hetero-zygotes for Wilson's disease	Wilson's disease, untreated, symptomatic	Primary biliary cirrhosis
Serum Cu (μg/100 ml)	90–140	50–140	10–100	120–300
Serum caeruloplasmin (mg/100 ml)	25– 45	10– 45	0– 30	30– 75
Urine Cu (μg/24 h)	<40	<50	80–800	50–300
Liver Cu (μg/g wet weight)	<10	<40	>30	>30
Urine Cu after 500 g D-penicillamine (μg/6 h)	<400	<450	>1000	300–700

MANAGEMENT

If it is accepted that Wilson's disease results from excessive deposition of copper in the tissues, principally the liver and brain, then whatever the pathogenic mechanism of this may be, it follows logically that treatment must be directed towards removal of the excess metal. Cumings[5] was the first to point this out, but his attempts to achieve this end with the then only available chelating agent dimercaptopropanol (British anitlewisite (BAL), Dimercaprol; The Boots Company Ltd, Nottingham, England) proved somewhat disappointing. There can now be no doubt that penicillamine (Distamine; Dista Products Ltd, Liverpool, England: Cuprimine; Merck, Sharp and Dohme, West Point, Pennsylvania: Metalcaptase; Heyl, Berlin) is now the drug of choice for the management of patients with Wilson's disease, a fact which is amply borne out by the evidence in the literature[9,14-18].

Penicillamine
Penicillamine, β, β-dimethyl cysteine, is a derivative of penicillin; its first clinical association was the observation that it could be found in

the urine of patients with liver damage who were receiving penicillin therapy[19]. The two methyl groups on the β carbon atom appeared to protect the —SH group from readily undergoing auto-oxidation, thus permitting the amino acid to be excreted in the urine in the reduced state. The site of degradation of penicillin in the body was not determined. Having an asymmetric carbon atom penicillamine can exist in both D and L forms, perhaps surprisingly the former is the naturally occurring one. The point is of importance as the L isomer is much more likely to give rise to toxic reactions when administered to man. In practice all penicillamine preparations marketed for therapy are in the D form* though in some early studies DL penicillamine was used and led to both renal damage[20] and to pyridoxine deficiency[21]. The relatively stable nature of the —SH group in penicillamine suggested to me that this might be available for copper chelation in patients with Wilson's disease[8]. Thus the metal ion might form a ring with the thiol and either the —COOH or —NH$_2$ groups; an alternative possibility is that two molecules of penicillamine bind copper by forming both anionic and co-ordination linkages. In practice the exact nature and strength of the ligands has not been determined[22].

Biochemical monitoring

Penicillamine is a powerful metal binding agent. It will remove large quantities of copper from the body via the urine (up to 9 mg daily in the early stages of treatment) and this will result in depletion of the body stores of the metal. Evidence for this is found in a fall in the concentration of copper and caeruloplasmin in the serum, a return of the basal urine copper to normal, and a reduction in the amount of copper excreted in 6 hours following a standard test dose of penicillamine†. In view of this ability of penicillamine to reduce the body stores of copper and, consequently, to modify the handling of radio-copper[23] by the liver, it is clear that certain base-line data must be obtained before treatment is started. Not only is it essential to obtain such pretreatment information about copper transport but it is also desirable to document those other facets of the disease which can reasonably be expected to improve with treatment, for without such

* Penicillamine used in therapy is assumed, throughout this chapter, to be D-penicillamine

† By basal urine copper excretion I mean the rate of copper excretion in the urine when no penicillamine is given or has been given for at least 72 hours. A standard test dose of 500 mg D-penicillamine base is given at the end of this basal urine collection and a further collection is made over a period of six hours, see Table 5.1

information long-term monitoring, both biochemical and clinical, becomes little more than guess work. Table 7.2 lists the tests which have been grouped as those considered essential and those desirable. Certain tests, the blood count and presence or absence of proteinuria are needed as much for the monitoring of penicillamine toxicity as for measuring possible improvement with treatment.

Table 7.2. Data to be obtained before starting treatment

Essential
  Serum copper
  Serum caeruloplasmin
  Urine copper 1. basal
                    2. after a test dose of 500 mg D-penicillamine
  Liver function tests
  Full blood count, ESR, platelets, antinuclear factor
  Renal function studies—sugar, protein, 24 h calcium
                    —ability to secrete acid urine after NH_4Cl load
Desirable
  Radiocopper studies; liver uptake, % dose injected at 2, 24, 48 h
                    Liver/thigh ratio, normalised, at 5, 10, 15 min and 2 h
                    Plasma radiocopper, ratio of concentration 2 h/24 h; 2 h/48 h
  Electroencephalogram
  Skeletal X-rays for osteoarticular changes—bone density

Besides laboratory studies it is necessary to document fully the patient's clinical condition, noting particularly changes of speech which can be recorded on tape and abnormalities of movement which can be simply illustrated on a single photographic plate[9] (Figure 7.3) or as handwriting samples (Figure 7.4).

Once all the base line data have been gathered they can be used to form a rough estimate of the degree of copper overload. Factors which suggest that the normal binding sites for copper have become saturated are (1) a relatively high serum copper concentration (in excess of 60 μg/100 ml), (2) a high basal urine copper excretion (in excess of

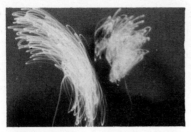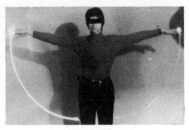

Figure 7.3. (left) Taxogram, a single 30 second exposure on a photographic plate with the patient asked to hold her hands still, outstretched, for 30 seconds. (right) taxogram repeated after 14 months' treatment with penicillamine, movements are now completely steady and controlled

400 µg/day), and (3) a wide discrepancy between the total serum copper and the caeruloplasmin-bound copper (in normals this is less than 10 µg/100 ml). Studies with radiocopper, when possible, will give additional information; for instance the finding of a very low uptake of radiocopper by the liver at 24 hours (less than 40% of the dose) and a liver/thigh ratio of less than unity at 15 minutes[23] together with a marked excretion of radiocopper in the urine (more than 5% of the dose at 24 hours); this is usually associated with a large cupruresis in response to a test dose of penicillamine[24]. All the findings point to

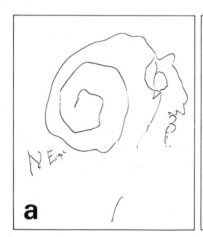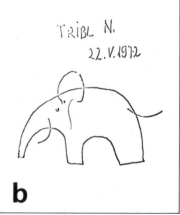

Figure 7.4. Handwriting of Tribl N.
(a) June 1970, scarcely able to put pen to paper, unable to write his name
(b) May 1972, writes neatly and able to draw

saturation of the normal binding sites for the metal. Such radioisotope studies are not easily carried out and are best done at centres with experience in the various techniques involved; they may be usefully repeated in 3 or 4 years' time.

Dosage
There is no standard dose of penicillamine, the requirements of each patient differ. Obviously it is desirable to reduce the body stores of copper quickly in a patient who is severely ill, who has a short history of rapidly progressing disability and who shows biochemical evidence suggesting heavy saturation of the binding sites for the metal. In an adolescent or adult a maximum starting dose of penicillamine is 1 g, 3 times a day to be taken about half an hour before food. Penicillamine is the most effective as a cupruretic when it is present in the plasma at the time of arrival of newly absorbed copper[9], that is before the metal can become firmly attached to protein. This relatively large dose of penicillamine is usually well tolerated for a short period only and should be reduced at around 3 months to 2 g daily and again after 6 months further reduced to 1·5 g/day. My own experience does not suggest that patients with Wilson's disease need to start with a small dose of penicillamine and work this up gradually as do patients with rheumatoid arthritis and those with cystinuria. When penicillamine is used in a large dose, such as 2 or 3 g daily, it is wise to keep a careful watch on the platelet and white cell counts, particularly in patients with liver damage and hypersplenism; it is also desirable to give supplementary pyridoxine; 50 mg weekly will prevent the development of a deficiency of this vitamin[25].

Response to treatment
In the first few weeks after starting treatment there is often an increase in neurological signs, tremor may well become worse and the patient should be warned of this or it may be a source of great concern. By 3 months there should be a fall in the blood and urine copper levels, soon to be followed by evidence of clinical improvement. The response in some patients will be early and dramatic, in others it may be slow and, at first, scarcely perceptible; hence the collection of good pretreatment records showing the severity of movement and speech disturbances; these will be of great value to demonstrate improvement to such patients. Fortunately the great majority who have predominantly neurological involvement will eventually get better and return to

normal life, any remaining functional deficit being minimal and often only detectable on detailed clinical examination; but such a state of affairs may take 2 years or more to achieve.

Liver function is apt to be slow to improve as are haematological changes so that correction of the serum proteins and a return to normal of elevated serum transaminases may take a year or more. Fluid retention, when present, will need the usual management with salt restriction and diuretics but this too will eventually recover so that dietary restrictions of sodium intake will cease to be necessary.

The concept that liver damage in patients with Wilson's disease is irreversible[26] is no longer tenable. However as with neurological involvement, so with liver damage some patients, when first seen, will have suffered a structural lesion from which there is no recovery: it is not always easy to assess whether or not this be the case when the patient is first seen. Jaundice, ascites and large oesophageal varices do seem to be associated with a particularly poor prognosis[27].

Time was when a copper restricted diet was advocated in the management of Wilson's disease together with the administration of potassium sulphide to reduce copper absorption from the gut; it is my view that, provided the patient takes his penicillamine regularly and in adequate dosage, such additional measures are quite unnecessary. Each individual should be encouraged to lead as normal and unrestricted a life as possible.

Follow up

Once a good clinical response has been achieved the question arises as to what maintenance dose of penicillamine will be needed to prevent reaccumulation of copper stores and the recurrence of symptoms. As a general rule it is undesirable to keep a patient on 2 g or more of penicillamine for longer than one year as this commonly leads to breakdown in collagen cross linkages and increased skin fragility[28]. For most patients 1·0–1·5 g daily is enough; the adequacy of this dose can be judged by periodic measurement of the basal urine copper excretion and the serum copper and caeruloplasmin concentrations.

The frequency with which these determinations are done will depend in part on the distance the patient lives away from the follow up centre and in part upon clinical judgment of his needs and his reliability in taking his treatment. It is my custom to aim at repeat determinations in 6 months and then yearly as a compromise between what may be desirable and what is practicable.

The object of treatment should be to reduce the basal urine copper excretion to 50 μg a day or less, the serum copper to 15 μg/100 ml or less and the caeruloplasmin to a corresponding concentration. The cupruretic response to 500 mg penicillamine is also of value and should be less than 400 μg in 6 hours. In a few patients, particularly those with an initially relatively high serum caeruloplasmin concentration (above 15 mg/100 ml) it may be difficult to depress the blood level of this protein and even if this is achieved it may later return to the pretreatment concentration even though the other available evidence all points to depletion of the body stores of copper.

If, during maintenance therapy, copper excretion starts to rise, then either the dose of penicillamine is not adequate or the patient has ceased to take his drug regularly. This is not an uncommon finding in a patient who has been taking tablets for many years (and ones with a particularly nasty taste) and who has become bored with the process, who does not notice any return of symptoms if he misses a few doses and who has long since forgotten just how seriously disabled he was before treatment was started. Fortunately biochemical relapse occurs some months before clinical relapse so that the dose can be stepped up before too much damage has been done.

Once treatment of Wilson's disease has been started, and this should be done as soon as possible after the diagnosis has been established beyond doubt, it must be realised that this is a life-long procedure. The biochemical defect underlying the accumulation of copper in the tissues is genetically determined and therefore should treatment be interrupted or, worse still, discontinued, the patient will again go into positive copper balance and be in danger of tissue damage. It can be stated quite simply that, in the present state of knowledge, treatment is for life.

Toxicity of penicillamine

The list of toxic reactions which have been reported in association with the use of penicillamine is indeed formidable and might well deter a cautious physician from using such a potentially poisonous drug. Fortunately most of the reactions are rare in patients with Wilson's disease and in any case, as the disease untreated is invariably fatal, the degree of acceptable risk is higher than it would be in a less lethal illness.

An analysis of over 100 cases seen during the past 18 years reveals that in only 9 was it necessary to discontinue penicillamine. The reasons for interrupting therapy were as follows; the nephrotic syndrome; thrombocytopoenia; rheumatoid-like arthritis with LE cells and a positive antinuclear factor; very severe mouth ulceration; fever with skin rash and respiratory embarrassment; fever with malaise, steatorrhoea and jaundice. Two of these patients were later able to restart penicillamine, one had suffered from a severe febrile illness with LE cells, the other from thrombocytopoenia.

In an additional 7 patients it became necessary to reduce the penicillamine dose by approximately half; 2 because of thrombocytopoenia; 2 because of increased skin fragility with haemorrhages and in the remaining 3 because of the development of a positive test for antinuclear factor with joint pains. Two of these 3 patients had, in addition a positive LE cell test with raised sedimentation rates while the third had a positive Rose Waaler reaction. A positive antinuclear factor was found in 3 further patients, 2 had no symptoms, the third had joint pains affecting the wrists and metacarpophalangeal joints but neither cessation nor restarting treatment affected these symptoms, thus their relationship to therapy is not clear.

Four patients were seen in whom an urticarial reaction developed shortly after starting treatment, 2 responded to an antihistamine, the third required desensitisation under steroid cover whilst the fourth patient received no specific treatment. It may be significant that this later patient, 6 years later developed the nephrotic syndrome[29] whilst the 2 who were treated with antihistamines later developed a positive test for antinuclear factor. The fourth patient who had received steroids has, to date, shown no signs of drug toxicity.

Attention has already been drawn to the antipyridoxine action of penicillamine, much more marked with the L than the D isomer. Clinical, as opposed to biochemical, evidence of pyridoxine deficiency has not been reported with D-penicillamine although optic neuritis has been described following the use of the DL form[21]. Gibbs and Walshe[30] analysed their experience in 32 cases of Wilson's disease and found biochemical evidence of pyridoxine deficiency, after a tryptophan load, in 13; the principal abnormalities were an increase in the urinary excretion of xanthurenic and kynurenic acid and their conjugates. This was rapidly corrected by the administration of 50 mg of the vitamin on 2 consecutive days. In all cases showing this biochemical abnormality there was always an additional factor such as pregnancy, a growth spurt or intercurrent illness. In adults, under stable conditions and taking less than 2 g penicillamine daily evidence of pyridoxine deficiency was not found.

Penicillamine has been incriminated as a cause of general marrow hypoplasia and also selective depression of white cell and platelet production. It is therefore essential to know before starting treatment, as already stated, the full blood count especially as leucopoenia and thrombocytopoenia are common in untreated patients with Wilson's disease. Thus, if these parameters are not recorded in advance the drug may, at some later date, be unfairly incriminated and hence unnecessarily withdrawn to the great detriment of the patient.

Penicillamine toxicity may be summarised as follows:

Chemical toxicity; the effect on collagen leading to breakdown of cross linkages, thinning and fragility of the skin and haemorrhages over pressure areas, this is dose-dependent at around 2·0 g/day for a year; the antipyridoxine effect, usually in association with an additional factor resulting in increased vitamin requirements as described above.

Immunological toxicity, presumably secondary to protein binding of penicillamine with the formation of antigens. The reactions under this heading probably include the nephrotic syndrome, urticarial reactions, thrombocytopoenia and leucopoenia, joint involvement with positive antinuclear factor and LE cells. Generalised marrow depression is fortunately rare so that there may be other factors involved, perhaps this is an example of pharmacogenetics.

The pathogenesis of mouth ulceration is quite obscure, first described by Sumner[31] it is a very rare complication but one case has been seen in whom it was so severe that penicillamine had to be stopped and this was followed by slow healing of the ulcers.

ALTERNATIVE TREATMENT

The toxic reactions to penicillamine just listed make it clear that occasionally this drug must be discontinued even though untreated Wilson's disease is invariably fatal. Alternative treatment is therefore essential for such patients. The various chelating agents at present in use in clinical medicine have recently been reviewed[22]. The first of these to be introduced was dimercaptopropanol, this was designed by Sir Rudolph Peters and his team in Oxford to combat the arsenical war gas Lewisite[32] and it still remains the drug of choice for arsenic intoxication forming a very stable 5-membered ring between the metal and the 2 thiol groups. As already stated its use in Wilson's disease, despite a few notable exceptions, has proved disappointing partly because of the great frequency of toxic reactions, partly because of the very painful nature of the injections and partly because of the tachyphylaxis so commonly associated with its use.

The powerful chelating agent ethylene diamine tetra-acetic acid (EDTA. Calcium disodium versenate, Riker) introduced by Bessman and his colleagues[33] from industry for the treatment of lead poisoning has also failed to make a significant contribution to the therapy of Wilson's disease[34] and, like BAL, this compound also suffered from the major disadvantage that it required parenteral administration. The analogous compound, diethylene triamine penta-acetic acid, though having an even higher affinity for copper, has also found no regular place in the treatment of Wilson's disease: furthermore it has the additional disadvantage that it is not readily available commercially.

The failure of the other therapeutic agents available for metal binding in medicine led to the hunt for an alternative chelating agent for the management of patients with Wilson's disease who had developed severe penicillamine intolerance. Of a wide variety of chemicals screened in the laboratory triethylene tetramine (trien) appeared the most promising[29]. This compound as the dihydrochloride has now been in use in my clinic since 1968, given in doses of 400 mg 3 or 4 times a day it has not been associated with any toxic reactions. During this time its cupruretic action has been studied in all new patients[24] and shown to be comparable to that of penicillamine; it has been used as the sole therapy in 4 patients. Three of these patients had symptoms of neurological damage including disturbances of speech and movement and all have improved significantly if perhaps more slowly than might have been expected on treatment with penicillamine. The fourth patient was symptom free when the change in treatment was made: she has remained so for the two years she has been taking trien and her blood and urine copper levels, like those of the other 3 patients taking this compound, have remained satisfactorily low. This, then, would appear to be a satisfactory alternative treatment for patients with Wilson's disease and on rather slender present evidence, to be free of the toxic reactions to which penicillamine so often gives rise.

Trien, unfortunately, is not commercially available and all that has been used over the past 5 years has been prepared from a crude commercial product in my laboratory[35]. In view of current attitudes, both official and public, to drug toxicity and also because of the expense involved in testing any new compound designed for use in man it seems improbable that this compound, for which the demand must be small, will ever pass the various bureaucratic baffles set in its way and thus achieve the commercial market. Unhappily this is probably also true for all potential new drugs designed especially for the benefit of sufferers from a rare disease. In the modern Welfare State well-meaning administrators, who deem it necessary to make all our decisions for us have, in a predictably futile quest for totally safe drugs, consigned the patient with a rare disease to a therapeutic never-never land. Should such a policy be followed to its logical conclusion it must inevitably result in complete arrest of all therapeutic advances. Fortunately, in this country at least, it is still permissible for a doctor to give an experimental therapy without a licence provided he can reasonably establish that he believes it to be for the good of the patient and provided also that he assumes for himself full responsibility. The mind boggles at the thought of what a learned judge might say should such an experiment prove a failure.

RESULTS OF TREATMENT

As has already been mentioned, whether penicillamine or trien 2HCl has been used, the results of treatment are usually very rewarding. It is reasonable to expect near complete remission of signs and symptoms of both neurological and hepatic disease. The *sine qua non* of such results is, obviously, diagnosis before irreversible damage has been done to either liver or brain; the development of oesophageal varices with haemorrhage is almost invariably associated with a bad prognosis. Further, on the debit side, it must be mentioned that very occasionally a patient is seen with neurological Wilson's disease in whom a useful recovery can reasonably be predicted yet who, despite apparently adequate treatment, goes steadily downhill and dies. Sometimes an additional factor which may have unfavourably influenced the situation can be defined but this is not always the case. Unfortunately it does not seem possible to identify these cases before treatment is started.

PREGNANCY IN PATIENTS WITH WILSON'S DISEASE

Now that Wilson's disease can be considered as a treatable condition it is not surprising to find that girls with the abnormal gene will grow up normally, get married and wish to procreate. This they usually do without seeking medical advice or genetic counselling until it is too late. However experience suggests that the risk of pregnancy in well-treated Wilson's disease is little greater than in normal women. Fifteen pregnancies have been observed of which 3 were terminated therapeutically at around 12 weeks for medicosocial reasons.

A brief analysis of the remainder shows that 9 patients had 12 pregnancies, there were 10 normal live births and 2 miscarriages, one at 16 and one at 26 weeks. The latter child was normal and lived about 12 hours. Three patients required caesarean section and 2 a forceps delivery. One patient, a bad risk *ab initio*, developed severe toxaemia of pregnancy and this clearly precipitated the fatal outcome of her illness. Had she sought advice she would certainly have been warned to postpone pregnancy at least until there had been a greater degree of restoration of liver function and a further decrease in the size of her oesophageal varices.

THE GENETICS OF WILSON'S DISEASE AND PRESYMPTOMATIC DIAGNOSIS

Wilson's disease is inherited as an autosomal recessive condition[36], the risk therefore to any sibling of a patient is 1 : 4. The risk to other close relatives is very much smaller unless there has been a quite remarkable amount of inbreeding as occurs occasionally in small isolated communities. A search should be made through all families in which a case of Wilson's disease has been identified for presymptomatic patients[37] so that prophylactic treatment may be started where necessary[38].

As a general rule the illness runs true to type in a family so that all affected children tend to present at the same age and with the same symptoms. Very occasionally the disease makes itself known first in a younger child and only then does biochemical analysis and clinical examination show that an elder sibling has indeed developed early signs of the disease that had hitherto passed unnoticed. Three such sibships have been studied.

Whilst presymptomatic diagnosis may be relatively straightforward on biochemical evidence alone[37] it can be one of the most difficult differential diagnoses in medicine. When other methods have failed reliance can usually be placed on a chemical analysis of the liver tissue for copper and a figure in excess of 250 µg copper per g dry weight of liver can be considered diagnostic[38]. Radiochemical methods may also be of help though they can be deceptive[39] and it is my policy now to rely on them as no more than confirmatory evidence; nevertheless the absence of incorporation of labelled copper into caeruloplasmin is a very valuable pointer to the diagnosis.

A useful first screening procedure is to determine the serum oxidase activity for dimethyl-p-phenylenediamine[40] as a rough estimate of caeruloplasmin concentration. Provided that the propositus has a low level of this protein, less than 20% of normal, the method is reasonably reliable since any other case in the same family will have a similarly low concentration. In such families concentrations of around 50% of normal probably indicate the heterozygous state. The diagnosis of Wilson's disease can be confirmed by determining serum copper and by showing a wide discrepancy between this and the concentration of caeruloplasmin-bound copper; the difference between these two is around 10 µg/100 ml in normal individuals. Further confirmation is obtained by finding an increased excretion of copper in the urine, though this is not invariable in presymptomatic patients, and by finding a very large cupruresis in response to a test dose of penicillamine.

However it is in those sibships in which the propositus has a relatively high caeruloplasmin concentration that the greatest difficulty occurs. Unquestionably the finding of excess urine copper, abnormal liver function tests, reduced incorporation of radiocopper into caeruloplasmin and reduced radiocopper uptake by the liver are all of great help when present but any or all may give inconclusive results. As has already been stated such cases present a most difficult diagnostic problem. Clearly it is as undesirable to use, for a life time, a potentially toxic drug such as penicillamine when it is not needed; but it would be equally wrong to withhold treatment from a patient accumulating copper and liable to severe occult liver damage before clinical signs have appeared. In cases of doubt, therefore, it is wise to determine the copper content of the liver and to study the histology (Figure 7.2), the early changes to be sought are inflammation in the portal tracts, fatty droplets in the hepatocytes and glycogen nuclei. In the last instance the finding of Kayser Fleischer corneal pigment by an experienced observer is diagnostic, but this is rare in presymptomatic patients.

Once potential cases have been identified prophylactic treatment should be started with penicillamine. A dose of 1 g daily usually suffices in these cases but the same base-line biochemical data as for symptomatic cases are needed so that both progress and treatment over the years can be satisfactorily controlled. There are no logical grounds for withholding treatment until symptoms develop; prevention is always better than cure.

CONCLUSIONS

Wilson's disease is one of the first of the metabolic disorders for which a specific and effective treatment has been devised based upon an understanding of the biochemical lesion. This being the case it is important that the disease, rare though it is, should be widely recognised so that diagnosis can be made and treatment started before irreversible damage has been done to either brain or liver. It is probably true to say that only those cases are lost which are subjected to unnecessary delay in diagnosis or are given inadequate therapy. However, as with all rare diseases, when detailed biochemical monitoring is necessary to obtain the best results these are only achieved at specialist centres where both time and experience are available. While the results of good treatment are most rewarding the consequences of error can be both disastrous and tragic.

If it is true, as Samuel Butler said that 'genius has been defined as a supreme capacity for taking trouble', then the best management of Wilson's disease surely requires a touch of genius.

REFERENCES

1. Wilson, S. A. K. (1911/12). Progressive lenticular degeneration: a familial nervous disease associated with cirrhosis of the liver. *Brain*, **34**, 295
2. Rumpel, A. (1913). Über das wesen und die bedeutung der leberveränderungen und der pigmentierungen bei den damit verbundenen fällen von pseudosklerose, zugleich ein beitrag zur lehre von der pseudosklerose (Westphal-Strümpell). *Dtsh. Z. Nervenheilk*, **49**, 54
3. Siemerling, E. and Oloff, H. (1922). Pseudosklerose (Westphal-Strümpell) mit Cornealring (Kayser–Fleischer) und doppelseitiger Scheinkatarakt, die

nur bie seitlicher Beleuchtung sichtbar ist und die der nach Verletzung durch Kupfersplitter entstenhenden Katarakt ähnlich ist. *Klin. Wschr.*, 1, i, 1087

4. Glazebrook, A. J. (1945). Wilson's disease. *Edinburgh med. J.*, **52**, 83
5. Cumings, J. N. (1948). The copper and iron content of brain and liver in the normal and in hepato-lenticular degeneration. *Brain*, **71**, 410
6. Bearn, A. G. (1957). Wilson's disease: an inborn error of metabolism with multiple manifestations. *Am. J. Med.*, **22**, 747
7. Bickel, H., Neale, F. C. and Hall, G. (1957). A clinical and biochemical study of hepatolenticular degeneration (Wilson's disease). *Quart. J. Med.*, **26**, 527
8. Walshe, J. M. (1956). Penicillamine. A new oral therapy for Wilson's disease. *Am. J. Med.*, **21**, 487
9. Walshe, J. M. (1967). The physiology of copper in man and its relation to Wilson's disease. *Brain*, **90**, 149
10. Cairns, J. E. and Walshe, J. M. (1970). The Kayser Fleischer ring. *Trans. ophthal. Soc. U.K.*, **90**, 187
11. Scheinberg, I. H. and Sternlieb, I. (1963). Wilson's disease and the concentration of caeruloplasmin in serum. *Lancet*, **i**, 1420
12. Walshe, J. M. and Briggs, J. (1962). Caeruloplasmin in liver disease, a diagnostic pitfall. *Lancet*, **ii**, 263
13. Walshe, J. M. (1970). Wilson's disease: its diagnosis and management. *Brit. J. Hosp. Med.*, **4**, 91
14. Walshe, J. M. (1960). The treatment of Wilson's disease with pencillamine. *Lancet*, **i**, 188
15. Sternlieb, I. and Scheinberg, I. H. (1964). Pencillamine therapy for hepatolenticular degeneration. *J. Am. med. Ass.*, **189**, 748
16. Goldstein, N. P., Tauxe, W. N., McCall, J. T., Gross, J. B. and Randall, R. V. (1969). Treatment of Wilson's disease (Hepatolenticular degeneration) with penicillamine and low copper diet. *Trans. Am. neurol. Ass.*, **94**, 34
17. Richmond, J., Rosenoer, V. M., Tompsett, S. L., Draper, I. and Simpson, J. A. (1964). Hepato-lenticular degeneration (Wilson's disease) treated by penicillamine. *Brain*, **87**, 619
18. Strickland, G. T., Frommer, D., Leu, M.-L., Pollard, R., Sherlock, S. and Cumings, J. N. (1973). Wilson's disease in the United Kingdom and Taiwan. *Quart. J. Med.*, **42**, 619
19. Walshe, J. M. (1953). Disturbances of amino acid metabolism following liver injury. *Quart. J. Med.*, **22**, 483
20. Sternlieb, I. (1966). Penicillamine and the nephrotic syndrome. *J. Am. med. Ass.*, **198**, 1311
21. Tu, J. B., Blackwell, R. Q. and Lee, P. F. (1963). DL-Penicillamine as a cause of optic axial neuritis. *J. Am. med. Ass.*, **185**, 83
22. Anon. (1971). Chelating agents in medicine. *Brit. Med. J.*, **ii**, 270

23. Osborn, S. B. and Walshe, J. M. (1967). Studies with radioactive copper (^{64}Cu and ^{67}Cu) in relation to the natural history of Wilson's disease. *Lancet*, **i**, 346

24. Walshe, J. M. (1973). Copper chelation in patients with Wilson's disease, a comparison of penicillamine and triethylene tetramine dihydrochloride. *Quart. J. Med.*, **42**, 441

25. Gibbs, K. and Walshe, J. M. (1966). Penicillamine and pyridoxine requirements in man. *Lancet*, **i**, 175

26. Denny-Brown, D. (1964). Hepatolenticular degeneration (Wilson's disease). Two different components. *New. Engl. J. Med.*, **270**, 1149

27. Sternlieb, I., Scheinberg, I. H. and Walshe, J. M. (1970). Bleeding oesophageal varices in patients with Wilson's disease. *Lancet*, **i**, 638

28. Harkness, R. D. (1968). *In vitro* and *in vivo* observations on the effect of penicillamine on collagen. *Postgrad. med. J.* Supplement, October 1968, p. 31

29. Walshe, J. M. (1969). Management of penicillamine nephrophathy in Wilson's disease: a new chelating agent. *Lancet*, **ii**, 1401

30. Gibbs, K. and Walshe, J. M. (1969). Interruption of the tryptophan-nicotinic acid pathway by penicillamine-induced pyridoxine deficiency in patients with Wilson's disease and in experimental animals. *Ann. N.Y. Acad. Sci.*, **166**, 158

31. Garland, H. and Sumner, D. (1961). *Wilson's Disease Some Current Concepts.* (J. M. Walshe, and J. N. Cumings, editors) (Oxford: Blackwell Scientific Publications)

32. Peters, R. A., Stocken, L. A. and Thompson, R. H. S. (1945). British anti-lewisite (BAL). *Nature (London)*, **156**, 616

33. Bessman, S. P., Reid, H. and Rubin, M. (1952). *Med. Ann. Distr. Columbia*, **21**, 312

34. Bickel, H., Neale, F. C. and Hall, G. (1957). A clinical and biochemical study of hepatolenticular degeneration (Wilson's disease). *Quart. J. Med.*, **26**, 527

35. Dixon, H. B. F., Gibbs, K. and Walshe, J. M. (1972). Preparation of triethylene tetramine dihydrochloride for the treatment of Wilson's disease. *Lancet*, **i**, 853

36. Bearn, A. G. (1960). A genetical analysis of thirty families with Wilson's disease (hepatolenticular degeneration). *Ann. Hum. Genet. (London)*, **24**, 33

37. Sternlieb, I. and Scheinberg, I. H. (1963). The diagnosis of Wilson's disease in asymptomatic patients. *J. Am. med. Ass.*, **183**, 747

38. Sternlieb, I. and Scheinberg, I. H. (1968). Prevention of Wilson's disease in asymptomatic patients. *New Engl. J. Med.*, **278**, 352

39. Sternlieb, I. and Scheinberg, I. H. (1972). Radiocopper in diagnosing liver disease. *Seminars in Nuclear Medicine*, **2**, 176

40. Broman, L. (1958). Separation and characterization of two caeruloplasmins from human serum. *Nature (London)*, **182**, 1655

CHAPTER 8

Organic Acidaemias

D. Gompertz

The organic acidaemias and acidurias are a recently discovered group of inborn errors of metabolism that are associated with the accumulation in the blood and/or the excretion of small molecular-weight organic acids[1]. Their clinical presentation varies from an acute neonatal episode of metabolic acidosis and ketosis to an intermittent condition, the initial episodes of which may not present until school age. Several

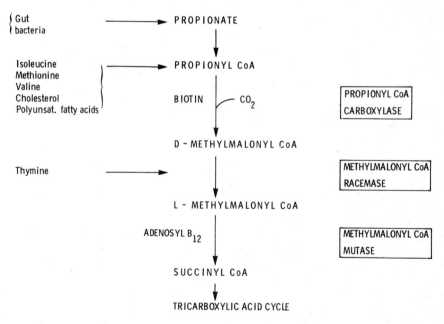

Figure 8.1. The propionate-methylmalonate pathway. The role of biotin and the co-enzyme form of vitamin B_{12} (adenosylcobalamin) as cofactors for propionyl CoA carboxylase and methylmalonyl CoA mutase respectively is indicated

distinct organic acidaemias have now been described and two important features have emerged; namely, 1. these conditions cannot be distinguished from each other by clinical criteria and 2. some of the individual organic acidaemias are secondary to inborn errors of vitamin metabolism rather than a primary defect of an enzyme involved in organic acid interconversions.

The majority of these disorders so far described are associated with derangements of two metabolic pathways; the propionate–methylmalonate pathway (Figure 8.1) and that by which the branched chain amino acids are degraded (Figure 8.2). Current experience suggests that defects of propionate and methylmalonate metabolism are more frequent. Although the clinical presentation and biochemical diagnosis of several organic acidaemias will be described, the treatment of propionic acidaemia and the methylmalonic acidurias will receive special attention.

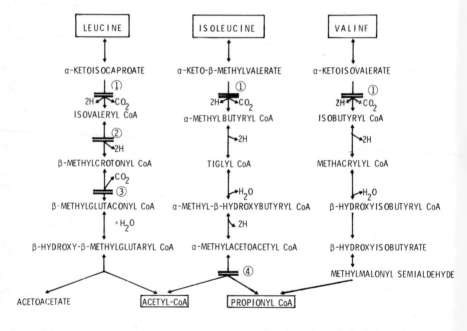

Figure 8.2. The degradation pathways of the three branched-chain amino acids. Metabolic blocks in (1) maple syrup urine disease, (2) isovaleric acidaemia, (3) β-methylcrotonyl CoA carboxylase deficiency and (4) α-methylacetoacetic and α-methyl-β-hydroxybutyric aciduria

The pathways of propionate and branched-chain amino acid metabolism are associated with five organic acidaemias and three of these have vitamin-responsive variants (Table 8.1). Several detailed mechanisms have been described or postulated to account for vitamin responsiveness (see Scriver, 1973[2]). The mechanisms involved in any specific inborn error of metabolism will depend on the exact bio-chemical role of the vitamin; whether it acts as a co-enzyme or a prosthetic group and also on its metabolic interconversions. The

Table 8.1. Organic acidaemias and acidurias

Condition	Vitamin responsive variants	Vitamin
1. Propionic acidaemia	+	Biotin
2. Methylmalonic acidaemias	+	B_{12}
3. β-Hydroxyisovaleric aciduria and β-methylcrotonylglycinuria	+	Biotin
4. Isovaleric acidaemia	−	−
5. α-Methylacetoacetic and α-methyl-β-hydroxybutyric aciduria	−	−

vitamins associated with the organic acidaemias described here are vitamin B_{12} and biotin. Their mode of action is different and they will be described separately.

Disorders responsive to vitamin B_{12}

Vitamin B_{12} occurs in the diet as hydroxycobalamin and it is converted enzymically to its co-enzyme forms, adenosyl cobalamin (co-enzyme B_{12}) and methyl cobalamin (methyl B_{12}) (Figure 8.3). Adenosyl cobalamin is the co-enzyme of methylmalonyl CoA mutase and so far no other function has been described for it in mammalian tissues. Inborn errors of cobalamin metabolism have been discovered during investigation of various children with methylmalonic acidaemia. These children have normal methylmalonyl CoA mutase activity *in vitro*

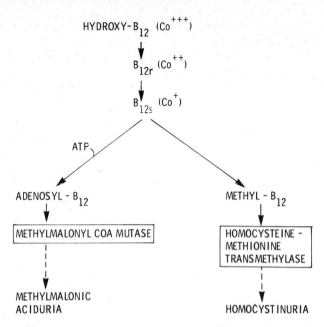

Figure 8.3. Metabolic conversion of hydroxycobalamin (HO-B_{12}) to the co-enzyme forms of B_{12}. Adenosyl cobalamin (co-enzyme B_{12}) and methyl-cobalamin (Me-B_{12}) are shown in relation to the enzymes involved in methylmalonic acid and homocysteine metabolism

only on addition of saturating amounts of co-enzyme B_{12}, showing that the methylmalonic acidaemia is secondary to a failure to synthesise co-enzyme B_{12} rather than a lack of the enzymes acting on methyl malonyl CoA. Thus methylmalonic acidaemia may be either due to impaired synthesis of enzymes of the propionate–methylmalonate pathway or to failure of co-enzyme B_{12} formation.

The defect in co-enzyme B_{12} synthesis may involve the enzyme converting B_{12s} to co-enzyme B_{12} (Figure 8.3); this leads to an impaired methylmalonyl CoA mutase activity and no other metabolic effects. Earlier defects in the pathway of cobalamin metabolism, before B_{12s}, produce a failure of both methylmalonyl CoA mutase and homo-cysteine-methyltetrahydrofolate transmethylase (homocysteine-methi-onine transmethylase). The defect in the latter enzyme is associated with a homocystinuria paralleled by a hypomethioninaemia.

Methylmalonic acidaemia secondary to defects in co-enzyme B_{12}

biosynthesis may be responsive to massive doses of vitamin B_{12} or hydroxy vitamin B_{12} (1 mg/day). Inborn errors are frequently associated with diminished rather than absent enzyme activity, and these have been described as 'leaky mutations'. It is assumed that B_{12}-responsiveness is due to 'leaky mutations' of the enzymes involved in co-enzyme B_{12} synthesis, and that the administration of massive amounts of B_{12} is associated with an enhanced formation of co-enzyme B_{12} sufficient to cause a significant increase in methylmalonyl CoA mutase activity.

Inherited defects of vitamin B_{12} absorption and transport are other possible causes of methylmalonic acidaemia discovered in childhood. The congenital form of pernicious anaemia has been shown to be associated with methylmalonic acidaemia and homocystinuria. Defects of the B_{12} carrier protein, transcobalamin II, have been described. Methylmalonic acidaemia has not been found in this condition perhaps because the child involved had already received vast amounts of parenteral B_{12} before the determinations were performed. It is possible, however, that transcobalamin II defects might first be detected as a methylmalonic acidaemia.

The investigations of methylmalonic acidaemia described later are designed to establish whether the child is B_{12}-responsive and also the underlying biochemical defect responsible for the methylmalonic acidaemia. The methylmalonic acidaemias and their relationship to inborn errors of vitamin B_{12} absorption, transport and metabolism have been reviewed in detail[3].

Disorders responsive to biotin
Biotin is the prosthetic group for two enzymes, propionyl CoA carboxylase (Figure 8.1) and β-methylcrotonyl CoA carboxylase, an enzyme involved in leucine degradation (Figure 8.2). This vitamin has to be activated and attached to the inactive carboxylase by another enzyme, the holoenzyme synthetase (Figure 8.4). It is apparent that defective synthesis of either the carboxylase enzyme protein or of the enzyme responsible for attaching biotin will result in diminished carboxylase activity. It is not clear as yet whether there are separate holoenzyme synthetases responsible for attaching biotin to each individual carboxylase. However, both biotin-responsive propionyl CoA carboxylase deficiency and also biotin-responsive β-methylcrotonyl CoA carboxylase deficiency have been reported although the mechanism for the responsiveness has not yet been defined[1].

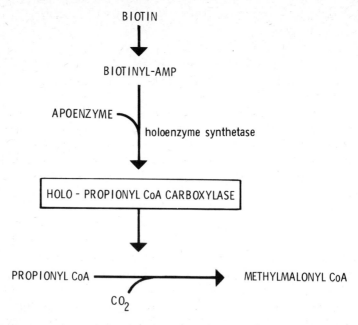

Figure 8.4. The synthesis of active propionyl CoA carboxylase (holoenzyme) from biotin and inactive carboxylase (apoenzyme). This reaction is mediated by the enzyme, holocarboxylase synthetase (apoenzyme-biotin ligase)

CLINICAL PRESENTATION

Acute neonatal metabolic acidosis

The first type of presentation is associated with a severe neonatal metabolic acidosis frequently accompanied by ketosis. The first signs develop within a few days of birth and are frequently those of a respiratory disturbance. The children present with tachypnoea; respiratory difficulty may be indicated by a grunting respiration. However, the child may have increasingly frequent apnoeic attacks needing artificial ventilation. Blood–gas analysis shows a severe base deficit and a low pCO_2. This latter finding may have been ascribed to over-ventilation.

Severe ketonuria in the neonatal period is an unusual clinical finding and is, therefore, a useful diagnostic indicator to these conditions. Besides the metabolic acidosis and ketosis there are characteristic neurological changes. There is frequently a marked hypotonia with almost total areflexia.

Failure to thrive and vomiting in the first year
The second type of presentation is of a child between 2 and 12 months with failure to thrive, lethargy, hypotonia, persistent vomiting and developmental retardation. There may be a continual metabolic acidosis. A history of protein intolerance is frequently given. Inter-current infections may have had an effect on the child's status out of all proportion to their severity and the child may have become severely acidotic and ketotic with a diminished degree of consciousness during these episodes.

Late-onset intermittent presentations
In this type of presentation the child is seen in an acute acidotic and ketotic state which has followed a minor intercurrent infection. A typical presentation is of a child with an otitis media who has been vomiting persistently and has become increasingly lethargic, finally lapsing into coma. Occasionally the precipitating cause is surgical intervention, such as tonsillectomy or appendicectomy. The operation is followed by unexplained coma, severe metabolic acidosis and ketosis. The patient may have been slow to develop but this has not been considered sufficient to require investigation. There may have been previous episodes of acidosis and ketosis that have not been explained and perhaps the history of a previous sibling dying during such an attack. Patients who have had several previous episodes may be developmentally retarded. The possibility of poisoning by agricultural or domestic chemicals has been considered on several occasions. Although some children may have had their first attack during the first year of life, some may be of school age before the first attack or before the biochemical diagnosis is finally made.

These clinical presentations are not unique to any of the organic acidaemias, and in fact parallel the presentations described for the classical and variant forms of maple syrup urine disease. The initial emergency supportive therapy is the same in all conditions; rehydra-tion, treatment of the metabolic acidosis and stopping protein intake. However, the earlier the biochemical diagnosis can be made, the sooner specific therapy can be instituted and the effect of vitamin-therapy can be investigated in those organic acidaemias which have vitamin-responsive variants.

BIOCHEMICAL DIAGNOSIS

In propionic acidaemia, in the methylmalonic acidaemias and in
α-methylacetoacetic and α-methyl-β-hydroxybutyric aciduria, there
are secondary biochemical changes that may be recognised before an
organic acidaemia is suspected. These three conditions may all be
associated with hyperglycinaemia and long-chain ketonuria, i.e. they
may present with the 'ketotic hyperglycinaemia' syndrome. This
syndrome was described as an association of metabolic acidosis, long-
chain ketonuria characterised by the excretion of butanone and
hexanone, hyperglycinaemia with secondary increases in other plasma
amino acids and intolerance to branched-chain amino acids[4]. It has
now been demonstrated that these changes are secondary phenomena
in methylmalonic aciduria[5], in propionic acidaemia[6,7], and in α-methylacetoacetic and α-methyl-β-hydroxybutyric aciduria[8].

These three organic acidurias may first be detected by finding
hyperglycinaemia or hyperglycinuria on amino acid screening. The
presence of long-chain ketones may have been demonstrated by thin-
layer chromatography of their dinitrophenylhydrazine derivatives. The
presence of a raised glycine concentration in blood and urine and/or
long-chain ketones must be followed by investigation of organic acid
excretion.

Diagnosis using gas chromatography

Gas chromatography is the method of choice for the diagnosis of the
organic acidaemias. Inborn errors of the propionate-methylmalonate
pathway and of branched-chain amino acid degradation give rise to
the accumulation of volatile and/or non-volatile organic acids.
Volatile fatty acids can be detected simply by steam distillation of
plasma or urine and gas chromatography of the free acids collected in
the distillate[9]. The branched-chain ketoacids of maple syrup urine
disease are also detectable using this method[10].

Methylmalonic acid and the non-volatile metabolites from the
pathways of branched-chain amino acid degradation must be converted to volatile derivatives before gas chromatography. They are
usually analysed as their methyl or trimethylsilyl derivatives. A two-
stage analytical system is frequently employed, the volatile acids being
analysed separately from those requiring derivative formation.
Numerous methods for these analyses have been described[10-13].

One of the major problems associated with the gas-chromatographic diagnosis of the organic acidurias is the complexity of the metabolite pattern that may be found. Many patients in an acute attack are ketotic and the ketone bodies and secondary metabolites detected during ketosis may obscure the metabolites due to the enzymic block itself. Metabolites detected in abnormal amounts in extracts of urine from ketosed patients are listed in Table 8.2.

Table 8.2. Urinary metabolites detected in ketosis secondary to any metabolic defect [49, 50]

β-Hydroxybutyric acid
Acetoacetic acid
Cis and *trans* enol forms of acetoacetic acid
C_6 dicarboxylic acid
C_8 dicarboxylic acids, saturated and monounsaturated
C_{10} dicarboxylic acid, saturated and monounsaturated

Metabolites produced by artefact may also be a problem; β-hydroxy-butyric acid may be converted to crotonic acid during steam distillation[14] and hippuric acid may be broken down to benzoic acid by bacterial action in infected urine[15]. In methylmalonic aciduria there is a significant production of propionic acid which may be increased by chemical decarboxylation of methylmalonic acid during steam distillation[16]. The presence in urine of propionic acid is not diagnostic of propionic acidaemia unless methylmalonic acid is shown to be absent.

A major problem associated with gas-chromatographic diagnosis is the identification of the abnormal compounds appearing in the gas-chromatographic profile of urinary metabolites. The availability of the combined technique of gas chromatography–mass spectrometry (GC–MS) is important in the identification of unknown metabolites and Nyhan and his colleagues[17] have revealed that incorrect diagnoses have been made and published when sole reliance was placed on gas chromatography without the identity of the abnormal metabolite being confirmed by mass spectrometry or some other method. However, GC–MS is an expensive and specialised technique only likely to be available in a few centres, and the interpretation frequently requires considerable experience.

Although sophisticated methods have been devised to establish quantitative patterns of organic acids in urine it is essential to compromise between detailed quantitation and speed. In the acute acidotic attack it is important for the clinician to have a diagnosis within a few hours. The quantitation of abnormal metabolites is not necessary in the first instance. However, only if the identity of the abnormal metabolites is known can a rational approach to therapy be made.

A simple chemical screening test has been developed for methyl-malonic acid in the urine[18] but this test lacks specificity as acetoacetate in ketotic urine interferes with the reaction and α-methylacetoacetate (formed from isoleucine, Figure 8.2) also gives a colour with this reaction. A specific thin-layer chromatographic method has been described for methylmalonic aciduria[19] but this method used alone precludes detection of the other organic acidurias. Thin-layer chromatography has been recommended for the glycine conjugates of organic acids excreted in some of the organic acidaemias but the extent of conjugate formation differs widely between the various organic acids[20]. Simple colour reactions and thin-layer chromatographic methods should be retained only for confirmation of diagnoses obtained by gas chromatography.

Investigation of a suspected case of an organic acidaemia
Individual urine specimens are collected as they are passed and immediately deep frozen without a preservative[15]. Frequently the abnormal metabolites disappear from the urine as initial treatment is commenced (withdrawal of protein, treatment of intercurrent infections and increase in carbohydrate intake). The first specimen of urine passed after the diagnosis of an organic acidaemia is suspected may be the only one containing the characteristic metabolites. The whole of these early urine specimens should be saved. 10–20 ml of urine may be required to identify abnormal metabolites if several gas-chromatographic analyses and chemical estimations have to be performed. Each urine specimen should be tested for ketones (Acetest) and the results recorded. This is one of the best parameters for following the clinical progress of the patient.

Urine is usually used for diagnostic purposes, as many organic acids are efficiently cleared by the kidney, but plasma is also required in propionic acidaemia. The severity of this condition may be assessed by the plasma propionate concentration. Blood should also be taken for vitamin B_{12} estimations to exclude B_{12} deficiency states as a cause of methylmalonic acidaemia.

Amino acid screening is an essential part of the investigation of an organic acidaemia, and blood and urine should be provided for these analyses.

TREATMENT AND MANAGEMENT

In an acute acidotic episode supportive therapy will probably have been started before the possibility of an organic acidaemia has been considered. The patient may be having assisted ventilation to treat apnoeic episodes as they occur. Metabolic acidosis, due to an organic acidaemia, is treated no differently from other forms of metabolic acidosis. Although THAM has been used, the treatment of choice is intravenous bicarbonate. The progress of this alkali therapy is monitored by frequent blood gas analysis.

Protein intake is stopped immediately and an adequate caloric intake is maintained with carbohydrate, either intravenously, orally or via a nasogastric tube according to the clinical state of the patient. A high fluid intake appears to help the excretion of the abnormal metabolites produced in the organic acidaemias, and as dehydration is frequently present following a period of vomiting and perhaps diarrhoea, it is probable that the administration of intravenous fluids will have been already started.

Many of the acidotic episodes in the organic acidaemias are secondary to some minor intercurrent infections. Such an infection should be sought for and treated actively.

Once acid–base balance is restored and ketonuria has disappeared, protein should be introduced at the level of 0·5 g/kg body weight. This reintroduction of protein can be started while awaiting accurate biochemical diagnosis, but must be monitored by blood gas analysis and by looking for ketonuria in each urine specimen passed (Acetest tablets). If this protein intake is tolerated it can be increased within a few days by increments of 0·5 g/kg body weight.

If the acidosis and ketosis do not respond to alkali therapy and withdrawal of protein, and the blood pH remains between pH 6·9 and 7·2, peritoneal dialysis can be considered. This has been shown to be a considerable help in the management of maple syrup urine disease[21-23], propionic acidaemia[24] and methylmalonic acidaemia[25].

The maintenance therapy in the organic acidaemias usually involves a restricted protein intake. In some severe cases an artificial amino acid mixture is required. The use of either long-term vitamin treatment and/or specific artificial amino acid diets depends on the diagnosis, and is discussed in the following sections describing the individual organic acidaemias.

ORGANIC ACIDAEMIAS WITH VITAMIN-RESPONSIVE VARIANTS

Propionic acidaemia

The initial diagnosis of propionic acidaemia may either be made in a child acutely ill with a severe metabolic acidosis and ketosis, or in a relatively well child with a modified form of the disease who has survived numerous ketotic acidotic attacks, and is reinvestigated at a later date. The management and investigation of propionic acidaemia in these two situations is obviously different. The first priority in a child in an acute attack is treatment and detailed investigation is postponed until the child has recovered and appears reasonably well.

Biochemical diagnosis
Propionic acidaemia is usually diagnosed by the demonstration of raised propionate concentrations in plasma and urine in the absence of methylmalonic aciduria. The concentration of propionic acid in plasma may be between 0·3mmol/l and 5 mmol/l. The latter concentration is 1000 times normal. The definitive diagnosis is made by demonstrating a defective propionyl CoA carboxylase activity in leucocyte or fibroblast preparations: this assay is only available at a few specialised centres. Other biochemical changes that help in the initial diagnosis before the enzyme assay has been performed are hyperglycinaemia and hyperglycinuria, long-chain ketonuria, and the presence of C_{17} long-chain fatty acids in red cell lipids. These acids are usually present in trace amounts but are greatly increased in propionic acidaemia[6,26].

Treatment of the acute neonatal disease
By the time propionic acidaemia is diagnosed active treatment of the metabolic acidosis, apnoeic attacks and changes in fluid and electrolyte balance are usually well under way. The diagnosis of propionic acidaemia in no way alters the requirement to continue with this

policy. Plasma propionate can be lowered effectively using peritoneal dialysis[24]. Peritoneal dialysis has the added advantages, that it helps to lower the concentration of circulating ketone bodies, to reduce the hyperammonaemia seen in this condition, and to correct the acidosis.

The other treatment that can be tried as soon as the diagnosis of propionic acidaemia is made is to give D-biotin in massive doses (10 mg orally in the first instance and then 5 mg twice daily). This dose is over one hundred times the estimated maintenance dose for an adult, and does not have to be adjusted for the child's size. In some severe non-biotin responsive forms of propionic acidaemia there is a continual rise in plasma propionate in spite of any form of therapy, and death may be inevitable[6]. However, in other cases, the plasma propionate falls after the peritoneal dialysis and the effect of biotin is to greatly reduce the rate of production of propionate.

Propionate has numerous metabolic precursors, these include the amino acids, valine, isoleucine, methionine and threonine. Protein intake should be stopped as soon as the diagnosis of an organic acidaemia is suspected and sufficient calories provided in the form of carbohydrate to restrict protein catabolism. Protein intake is gradually reintroduced once the child's plasma propionate has fallen to less than 0·1 mmol/l. This concentration is an arbitrary figure based on experience of only a few cases and may have to be modified later. Artificial amino acid mixtures low in isoleucine, valine, methionine and threonine may be of value in this condition[27]. The gradual increase of protein intake using milk from 0·5 g/kg body weight per day with daily monitoring of plasma propionate concentrations is an alternative policy that has proved effective.

Once plasma propionate has stabilised at a low level and protein intake has gradually been increased, so that there is a resumption of weight gain in the neonate, it is necessary to decide whether the child is biotin responsive or whether the control of propionate concentration is solely due to restriction of protein intake. A child with propionic acidaemia should not be treated in the long term with daily biotin, if the condition is not biotin responsive. When the child is in a satisfactory clinical condition biotin therapy is discontinued and plasma propionate monitored daily. As biotin is bound covalently to propionyl CoA carboxylase enzyme there is a long half-life of the biotin–enzyme complex. Recent experience with two cases suggests that plasma propionate concentrations may take as long as 15 days to rise after biotin therapy is stopped. Once it has been established that plasma propionate concentrations have risen significantly, biotin is reintroduced and if the plasma propionate falls over the next few days to the earlier level, biotin therapy is continued indefinitely.

Throughout the initial period, from the time of diagnosis up to and including the attempt to withdraw biotin, plasma propionate concentrations should be monitored daily but later can be measured at weekly and then monthly intervals.

Management of the disease in the older child
Propionic acidaemia may be diagnosed in older children either during an acute acidotic episode or during investigation of a child previously known to suffer from acidotic-ketotic attacks. Acute attacks in older children are managed in the same way as neonatal propionic acidaemia. Intravenous bicarbonate is the treatment of choice for the metabolic acidosis. It is possible that peritoneal dialysis could be used but so far it has not been used in our older patients. If the child has not been investigated for biotin responsiveness, biotin should be given (5 mg twice daily) and the response assessed once the acute episode has subsided. Intercurrent infections should be treated actively. Protein intake is stopped during the initial period and gradually increased as the child recovers. Daily assessment is made using plasma propionate concentrations as a guide to protein intake.

In a child with newly diagnosed propionic acidaemia who is already controlled on a protein restricted diet, biotin responsiveness can be assessed by performing isoleucine loading tests (100 mg/kg or 0·75 mmol/kg body weight) before and on biotin therapy[28].

Long-term management
Children with either biotin responsive or non-responsive propionic acidaemia are in continual danger from intercurrent infections, and it is important that both the parents and the family doctor should be aware that even a relatively mild upper respiratory tract infection or a gastrointestinal disturbance may precipitate an acute acidotic episode. A useful method of monitoring the child's progress at home is to provide the parents with test papers or tablets for urinary ketones. A significant ketonuria associated with a minor infection is an indication for immediate admission to hospital. The importance of maintaining a restricted protein diet should be emphasised, as well as the necessity to continue to take biotin in the biotin-responsive cases.

Prognosis
Although propionic acidaemia was not described as a clinical entity until 1968[26], a few children with propionic acidaemia who had been diagnosed as having 'ketotic hyperglycinaemia' have been followed from before this time. There is a complete range in the intellectual development of these children. A child studied by Hsia and his colleagues[27] has a normal intelligence whereas many others are severely handicapped mentally. It is not known whether the degree of handicap is related to the frequency and severity of the acidotic attacks or to phenotypic differences in the ability to deal with abnormal metabolites of propionic acid.

The methylmalonic acidurias
The detection of an abnormal excretion of methylmalonic acid in the urine is only the first stage in the investigation of methylmalonic aciduria. The presence of this metabolite may be due to either methylmalonyl CoA mutase or perhaps racemase defects in the propionate–methylmalonate pathway (Figure 8.1) or to defects in co-enzyme B_{12} biosynthesis (Figure 8.3) (Rosenberg and Mahoney[3]). Irrespective of the basic enzyme defect methylmalonic aciduria may present as an acute metabolic acidosis and ketosis or as failure to thrive. As with propionic acidaemia, the severity of the clinical state of the patient dictates whether active treatment should be started before detailed investigation has established the nature of the enzyme defect or whether investigations may be performed in a logical sequence. It is more convenient, in investigating a patient with methylmalonic aciduria, to institute therapeutic trials in an ordered sequence, but in an acute situation this is usually impossible and all measures that may be useful have to be tried concurrently.

Initial diagnosis
This is made by the detection of methylmalonic acid in the urine. Simple colour tests have been described for methylmalonic aciduria[18], but two children with α-methylacetoacetic aciduria have been incorrectly diagnosed as having methylmalonic acidaemia using such techniques. A specific thin-layer chromatography technique can be used to make the diagnosis[19], but this will not assist in the diagnosis of the other organic acidaemias. A full gas-chromatographic analysis of the urine is the method of choice.

Treatment of the acute and neonatal disease

In the acute episode, treatment of the metabolic acidosis, rehydration and correction of electrolyte disturbances are usually being performed before methylmalonic aciduria is diagnosed. Once methylmalonic acid is detected in the urine, all protein intake is stopped, and calories are supplied solely as carbohydrate. Although there will be no evidence to show whether the methylmalonic aciduria is due to an error in the propionate–methylmalonate pathway, or of vitamin B_{12} inter-conversions, treatment with hydroxycobalamin (1 mg intramuscularly daily) is started immediately.

Experience suggests that peritoneal dialysis may also be useful[25]. Routine monitoring of acid–base parameters is essential. Urine is collected continuously, as the daily methylmalonic acid excretion is an important measure of biochemical control. Individual urine collections are tested for ketones (Acetest tablets) and the total collections pooled for measurement of methylmalonic acid excretion.

It is essential that blood samples are taken for measurement of the various parameters of B_{12} metabolism before the first injection of B_{12} is given. A normal specimen of blood is taken for a total B_{12} estimation, and plasma (0·5 ml) is collected for transcobalamin assay (with NaF–heparin). These two measurements will exclude inborn errors of vitamin B_{12} absorption and transport that might give rise to methylmalonic aciduria. Blood may also be taken for the analysis of individual cobalamins[29]. These compounds are light-sensitive, and the blood is taken into a syringe wrapped in aluminium foil to exclude light. The cobalamins are relatively stable in whole blood, but separation of cells and plasma must be performed in a dark room (dim red light) and without undue delay. The separated red cells and plasma are stored in light-tight containers in the deep freeze until analysis. Measurement of transcobalamins and individual cobalamins are only available at a few specialised centres. Measurement of the individual cobalamins is, at the moment, of research interest only but may in the future be of prognostic significance.

All urine specimens collected before treatment is started are saved for methylmalonic acid and amino acid analysis. Homocystinuria should be looked for in these early samples, as its presence indicates an early defect in vitamin B_{12} interconversions[3].

Once the metabolic acidosis and ketosis are controlled and urinary methylmalonic acid excretion has fallen appreciably (for example from 1500 mg (15 mmol) to about 100 mg (1 mmol) per day), protein is introduced at the level of 0·5 g/kg body weight per day. The re-introduction of protein should be as soon as the child is well enough to consider increasing the metabolic load. Daily monitoring of methylmalonic acid excretion will indicate the degree of biochemical control, and protein intake is increased in increments of 0·5 g/kg body weight up to 2·0 g/kg body weight. If at any stage ketonuria recurs and there are changes in acid–base parameters suggesting a return of the metabolic acidosis, the protein intake is reduced by 0·5 g/kg body weight, and attempts are made to stabilise the child at this lower level.

During this period the child will have been receiving hydroxycobalamin (1 mg/day IM). Assay of methylmalonyl CoA mutase in leucocytes or cultured fibroblasts will indicate if there is a primary defect of this enzyme. If there is no enzyme activity in the presence of an excess of co-enzyme B_{12} *in vitro*, there is no likelihood that the disease will be responsive to B_{12} and the treatment with hydroxy B_{12} may be stopped. Even if laboratory evidence points towards the defect being in B_{12} interconversions, there is no certainty that massive doses of hydroxy B_{12} will be effective in increasing methylmalonyl CoA mutase activity. At this stage, therefore, it is useful to withdraw B_{12} treatment and monitor methylmalonic acid excretion daily. Evidence suggests that if the child is B_{12}-dependent, methylmalonic acid excretion will rise within 20 days[30]. If methylmalonic acid excretion increases on withdrawal of B_{12} therapy, treatment with hydroxycobalamin is restarted, and the excretion of methylmalonic acid is monitored daily until it falls once more.

Management of the disease presenting as failure to thrive
Under these circumstances, the therapeutic role of protein restriction and of massive doses of hydroxycobalamin can be investigated independently. Blood samples are taken as before for assay of total vitamin B_{12}, transcobalamins, and individual cobalamins. A leucocyte preparation is made or a skin biopsy is taken for cell culture, for enzymic diagnosis and sent to a centre equipped for these analyses.

If the child appears relatively well on a normal protein intake, urine is collected for 3 days to establish the child's normal methylmalonic acid excretion, and then protein intake is reduced to 1·5 g/kg body weight per day. A fall in methylmalonic acid excretion should be seen, and once a new stable level of methylmalonic acid excretion has been established a trial of hydroxycobalamin can be performed (1 mg IM daily). If there is a further fall in methylmalonic acid excretion, a gradual increase in protein intake can be tried. Under ideal circumstances it should be possible to differentiate between the effects of protein restriction and vitamin B_{12} therapy. It must be noted that even in B_{12}-responsive cases it is frequently not possible to lower methylmalonic acid excretion below 100–300 mg (1–3 mmol) per day. Attempts should be made to lower methylmalonic acid excretion as far as possible, although there may be considerable clinical improvement with only a limited fall in excretion. The effects of a raised methylmalonic acid excretion have not been established over a long enough period to specify a safe level of excretion.

Nyhan and his colleagues[31] have reported a child with vitamin B_{12}-non-responsive methylmalonic acidaemia, in whom such a severe protein restriction was required that the child was permanently verging on protein malnutrition. However, on this restricted diet, the patient's development quotient doubled between the ages of 17 and 42 months.

At the conclusion of a trial of protein restriction and then hydroxycobalamin treatment, the patient should be excreting lower amounts of methylmalonic acid, even if enzymic data and measurements of individual cobalamins are not available he can, if necessary, be managed empirically without further information about the nature of the metabolic defect.

Long-term management
A protein-restricted diet requires supervision by a dietician experienced in paediatric problems, and the degree of restriction may well have to be a compromise between lowering methylmalonic acid production and providing an adequate intake of essential amino acids[31]. Many of these children border on protein malnutrition. The role of artificial amino acid mixtures to increase the intake of non-toxic essential amino acids has not been established. Adequate calorie intake is essential, and this may be supplied as glucose polymers and fat emulsions.

Methylmalonic acid excretion should be monitored at frequent intervals. The effect of protein restriction is best assessed by measuring plasma amino acid and plasma albumin concentrations in those children receiving less than 1·5 g of protein/kg/day. The dietetic lessons learnt from the management of maple syrup urine disease and phenylketonuria apply here. It is important not to restrict protein intake unnecessarily, as this may also give rise to developmental retardation.

In vitamin-B_{12}-responsive cases, 1 mg hydroxycobalamin, intramuscularly, daily is the treatment of choice. Adenosylcobalamin seems no more effective. It may be possible to reduce the vitamin B_{12} injections to two a week instead of daily[32].

These children are all at risk from intercurrent infections, and both the family doctor and the parents must be aware of this. Significant ketonuria (a strongly positive reaction with Acetest tablets) indicates the need for admission to hospital and it may be helpful to have the parents test the child's urine for ketones when he appears unwell.

Prognosis
As with propionic acidaemia, patients are known with normal intelligence, and others with severe mental retardation. The relationship between methylmalonic acid excretion and/or the frequency of acidotic attacks and the developmental progress of these children has not been established.

Summary of investigation and treatment
The methylmalonic acidurias include a wide range of enzyme defects[3]. The most important investigation is to establish whether the condition is vitamin B_{12}-responsive. However, in both responsive and non-responsive variants, protein restriction is usually required. This restriction may have to be very much more rigorous in the non-responsive variants[31]. Full biochemical investigation of individual cases is required before the range of prognoses in the different enzymic forms of methylmalonic aciduria can be stated with certainty. The measurement of methylmalonyl CoA mutase activity will indicate whether there is the possibility of vitamin B_{12}-responsiveness in an individual case.

β-Hydroxyisovaleric aciduria and β-methylcrotonylglycinuria
These metabolites occur in the urine as a consequence of an impaired β-methylcrotonyl CoA carboxylase activity: this enzyme is involved in the leucine degradation pathway (Figure 8.2). Three children have been reported with this condition. The first child has a condition similar to Werdnig–Hoffman's disease[33]. Modification of her daily leucine intake reduced the excretion of these abnormal metabolites but had little effect on the clinical course of the disease. β-methylcrotonyl CoA carboxylase is a biotin-requiring enzyme, and a dose of 0·25 mg biotin per day was tried but without success[34].

The next two patients presented with entirely different clinical pictures. The first J.R. presented with an acute metabolic acidosis and ketosis and responded to severe protein restriction in the first instance and then dramatically to biotin 5 mg twice daily[35]. Subsequent investigations suggest that this child also had a propionyl CoA carboxylase deficiency, and was suffering from at least two mitochondrial carboxylase deficiencies possibly secondary to a failure of biotin metabolism[1].

The third child (M.K.) presented with an upper lobe pneumonia, diminished consciousness and neurological changes. The abnormal metabolites started to disappear from his urine during initial antibiotic therapy, before the diagnosis was made and before biotin therapy (5 mg twice daily) was started. After he had recovered from his respiratory tract infection and while on biotin therapy he did not excrete the abnormal metabolites[36].

Both J.R. and M.K. stopped receiving biotin therapy when their families moved to other areas. When they were next seen several months later, the abnormal urinary metabolites derived from β-methylcrotonyl CoA had returned. Biotin treatment was reintroduced, and the metabolites disappeared from the urine, confirming the initial biotin responsiveness.

This limited experience with three children with entirely different clinical presentations does not give an adequate basis to indicate detailed treatment of any new cases or to suggest an overall prognosis. One child is dead, one mentally retarded and the third appears to be developing normally. The combined experience of these three children does suggest, however, that leucine or protein restriction will reduce the excretion of abnormal metabolites, and that biotin treatment, to be effective, should be tried at the dose level of 5 mg twice daily.

ORGANIC ACIDAEMIAS AND ACIDURIAS WITHOUT VITAMIN-RESPONSIVE VARIANTS

Isovaleric acidaemia
Isovaleric acid is derived from isovaleryl CoA, an intermediate in leucine degradation (Figure 8.2). This volatile acid has a characteristic and unpleasant smell, and the diagnosis may be suggested by the abnormal smell of the patient's breath, sweat and urine. The smell has been likened to that of 'sweaty feet' or 'a locker-room'[37]. The clinical presentations of isovaleric acidaemia do not differ from the other

organic acidaemias except for the presence of this offensive smell during acute acidotic episodes.

Biochemical diagnosis
During acute episodes isovaleric acidaemia is diagnosed by the finding of extremely high concentrations of free isovaleric acid in blood and urine[37]. Isovaleric acid is detected during analysis of volatile fatty acids by gas chromatography. However, during remission isovaleric acid does not accumulate, and is excreted as its glycine conjugate, isovalerylglycine[37]. Isovalerylglycine is detected during the analysis of the non-volatile organic acid fraction isolated from urine.

Treatment
The acute neonatal form and later acidotic episodes of isovaleric acidaemia are treated in the same way as the other organic acidaemias. Alkali therapy, rehydration and correction of electrolyte disturbances are of prime importance. Protein intake is stopped and a high carbohydrate intake is instituted to reduce protein catabolism during the acute phase. Levy and his colleagues[38] have reported successful treatment of a second child in a family with isovaleric acidaemia. This child was treated with a low leucine diet from 17 days of age. Within one day of treatment the excretion of isovaleric acid and its conjugate, isovalerylglycine, fell considerably. At $3\frac{1}{2}$ years he is considered to have developed as well as his unaffected brother. However, his $11\frac{1}{2}$-year-old sister who was not diagnosed until 8 years of age is mentally retarded.

α-Methylacetoacetic and α-methyl-β-hydroxybutyric aciduria
Daum and colleagues[39,40] have described four children from two families with α-methylacetoacetic and α-methyl-β-hydroxybutyric aciduria due to a defect in isoleucine metabolism (Figure 8.2). These children presented between 12 and 22 months of age with severe episodes of metabolic acidosis and ketosis. Two of these children have normal intelligence: one suffered a cardiac arrest during an acute episode and has psychomotor retardation and one has died. The three surviving patients have been controlled on a restricted protein diet (2 g/kg body weight per day) with early and effective management of incipient acidotic attacks.

Keating and his colleagues[41] described another patient with this condition who presented with vomiting within the first four weeks of

life. This child showed all the characteristics of the 'ketotic hyperglycinaemia' syndrome, i.e. vomiting, metabolic acidosis, long-chain
ketonuria, hyperglycinaemia and hyperglycinuria. Subsequently,
Hillman and Keating[42] demonstrated that this was associated with
α-methylacetoacetic and α-methyl-β-hydroxybutyric aciduria. This
child was treated with a restricted protein diet (1·5 g of protein/kg
body weight), with satisfactory somatic growth. Motor development
was retarded to some extent.

The treatment of these children has not differed from those with
other organic acidaemias. The acute acidotic and ketotic episodes have
been treated with alkali therapy and withdrawal of protein while
long-term maintenance on a restricted protein diet has reduced the
frequency of acute acidotic attacks.

The enzyme defect in this condition is thought to be associated with
a β-ketothiolase deficiency (Figure 8.2). This enzyme requires
coenzyme A as its co-factor, and it is difficult to visualise ways in which
the activity of the enzyme could be enhanced by vitamin therapy.

GENETIC COUNSELLING

Evidence from family studies suggests that the organic acidaemias
are inherited as autosomal recessive conditions. Evidence from fibroblast studies have shown that the heterozygote can be detected in
propionic acidaemia, but with difficulty[43]. The only other organic
acidaemia in which the heterozygous state has been detected is
α-methylacetoacetic and α-methyl-β-hydroxybutyric aciduria. In this
condition the heterozygotes excrete abnormal amounts of α-methyl-
β-hydroxybutyric acid[40]. The detection of the heterozygous state in
the other organic acidaemias requires improvement in the sensitivity
of specific enzyme assays.

PRENATAL DIAGNOSIS

The prenatal diagnosis of propionic acidaemia has been reported[44] but
there is great variability in enzyme activity from normal cultured
amniotic cells. The diagnosis can only be made with any confidence
if *no* activity is detected in the cultured cells from the pregnancy at
risk. The problems of culturing enough cells for enzyme assay between

the time of amniocentesis and the latest time for safe termination of pregnancy raises special difficulties in this condition.

Preliminary results suggest that methylmalonic acidaemia may be diagnosed prenatally by finding a raised concentration of methylmalonic acid in amniotic fluid[45-47]. If this can be confirmed in a large enough series it obviates the need to culture and perform metabolic studies on amniotic cells. However, the combination of a raised concentration of methylmalonic acid in the amniotic fluid with an impaired methylmalonic acid metabolism in cultured amniotic cells has been used successfully as an indication for the termination of an affected pregnancy[46].

Shih, Mandell and Tanaka[48] have demonstrated the possibility of diagnosing isovaleric acidaemia in cultured fibroblasts, and have suggested, therefore, that this condition can also be diagnosed prenatally.

CONCLUSIONS

The clinical presentations of the organic acidaemias do not allow their biochemical differentiation. Identification of the abnormal metabolites excreted in these conditions will indicate whether specific restriction of certain amino acids or a more generalised protein restriction is required. In propionic acidaemia, in methylmalonic aciduria and in β-methylcrotonyl CoA carboxylase deficiency there is the possibility of massive vitamin therapy. In the acute presentations of these three conditions, vitamin therapy is started as soon as the initial biochemical diagnosis is made, and at a later date this therapy is withdrawn to establish whether the child is vitamin responsive. In children in whom these defects are diagnosed while they are relatively well, vitamin responsiveness can be investigated under carefully controlled conditions. The children with vitamin-responsive variants appear to be at an advantage as a lesser degree of protein-restriction is required, and there appear to be fewer episodes of acute metabolic imbalance.

REFERENCES

1. Gompertz, D. (1974). Inborn errors of organic acid metabolism. *Clinics in Endocrinology and Metabolism*, Vol. 3, No. 1, p. 107. (H. Bickel, editor) (London: Saunders)

2. Scriver, C. R. (1973). Vitamin-responsive inborn errors of metabolism. *Treatment of Inborn Errors of Metabolism*, p.127 (J. W. T. Seakins, R. A. Saunders and C. Toothill, editors) (London: Churchill Livingstone)

3. Rosenberg, L. E. and Mahoney, M. J. (1973). Inherited disorders of methylmalonate and vitamin B_{12} metabolism. *Inborn Errors of Metabolism*, p. 301 (F. A. Hommes and C. J. Van den Berg, editors) (London: Academic Press)

4. Childs, B., Nyhan, W. L., Borden, M., Bard, L. and Cooke, R. E. (1961). Idiopathic hyperglycinaemia and hyperglycinuria: a new disorder of aminoacid metabolism. *Pediatrics*, **27**, 522

5. Stokke, O., Eldjarn, L., Norum, K. R., Steen-Johnsen, J. and Halvorsen, S. (1967). Methylmalonic Acidaemia. *Scand. J. of Clin. Lab. Invest.*, **20**, 313

6. Gompertz, D., Storrs, C. N., Bau, D. C. K., Peters, T. J. and Hughes, E. A. (1970). Localisation of enzymic defect in propionicacidaemia. *Lancet*, **i**, 1140

7. Hsia, Y. E., Scully, K. J. and Rosenberg, L. E. (1970). Inherited propionyl-CoA carboxylase deficiency in 'ketotic hyperglycinaemia'. *Pediat. Res.*, **4**, 439

8. Hillman, R. E., Feigin, R. D., Tenenbaum, S. M. and Keating, J. P. (1972). Defective isoleucine metabolism as a cause of the 'ketotic hyperglycinaemia' syndrome. *Pediat. Res.*, **6**, 394

9. Perry, T. L., Hansen, S., Diamond, S., Bullis, B., Mok, C. and Melançon, S. B. (1970). Volatile fatty acids in normal human physiological fluids. *Clin. Chim. Acta*, **29**, 369

10. Gompertz, D. and Draffan, G. H. (1972). Gas-chromatographic diagnosis of intermittent maple syrup urine disease. *Clin. Chim. Acta*, **40**, 5

11. Jellum, E., Stokke, O. and Eldjarn, L. (1971). Screening for metabolic disorders using gas-liquid chromatography, mass spectrometry, and computer technique. *Scand. J. Clin. Lab. Invest.*, **27**, 273

12. Mamer, O. A., Crawhall, J. C. and Tjoa, S. S. (1971). The identification of urinary acids by coupled gas chromatography—mass spectrometry. *Clin. Chim. Acta*, **32**, 171

13. Chalmers, R. A., Lawson, A. M. and Watts, R. W. E. (1974). Studies on the urinary acidic metabolites excreted by patients with β-methylcrotonylglycinuria, propionic acidaemia and methylmalonic acidaemia, using gas-liquid chromatography and mass spectrometry. *Clin. Chim. Acta*, **52**, 43

14. Gompertz, D. (1971). Crotonic acid, an artefact in screening for organic acidaemias. *Clin. Chim. Acta*, **33**, 457

15. Hansen, S., Perry, T. L., Lesk, D. and Gibson, L. (1972). Urinary bacteria: potential source of some organic acidurias. *Clin. Chim. Acta*, **39**, 71

16. Duran, M., Ketting, D., Wadman, S. K., Trijbels, J. M. F., Bakkeren, J. A. J. M. and Waelkens, J. J. J. (1973). Propionic acid, an artefact which can leave methylmalonic acidaemia undiscovered. *Clin. Chim. Acta*, **49**, 177

17. Ando, T., Nyhan, W. L., Bachmann, C., Rasmussen, K., Scott, R. and Smith, E. K. (1973). Isovaleric acidaemia: identification of isovalerate, isovalerylglycine and 3-hydroxyisovalerate in urine of a patient previously reported as having butyric and hexanoic acidemia. *J. Pediat.*, **82**, 243

18. Giorgio, A. J. and Luhby, A. L. (1969). A rapid screening test for the detection of congenital methylmalonic aciduria in infancy. *Amer. J. Clin. Pathol.*, **52**, 374

19. Gutteridge, J. M. C. and Wright, E. B. (1970). A simple and rapid thin-layer chromatographic technique for detection of methylmalonic acid in urine. *Clin. Chim. Acta*, **27**, 289

20. Bartlett, K. and Gompertz, D. (1974). The specificity of glycine-N-acylase and acylglycine excretion in the organic acidaemias. *Biochem. Med.*, **10**, 15

21. Gaull, G. E. (1969). Pathogenesis of maple syrup urine disease: observations during dietary management and treatment of coma by peritoneal dialysis. *Biochem. Med.*, **3**, 130

22. Rey, F., Rey, J., Cloup, M., Féron, J. F., Doré, F., Labrune, B. and Frézal, J. (1969). Traitement d'urgence d'une forme aigue de leucinose par dialyse péritonéale. *Archiv. Franç. Pédiat.*, **26**, 133

23. Sallan, S. E. and Cottom D. (1969). Peritoneal dialysis in maple syrup urine disease. *Lancet*, **ii**, 1423

24. Russell, G., Thom, H., Tarlow, M. J. and Gompertz, D. (1974). Reduction of plasma propionate by peritoneal dialysis. *Pediatrics*, **53**, 281

25. Saudubray, J. M., Fournet, J.-P. and Cloup, M. (1971). Intérêt de la dialyse péritonéale dans le traitment d'urgence des maladies métaboliques d'origine constitutionnelle révélées dans la période néonatale. *Ann. Med. Interne*, **122**, 1279

26. Hommes, F. A., Kuipers, J. R. G., Elema, J. D., Jansen, J. F. and Jonxis, J. H. P. (1968). Propionic acidaemia, a new inborn error of metabolism. *Pediat. Res.*, **2**, 519

27. Brandt, I. K., Hsia, Y. E., Clement, D. H. and Provence, S. A. (1974). Propionic acidaemia (ketotic hyperglycinaemia): dietary treatment resulting in normal growth and development. *Pediatrics*, **53**, 391

28. Barnes, N. D., Hull, D., Balgobin, L. and Gompertz, D. (1970). Biotin-responsive propionicacidaemia. *Lancet*, **ii**, 244

29. Linnell, J. C., Hussein, H. A.-A. and Matthews, D. M. (1970). A two-dimensional chromato-bioautographic method for complete separation of individual plasma cobalamins. *J. Clin. Pathol.*, **23**, 820

30. Rosenberg, L. E., Lilljeqvist, A.-C. and Hsia, Y. E. (1970). Methylmalonic aciduria: metabolic block localisation and vitamin B_{12} dependency. *Science*, **162**, 805

31. Nyhan, W. L., Fawcett, N., Ando, T., Rennert, O. M. and Julius, R. L. (1973). Response to dietary therapy in B_{12} unresponsive methylmalonic acidaemia. *Pediatrics*, **51**, 539

32. Mahoney, M. J. and Rosenberg, L. E. (1970). Inherited defects of B_{12} metabolism. *Amer. J. Med.*, **48**, 584

33. Eldjarn, L., Jellum, E., Stokke, O., Pande, H. and Waaler, P. E. (1970). β-Hydroxyisovaleric aciduria and β-methylcrotonyl-glycinuria: a new inborn error of metabolism. *Lancet*, **ii**, 521

34. Stokke, O., Eldjarn, L., Jellum, E., Pande, H. and Waaler, P. E. (1972). β-Methylcrotonyl CoA carboxylase deficiency: A new metabolic error in leucine degradation. *Pediatrics*, **49**, 726

35. Gompertz, D., Draffan, G. H., Watts, J. L. and Hull, D. (1971). Biotin-responsive β-methylcrotonylglycinuria. *Lancet*, **ii**, 22.

36. Gompertz, D., Bartlett, K., Blair, D. and Stern, C. M. M. (1973). A child with a defect in leucine metabolism associated with β-hydroxyisovaleric aciduria and β-methylcrotonylglycinuria. *Archiv. Dis. Childhood*, **48**, 975

37. Tanaka, K. (1973). Isovaleric acidaemia and its induction in experimental animals by hypoglycin A: *Inborn Errors of Metabolism*, p. 269 (F. A. Hommes and C. J. Van den Berg, editors) (London: Academic Press)

38. Levy, H. L., Erickson, A. M., Lott, I. T. and Kurtz, D. L. (1973). Isovaleric acidaemia: results of family study and dietary treatment. *Pediatrics*, **52**, 83

39. Daum, R. S., Lamm, P. H., Mamer, O. A. and Scriver, C. R. (1971). A 'new' disorder of isoleucine catabolism. *Lancet*, **ii**, 1289

40. Daum, R. S., Scriver, C. R., Mamer, O. A., Delvin, E., Lamm, P. and Goldman, H. (1973). An inherited disorder of isoleucine catabolism causing accumulation of α-methylacetoacetate and α-methyl-β-hydroxybutyrate and intermittent acidosis. *Pediat. Res.*, **7**, 149

41. Keating, J. P., Feigin, R. D., Tenenbaum, S. M. and Hillman, R. E. (1972). Hyperglycinaemia with ketosis due to a defect in isoleucine metabolism: a preliminary report. *Pediatrics*, **50**, 890

42. Hillman, R. E. and Keating, J. P. (1974). Beta-ketothiolase deficiency as a cause of the 'ketotic hyperglycinaemia syndrome'. *Pediatrics*, **53**, 221

43. Hsia, Y. E., Scully, K. J. and Rosenberg, L. E. (1971). Inherited propionyl-CoA carboxylase deficiency in 'ketotic hyperglycinaemia'. *J. Clin. Invest.*, **50**, 127

44. Gompertz, D., Goodey, P. A., Thom, H., Russell, G., Maclean, M. W., Ferguson-Smith, M. E. and Ferguson-Smith, M. A. (1973). Antenatal diagnosis of propionic acidaemia. *Lancet*, **i**, 1009

45. Morrow, G. III, Schwarz, R. H., Hallock, J. A. and Barness, L. A. (1970). Prenatal detection of methylmalonic acidaemia. *J. Pediat.* **77**, 120

46. Mahoney, M. J., Rosenberg, L. E., Waldenstrom, J., Lindblad, B. and Zetterstrom, R. (1973). Prenatal diagnosis of methylmalonic aciduria. *Pediat. Res.*, **7**, 342

47. Gompertz, D., Goodey, P. A., Saudubray, J. M., Charpentier, C., Chignolle, A. and Girard, S. (1974). Prenatal diagnosis of methylmalonic aciduria. *Pediatrics*, in press.

48. Shih, V. E., Mandell, R. and Tanaka, K. (1973). Diagnosis of isovaleric acidaemia in cultured fibroblasts. *Clin. Chim. Acta*, **48**, 437

49. Pettersen, J. E., Jellum, E. and Eldjarn, L. (1972). The occurrence of adipic and suberic acids in urine from ketotic patients. *Clin. Chim. Acta*, **38**, 17

50. Dosman, J., Crawhall, J. C., Klassen, G. A., Mamer, O. A. and Neumann, P. (1974). Urinary excretion of C_6-C_{10} dicarboxylic acids in glycogen storage disease types I and III. *Clin. Chim. Acta*, **51**, 93

CHAPTER 9

Treatment by Inhibition of Renal Tubular Reabsorption

D. N. Raine

The traditional approach to the treatment of the amino acidopathies is one of dietary restriction and the details for particular diseases are described in several of the preceding chapters. For this to be effective, however, it is necessary that the source of amino acid concerned is wholly or mainly dietary protein and that substantial amounts are not synthesised by the patient. Such amino acids have been termed 'essential' since the diet must contain adequate amounts for health and normal growth. Amino acids for which normal development is independent are termed 'nonessential'. Thus phenylalanine, methionine and the branched-chain amino acids, the subjects of the first three chapters, are included in the classical list of ten essential amino acids and the diseases in which they occur are, therefore, susceptible to management by dietary restriction.

Diseases characterised by the accumulation of non-essential amino acids include the several glycinaemias, sarcosinaemia, β-alaninaemia, cystinosis, ornithinaemia, argininaemia, citrullinuria, prolinaemia and hydroxyprolinaemia and theoretically, at least, these are not susceptible to dietary control.

Histidine is an interesting case for it is included in the ten essential amino acids and yet it is thought not to be essential in man. Nevertheless, it is easy to control the plasma concentration of histidine in infants with histidinaemia by dietary means. This illustrates the weakness of the concept of 'essential' and 'non-essential' for the degree to which a particular amino acid is 'essential' differs from one substance to another and it may also vary with age. Such variation can become important in managing children whose requirements are affected by their growth as well as a metabolic abnormality and in this context the concept is best disregarded.

In amino acidopathies that are not susceptible to dietary management an alternative approach is to inhibit reabsorption of the amino acid by the renal tubule. Plasma amino acids are filtered by the glomerulus and in normal circumstances are almost wholly reabsorbed by the tubules. The resultant renal clearances are generally low[1, 2], only aspartic acid, serine, glycine and histidine exceeding 2·0 ml/min/1·73 m² and the majority[3] less than 1·0 ml/min/1·73 m².

Tubular reabsorption of amino acids

The precise mechanism of absorption of amino acids in the renal tubule, in spite of extensive study, is still largely speculative[3, 4]. It is thought to involve several steps. However, for the present purpose it is convenient to consider five group transport systems, although at least two, those for the basic amino acids and cystine, and for the imino acids and glycine are known to be more complex. The five systems involve the following groups of amino acids:

1. Neutral amino acids

Leucine	Asparagine	Serine	Phenylalanine	Glycine	Cysteine
Isoleucine	Glutamine	Threonine	Tyrosine	Alanine	Methionine
Valine			Tryptophan		Histidine
					Citrulline

2. Basic amino acids and cystine

Cystine	Lysine	Arginine	Ornithine

3. Acidic amino acids

Aspartic acid   Glutamic acid

4. Imino acids and glycine

Proline   Hydroxyproline   Glycine

5. β-amino acids

β-Alanine   β-Amino isobutyric acid   Taurine

These systems have been defined partly by experiment but mainly by the recognition of specific defects of some part of the transport mechanism. The precise mechanism of transport is unknown and the defective component may be an enzyme, a carrier molecule or another constituent function.

A relatively complete failure of the first group transport mechanism occurs in Hartnup disease in which, but for the absence of proline and hydroxyproline, there is an almost generalised amino aciduria. The symptoms of Hartnup disease are thought to result from the wastage of tryptophan which is a precursor of nicotinic acid.

Failure of the second mechanism results in the condition cystinuria but already three varieties of cystinuria have been described, which illustrates the fact that the present description of tubular reabsorption is somewhat oversimplified. In some of the forms of cystinuria a corresponding defect in intestinal absorption has been demonstrated[5] and there are other examples of transport defects occuring in both kidney and intestine[6,7].

Inherited abnormalities of the third and fifth transport system have not been described but failure of the fourth system results in iminoglycinuria, which was at first thought to be associated with disease (Joseph's syndrome) but has now been established as benign[8].

Transport affinity and the effects of overloading

The common transport mechanism for glycine, proline and hydroxyproline has been demonstrated using slices of rat kidney tissue[9], hamster intestine[10] and fetal rat bone[11].

Patients with prolinaemia, in whom there is an endogenous overloading by proline of the transport mechanism in the renal tubule, excrete not only abnormal amounts of proline but also of glycine and hydroxyproline. As the plasma concentration of the latter amino acids is normal the increased excretion must result from inhibition of the grouped renal tubular reabsorption by proline[12]. The same phenomenon occurs when hydroxyproline is infused intravenously: the increased hydroxyproline in the plasma overflows into the urine and in so doing inhibits the reabsorption of proline and glycine[12]. In hydroxyprolinaemia, however, the overflow appears to be insufficient to produce this effect[13].

The discovery of families with inherited iminoglycinuria[14-16] allowed Scriver and his colleagues[17] to study the capacity of the transport process and its relative affinity for the three amino acids. Further information has been obtained by similar studies in a case of hyperglycinuria[18]. It is concluded that the group transport mechanism has a high capacity but is one of low affinity for the three amino acids, the lowest affinity being for glycine. In addition there are more specific transport mechanisms, one of which is exclusive for glycine, but is of low capacity. Glycine also shares the grouped transport mechanism for neutral amino acids, that which is defective in Hartnup disease. The imino acids are also transported by a separate mechanism of somewhat low capacity and for this hydroxyproline has the lower affinity of the two [17, 19, 20]. Thus, glycine is reabsorbed by at least three mechanisms, proline by two and hydroxyproline by two. The latter when present in high concentrations is reabsorbed mainly by the grouped transport mechanism, and when in normal concentrations mainly by the mechanism it shares with proline alone.

Homocystinuria

In a case of homocystinuria, Cusworth and his colleagues[21, 22] explored the feasibility of treating diseases characterised by a high concentration of one amino acid by facilitating the excretion of the offending substance. This was accomplished by inhibiting its reabsorption in the renal tubule after it had been filtered by the glomerulus.

Homocystine is carried by the cystine-dibasic amino acid mechanism and its reabsorption will be interfered with by arginine and lysine. Intravenous infusion of lysine and arginine glutamate did indeed promote the urinary excretion of homocystine but oral therapy had too little effect to be of long term therapeutic value. None the less, the opportunity remains for further attempts to be made with these substances and, if necessary, with synthetic compounds which are more specifically inhibitory.

Prolinaemia

There are two forms of prolinaemia: the first, designated type 1, is due to a deficiency of proline oxidase which converts proline to Δ^1pyrroline-5-carboxylic acid (PC); the other, type 2, is believed to be associated with a deficiency of the second enzyme in the pathway, a dehydrogenase which acts on PC. The two types can be distinguished by a convenient test for PC applied to urine[23].

Sufficient cases of type 1 prolinaemia detected in neonatal screening programmes appear to have developed normally without treatment to suggest that the genetic biochemical abnormality is not associated with disease. The association of the type 2 abnormality with disease may also be questioned on the evidence available at present. Six patients with type 2 prolinaemia in addition to the one we have studied have been reported. Two had no associated clinical features[24, 25] but the other four[23, 26-28] and ours are retarded mentally and have had fits. The higher concentration of plasma proline found in patients with type 2 prolinaemia, compared with type 1, suggests that it may be a more serious disorder and should be treated.

Proline is a non-essential amino acid and prolinaemia, theoretically, at least, should not be susceptible to management by dietary restriction of this amino acid. None the less, our experience with a type 2 patient that dietary restriction of proline has a definite, if insufficient, effect is shared by others who have studied type 1 patients[29, 30], although Similä's study of a type 2 patient[31] appears to have been more successful. The latter author maintained his patient for 3 years, with satisfactory growth and development, on a diet containing 90 mg proline/kg/day.

Our patient, (A.W.) showed signs of retarded development from the age of 8 months and was recognised as a case of type 2 prolinaemia at 18 months. Plasma proline on a normal diet (250–300 mg proline/kg/day) varied between 3·1 and 3·5 mmol/l (normal 0·07–0·23 mmol/l). Treatment with a diet containing 100 mg proline/kg/day resulted in a fall in plasma concentration to a mean of 2·8 mmol/l but the fluctuations were large (1·4–3·6 mmol/l) and further reduction of the proline intake to 10 mg/kg/day was barely more successful. At this stage glycine was added to the proline-reduced diet, three doses of 10 g being taken with the main meals, the last as late in the day as possible. The fall in plasma proline concentration was so dramatic (Figure 9.1) that an attempt was made to return to a normal and, later, a less restricted diet while continuing to administer glycine. This was not successful and the combination of proline restriction to 10 mg/kg/day and 30 g glycine daily was restored. This regime has been continued for more than 2 years and plasma proline is being maintained between 0·8 and 1·3 mmol/l.

The plasma glycine concentrations throughout this period have remained in the range 0·22–0·56 mmol/l (generally less than twice the upper limit of normal). The protein supplied by the diet was maintained at approximately 3 g/kg/day and the glycine load (30 g) was additional to this. The addition of this quantity of a single amino acid makes the apparent 'protein' intake higher than would normally be desired, but this is spurious since much of the glycine is excreted and it is also utilised less in this unbalanced form than it would be if accompanied by other amino acids in the pattern encountered in natural protein. It is interesting that the plasma urea concentration during the period of glycine supplementation never exceeded 23 mg/100 ml, except immediately after glycine was started, when it reached 40 mg/100 ml.

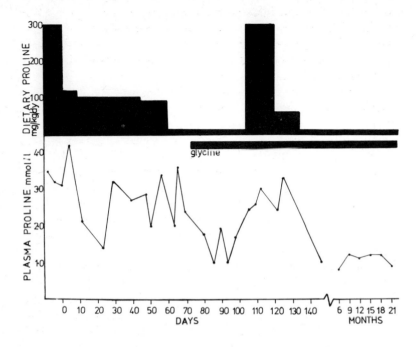

Figure 9.1. Response of plasma proline to dietary proline restriction and glycine administration (10 g three times daily) in a patient (A.W.), with prolinaemia type 2

The patient meanwhile has become a great deal easier to manage, but it is impossible to attribute this to the treatment alone since his parents are more experienced in his management, and have presumably benefited from clinical support and the child has passed through a stage in his development in which behaviour and skills develop rapidly. However, the biochemical management has proved entirely satisfactory and it will require a careful trial in unaffected patients showing the disorder to discover if there is any clinical benefit.

Hydroxyprolinaemia

Hydroxyproline is a constituent of collagen and it is formed by hydroxylation of proline after the latter has been incorporated into the collagen molecule. It is, therefore, a non-essential amino acid. Most studies of this amino acid in man have been concerned with hydroxyproline which is peptide bound, and the analyses are made after these substances, usually in urine, have been hydrolysed. As such the amino acid is a measure of collagen metabolism.

Hydroxyprolinaemia is presumed to be a defect of hydroxyproline oxidase, analagous with type 1 prolinaemia, and it is characterised biochemically by an increase in the concentration in plasma and urine of free hydroxyproline, a form in which the amino acid is normally absent from urine after the third month of life.

The first case, an 11-year-old mentally and physically retarded girl, described by Efron and her colleagues[13, 32] was discovered by screening hospital inmates for urinary amino acid abnormalities. The patient was hyperactive and agressive and although her mother was also mentally subnormal she did not have hydroxyprolinaemia. Another case[33, 34] was associated, probably coincidentally, with a nodular goitre, and in the same family another completely healthy subject also had the biochemical abnormality. The patient we have studied (B.P.) has not yet been described fully and has been only briefly referred to[35-38]. Like the first patient she was discovered at the age of 6 years by routine screening in a mental subnormality hospital and she too was hyperactive and very difficult to manage; although short, she was not under weight, and the degree of hydroxyprolinaemia was insufficient to induce an associated prolinaemia and glycinuria. Plasma hydroxyproline concentration was 0·53 mmol/l (normal, less than 0·02 mmol/l).

Hydroxyproline is a non-essential amino acid and Efron and her colleagues discovered that the plasma concentration in their patient was unaffected by dietary restriction of proline and hydroxyproline[13]. Their patient was also subject to a scorbutic diet in order to reduce collagen turnover, but this too failed to lower the plasma concentration of hydroxyproline[39].

Attempts to inhibit renal tubular reabsorption of hydroxyproline in our patient by giving 10 g of glycine with each of the three main meals in the day resulted in an immediate fall in plasma hydroxyproline to about 60% of that before treatment (Figure 9.2). Increasing the glycine to 15 g three times daily was no more effective. Even 30 g/day caused the previously normal plasma glycine concentration to rise to 2·7 mmol/l but without changing the treatment this fell within a few days to more acceptable levels between 0·22 and 0·81 mmol/l, while

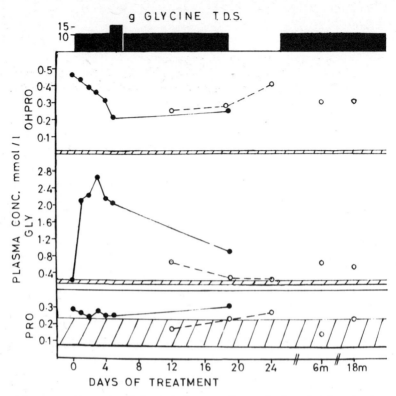

Figure 9.2. Response of plasma hydroxyproline to glycine administration in a patient (B.P.), with hydroxyprolinaemia

plasma hydroxyproline remained over a 2·5 year period between 0·22 and 0·28 mmol/l.

In order to lower the plasma hydroxyproline concentration further an attempt was made to block more of the tubular reabsorption by adding proline to the glycine supplements. At first 5 g L-proline was added to each dose of glycine, but this had little effect. When the dose of L-proline was increased to 10 g three times daily, however, the plasma hydroxyproline fell to 0·082 mmol/l in one day and was maintained at about this level for several weeks (Figure 9.3). Plasma proline increased from 0·24 mmol/l to 2·27 mmol/l and in order to reduce this the L-proline supplements were reduced from 10 g to 7 g. There was no consequent rise in plasma hydroxyproline and the glycine and

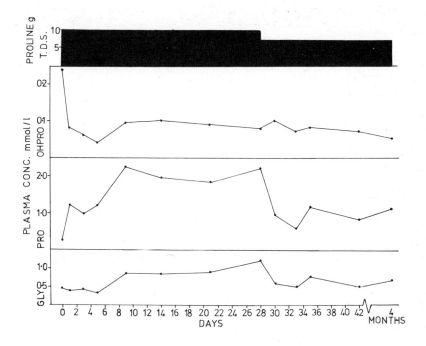

Figure 9.3. Response of plasma hydroxyproline to glycine (10 g three times daily) and proline administration in a patient (B.P.), with hydroxyprolinaemia

proline concentrations were maintained for several weeks at 0·48–0·72 mmol/l and 0·66–1·14 mmol/l respectively, that is three to four times the upper limit of normal. The requirements of individual patients can be expected to vary and it may be that the required dose of either glycine or proline, or both, will require adjustment to individual needs in this way.

The clinical state of the patient, who was severely abnormal when treatment began, did not improve and the treatment with both amino acids has now been withdrawn without any apparent deterioration. Again the value of this, or any other treatment, of hydroxyprolinaemia will require careful clinical studies to be made and in this

227

condition too there is still the possibility that the biochemical and clinical abnormalities are only coincidentally associated.

Conclusion

The attempts to treat the two patients with prolinaemia and hydroxy-prolinaemia should not be taken as prejudging the need for therapy in either disorder. However, until that question is decided the feasibility of treating either by renal tubular inhibition remains of interest. Perhaps more important is the principle that has been established and it may be that other amino acidaemias that prove resistant to dietary manipulation will be susceptible to a similar approach to their management and it is for this reason that the cases have been described in some detail.

APPENDIX

Details of Proline-Reduced Diet

The dietary intake of proline was controlled by the use of a proline-free synthetic amino acid mixture obtained from Scientific Hospital Supplies Ltd. (Code M.P.1. H.P.D.). This contains the essential amino acids together with a mixture of minerals and vitamins and provides 8 g 'protein' per 10 g. The required amount of proline was supplied by natural protein, and the additional protein required for adequate nutrition was provided by the amino acid mixture. Thus the initial diet which contained a total of 3 g protein/kg, but only 120 mg proline/kg was achieved by supplying 8·0 g protein as the amino acid mixture and the remaining 28 g from natural foods (Table 9.1). The remainder of the diet consisted of fat and carbohydrate to maintain the calorie intake. In addition a complete mineral supplement (Scientific Hospital Supplies Ltd.) and vitamin supplement in the form of Ketovite syrup and tablets were given.

In order to provide a diet which is virtually free of proline the amino acid mixture is used as the major protein source. The remainder of the diet consists of fruit, vegetables and special low-protein foods, such as bread, cakes and sweets. The amount of proline in these foods is minimal and can be calculated as 5% of the protein (Table 9.2).

The amino acid mixture was mixed with Prosparol milk and given to the child throughout the day.

Table 9.1   Diet suitable for a 12 kg child (approximately 2 years),
giving 120 mg proline/kg/day

	Protein (g)	Proline (mg)
BREAKFAST		
Cereal (e.g. 14 g Rice Crispies)	0·8	42
Egg (50 g)	6·8	271
Sugar, Jam, Low protein bread (1 slice)		
Prosparol Milk, Tomor Koshor Margarine.		
LUNCH		
Beef (30 g)	7·0	265
Potato (90 g)	1·2	60
Vegetable, Low-protein sweet.		
TEA		
Egg (50 g)	6·8	271
Crisps (14 g)	0·8	34
Low-protein bread (1 slice), Tomato,		
Fruit, Tomor Koshor Margarine.		
THROUGHOUT DAY		
Cows milk (130 ml)	4·4	506
Total natural goods	27·8 g/day	1449 mg/day
10 g amino acid mixture (in Prosparol)	8·0	—
TOTAL	35·8 g/day	1449 mg/day
	= 2·96 g/kg	120 mg/kg

Table 9.2   Diet suitable for a 12 kg child (approximately 2 years), giving 10 mg proline/kg/day

	Protein (g)	*Proline* (mg)
BREAKFAST		
2 Liga Aminex	0·26	22
Tomtao (30 g)	0·3	15*
Prosparol, Low-protein bread, Tomor Koshor Margarine, Jam.		
LUNCH		
Potato (90 g)	1·2	43
Vegetable (60 g)	0·42	21*
Low protein sweet.		
TEA		
Tomato (30 g)	0·3	15*
Apple (100 g)	0·2	10*
Butter, Salad, Low-protein bread, Low-protein cakes.		
THROUGHOUT DAY		
Prosparol, squashes as required		
Total natural foods	2·68 g/day	126 mg/day
40 g amino acid mixture (in Prosparol)	32	—
TOTAL	34·68 g/day	126 mg/day
	= 2·87 g/kg	10 mg/kg

* Based on protein containing 5% proline

REFERENCES

1. Brodehl, J., Gellissen, K. and Jäkel, A. (1968). Endogenous renal transport of free amino acids in infancy and childhood. *Pediatrics*, **42**, 395
2. Scriver, C. R. and Davies, E. (1965). Endogenous renal clearance rates of free amino acids in pre-pubertal children. *Pediatrics*, **36**, 592
3. Scriver, C. R. and Rosenberg, L. E. (1973). *Amino Acid Metabolism and its Disorders*. Philadelphia: W. B. Saunders Co.
4. Young, J. A. and Freedman, B. S. (1971). Renal tubular transfer of amino acids. *Clinical Chemistry*, **17**, 245
5. Rosenburg, L. E., Downing, S., Durant, J. L. and Segal, S. (1966). Cystinuria: biochemical evidence for three genetically distinct diseases. *J. Clin. Invest.*, **45**, 365
6. Morikawa, T., Tada, K., Ando, T., Yoshida, T., Yokoyama, Y. and Arakawa, T. (1966). Prolinuria: defect in intestinal absorption of amino acids and glycine. *Tohoku J. Exp. Med.*, **90**, 105
7. Goodman, S. I., McIntyre, C. A. and O'Brien, D. (1967). Impaired intestinal transport of proline in a patient with familiar iminoaciduria. *J. Ped.*, **71**, 246
8. Scriver, C. R. (1972). Familial iminoglycinuria. In Stanbury, J. B., Wyngaarden, J. B. and Fredrickson, D. S. *The Metabolic Basis of Inherited Disease*, p. 1520. (New York: McGraw Hill.)
9. Wilson, O. H. and Scriver, C. R. (1967). Specificity of transport of neutral and basic amino acids in rat kidney. *Amer. J. Physiol.*, **213**, 185
10. Lin, E. C. C., Hagihira, H. and Wilson, T. H. (1962). Specificity of the transport system for neutral amino acids in the hamster intestine. *Amer. J. Physiol.*, **202**, 919
11. Finerman, G. A. M. and Rosenberg, L. E. (1966). Amino acid transport in bone: evidence of separate transport systems for neutral amino acids and imino acids. *J. Biol. Chem.*, **241**, 1487
12. Scriver, C. R., Efron, M. L. and Schafer, I. A. (1964). Renal tubular transport of proline, hydroxyproline and glycine in health and in familial hyperprolinemia. *J. Clin. Invest.*, **43**, 374
13. Efron, M. L., Bixby, E. M. and Pryles, C. V. (1965). Hydroxyprolinemia II A rare metabolic disease due to a deficiency of the enzyme hydroxyproline oxidase. *New Eng. J. Med.*, **272**, 1299
14. Joseph, R., Ribierre, M., Job, J.-C. and Girault, M. (1958). Maladie familiale associant des convulsions à début trés précoce une hyper-albuminorachie et une hyperaminoacidurie. *Arch. Franc. Pediat.*, **15**, 374
15. Tada, K., Morikawa, T., Ando, T., Yoshida, T. and Minagawa, A. (1965). Prolinuria: a new renal tubular defect in transport of proline and glycine. *Tohoku J. Exp. Med.*, **87**, 133
16. Scriver, C. R. and Wilson, O. H. (1967). Amino acid transport: evidence

for genetic control of two types in human kidney. *Science*, **155**, 1428

17. Scriver, C. R. (1968). Renal tubular transport of proline hydroxyproline and glycine III Genetic basis for more than one mode of transport in human kidney. *J. Clin. Invest.*, **47**, 823

18. Green, M. L., Lietman, P. S., Rosenberg, L. E. and Seegmiller, J. E. (1973). Familial hyperglycinuria: new defect in renal tubular transport of glycine and imino acids. *Amer. J. Med.*, **54**, 265

19. Scriver, C. R. and Goldman, H. (1966). Renal tubular transport of proline hydroxyproline and glycine II Hydroxy-L-proline as substrate and as inhibitor in vivo. *J. Clin. Invest.*, **45**, 1357

20. Mohyuddin, F. and Scriver, C. R. (1970). Amino acid transport in mammalian kidney: multiple systems for imino acids and glycine in rat kidney. *Amer. J. Physiol.*, **219**, 1

21. Cusworth, D. C. and Gattereau, A. (1968). Inhibition of renal tubular reabsorption of homocystine by lysine and arginine. *Lancet*, **ii**, 916

22. Cusworth, D. C. and Dent, C. E. (1969). Homocystinuria. In *New Aspetcs of Human Genetics. Brit. Med. Bull.*, **25**, 42

23. Emery, F. A., Goldie, L. and Stern, J. (1968). Hyperprolinaemia type 2. *J. Ment. Def. Res.*, **12**, 187

24. Goodman, S. I. (1970). Personal communication to Scriver, C. R. Disorders of proline and hydroxyproline metabolism. In Stanbury, J. B., Wyngaarden, J. B. and Fredrickson, D. S. *The Metabolic Basis of Inherited Disease*, p. 351 (New York: McGraw Hill.)

25. Applegarth, D. A., Ingram, P., Hingston, J. and Hardwick, D. F. (1974). Hyperprolinemia type 2. *Clin. Biochem.*, **7**, 14

26. Efron, M. L. (1965). Familial hyperprolinaemia. *New Eng. J. Med.*, **272**, 1243

27. Similä, S. (1970). Hyperprolinaemia type 2. *Annals Clin. Res.*, **2**, 143

28. Jeune, M., Collombel, C., Michel, M., David, M., Guibaud, P., Guerrier, G. and Albert, J. (1970). Hyperleucinisoleucinémie par défaut partiel de transamination associée a une hyperprolinémie de type 2. *Ann. Pédiat.*, **17**, 85

29. Goyer, R. A., Mitchell, B. J. and Leonard, D. L. (1969). Dietary reduction of hyperprolinaemia. *J. Lab. Clin. Med.*, **73**, 819

30. Harries, J. T., Piesowicz, A. T., Seakins, J. W. T., Francis, D. E. M. and Wolff, O. H. (1971). Low proline diet in type 1 hyperprolinaemia. *Arc. Dis. Chidh.*, **46**, 72

31. Similä, S. (1974). Dietary treatment in hyperprolinaemia type 2. *Acta Paed. Scand.*, **63**, 249

32. Efron, M. L., Bixby, E. M., Palattao, L. G. and Pryles, C. V. (1962). Hydroxyprolinemia associated with mental deficiency. *New Eng. J. Med.*, **267**, 1193

33. Pelkonen, R., Lahdevirla, J., Visakorpi, J. K. and Kivirikko, K. I. (1969).

Hydroxyprolinaemia: a case without mental deficiency. *Scand. J. Clin. Lab. Invest.*, **23** Supplement 108, p. 21

34. Pelkonen, R. and Kivirikko, K. I. (1970). Hydroxyprolinemia: an apparently harmless familial metabolic disorder. *New Eng. J. Med.*, **283**, 451

35. Raine, D. N. (1969). Screening for inherited metabolic disease. *Annals of Clinical Biochemistry*, **6**, 29

36. Raine, D. N. and Cooke, J. R. (1971). The role of automatic amino acid analysis in screening for inherited metabolic disease in *Automation in Analytical Chemistry*, Technicon Instruments Co. Ltd., 105

37. Raine, D. N. (1971). Defects in renal tubular reabsorption of amino acids. In Benson, P. F. *Cellular Organelles and Membranes in Mental Retardation*, p. 43 (Edinburgh: Churchill Livingstone)

38. Cooke, J. R. and Raine, D. N. (1973). Competetive inhibition of renal tubular transport in the treatment of prolinaemia and hydroxyrpolinaemia. In Seakins, J. W. T., Saunters, R. A. and Toothill, C. *Treatment of Inborn Errors of Metabolism*, p. 97 (Edinburgh: Churchill Livingstone)

39. Efron, M. L., Bixby, E. M., Hockaday, T. D. R., Smith, L. H. and Meshorer, E. (1968). Hydroxyprolinemia. III The origin of free hydroxyproline in hydroxyprolinemia: collagen turnover: evidence for a biosynthetic pathway in Man. *Biochem. Biophys. Acta*, **165**, 238

CHAPTER 10

New and Experimental Approaches to Treatment

D. N. Raine

For diseases that present only once every two or three years, the average paediatrician may justly be satisfied if he recognises them for what they are and fumbles in the literature for the latest paper on the condition. However, it is likely that, in time, many countries will establish nationally co-ordinated systems, including referal centres, which will accumulate a meaningful amount of experience in the course of a few years[1,2]. Such centres can reasonably expect to follow some sort of progression, each patient benefiting from the experience obtained with those preceding him. As there will be very few referal centres, it is probable that any useful developments will be made by the centre in partnership with a more local paediatrician, and so it is useful if the latter is aware, not only that rational forms of therapy (other than special diets) can be contemplated, but also of the main directions in which these are developing.

Before new and unknown measures are embarked upon, however, a few cautionary words will not be out of place.

First be sure that the condition to be treated is a disease and not just a coincidental biochemical abnormality. Cystathioninuria, iminogly-cinuria, and the syndrome of mental retardation, hiatus hernia and sucrosuria have all been shown to be spurious diseases and prolinaemia type 1 may soon join them.

Secondly, consider how it is to be established that the proposed treatment is effective. It is probable that nothing short of a controlled trial, in which half the patients are left untreated, will satisfy the rigours of science, but this can pose difficult ethical questions with respect to individual patients. Certainly those who first established the treatment of phenylketonuria in 1952, after their first successes, did not consider withholding treatment from any infant subsequently shown to have the biochemical abnormality. The absence of a suitably controlled trial was used 15 years later (unwisely, and perhaps unjustly), to challenge the need to treat infants with persistent phenylalaninaemia.

Thirdly, consider how the effects of the treatment are to be monitored, whether or not a stringent trial is to be made, it is a fundamental requirement that all relevant observations are made and recorded, for only then can the case be reviewed retrospectively and lessons learned from it. Moreover, it may be undesirable to change the procedure after every patient, and instead to follow the same protocol for two or three subjects in order to decide whether to retain or change a particular feature of the proposed treatment. The best safeguard is for the clinician to communicate fully with an experienced investigator, even to the extent of sacrificing a little of the clinical freedom he normally enjoys. It is essential, of course, that the investigator understands the pressures and constraint that patient care imposes on the clinician.

Fourthly, it is necessary for an ethical framework to be established within which the work can proceed, the absence of any significant amount of case law has allowed the legal considerations with regard to minors to have an inhibitory effect on any experimental work involving children. But this must be balanced against the need of any branch of medicine, including paediatrics, to progress and any law that prevented this would be wholly unacceptable. These questions have been ventilated by, amongst others, Franklin, Porter and Raine[3].

The forms in which the treatment of inherited metabolic disease is developing range from simple improvements in dietary treatments already established in some form or other, to devices that border on the bizarre. Essentially two approaches can be made. In one the objective is to remove the noxious substance, usually that demonstrated to be present in increased concentration although this may not have been shown to be harmful and its return to normal may not be, by itself, beneficial. Removal of the accumulating substrate is mainly, and so far most effectively, achieved by manipulation of the diet so that the patient ingests only sufficient for his needs. However, an alternative is to prevent the reabsorption of the substance across the renal tubules and this has proved sufficiently practicable to be treated more fully in a separate chapter.

The second approach is, since these diseases are due to a defective enzyme, to introduce into the patient by various means a normally functioning enzyme. Attempts have been made to replace the defective

enzyme by intraperitoneal injection of normal enzyme, by transfusions of plasma and of leucocytes from normal subjects, and, more
recently, by infusion of normal enzymes embedded in liposomes.
Enzymes have been enclosed in permeable microcapsules with the
intention of passing the patient's arterial blood through a column of
these so that the accumulated substrate can be cleared before the blood
is returned to a vein. Problems arise from the instability of enzymes
and from their ability to act as antigens. Some of these are overcome
by causing normal cell lines to become established in the patient and
the most successful of these attempts have been with bone marrow
transplants. It is not impossible that this can be extended to implantation of normal cells in organs such as the liver and spleen. A gross form
of cell implantation is, of course, organ transplantation and this has
been attempted in more than one inherited metabolic disease with some
success. Other forms of genetic manipulation intended to result in an
endogenous increase in enzyme activity are still in the earliest stages of
development.

SPECIAL DIETS

Although dietary treatment of enzyme deficiency diseases has found
the widest application so far, this form of therapy has had to evolve,
and the several general points emphasised in Chapter 1, could only be
made in the light of clinical experience. The recent change from
hydrolysed casein and soya protein to mixtures of pure L-amino acids
has greatly improved the palatability of these special diets, but anyone
who has experience of these will agree that there is still room for
improvement in flavour as well as in the variety of preparations
available for the older child. Parents as well as dietitians will continue
to experiment and to share their experience on matters that, at
first sight, seem remote from medical care but which may be
crucial for the continuation of the treatment for the required number
of years.

For diseases other than phenylketonuria, galactosaemia and homocystinuria, there has been very little comparable development. Low
proline diets are still very difficult to achieve satisfactorily and very
little has been written on the low-protein diets that can be life-saving
in infants with the several hyperammonaemia syndromes. It is always
valuable if those with experience of such patients are as detailed in

their reports of these aspects of care as they are in describing the medical and scientific observations.

RENAL TUBULAR BLOCK

The concept that abnormally high concentrations of metabolites may be lowered by inhibiting their reabsorption in the renal tubule has been established for homocystine, proline and hydroxyproline. The principles involved and the methods adopted in the few patients studied so far are described in the previous chapter and the method is referred to again only because it is capable of extension to other diseases.

METABOLIC INTERFERENCE

The advent of cell culture techniques, particularly with cells grown from patients with storage diseases in which the product can be demonstrated in the fibroblasts, has led to the discovery that altering the environment of the cells can greatly influence the rate of accumulation of the stored material. Such changes in the environment may be as simple as changing the pH of the culture medium[4], but the effects of vitamins A and C, steroids and some synthetic chemicals on certain cultured cells have all been sufficiently encouraging for them to be used in clinical trials.

The *mucopolysaccharidoses* have been prominent subjects in these therapeutic attempts. This arose from the observation that *ascorbic acid* stimulated the already abnormal accumulation of dermatan sulphate in Hurler fibroblasts but did not do so in normal fibroblasts[5]. It was, therefore, argued that a Hurler patient deprived of ascorbic acid might accumulate less mucopolysaccharide and be better for this. Such has not proved to be so (see *Mucopolysaccharidosis type 1) and careful consideration of the basis of these studies, in fact, provides little hope of any real benefit[6,7].

The same approach has been made with *vitamin A* again on an ill-understood, if not confused, scientific basis, and again the clinical and even the biochemical effects have not been encouraging (see *Mucopolysaccharidosis types, 1, 2, 3 and 4). Treatment of the mucopolysaccharidoses with *corticosteroids* has been attempted with more encouraging clinical improvement (see *Mucopolysaccharidosis type 1) but possibly because of the harmful effects of the large doses needed, there are few reports with this treatment.

Metachromatic leucodystrophy has been treated by restricting *vitamin A* with equivocal results. At best, deterioration may be arrested but it is doubtful if any long-term benefit results from this treatment*.

In *cystinosis*, cystine crystals accumulate in cells both in the patient and in culture, and the latter at least have been shown to be affected by a soluble non-toxic SH compound *dithiothreitol**. Biochemical improvement has been reported in one patient who died from the advanced state of his disease after only four weeks' treatment. The basis of this treatment is similar to that with *penicillamine*, where occasional dramatic improvements have encouraged trials of this and similar drugs to continue*.

PARENTERAL ADMINISTRATION OF ENZYMES

Foreign proteins injected parenterally accumulate in lysosomal vacuoles by a process of pinocytosis[8-11]. Attempts to use this form of enzyme replacement were reported as much as a decade ago at a time when the role of lysosomes in the pathogenesis of storage diseases was barely established. Hers and his colleagues[12] gave eight intramuscular injections of a fungal α-glucosidase to a child with type 2 glycogen storage disease over the last three days of life. The effects of this were uncertain and somewhat unexpected and the possibility that the reduction in free rather than lysosomal glycogen was a post-mortem change could not be excluded.

Animal studies continued, and it was clearly established that fungal α-glucosidase, injected intraperitoneally into rats, is taken up by liver, kidney, spleen, heart and skeletal muscle and, in liver and spleen at least, remained for at least four days. The glycogen content of the liver in these normal animals was substantially reduced as a result of the injection[13]. In the same year (1967) intravenous injection, over 18 days, of fungal α-glucosidase into a patient with type 2 glycogen storage disease reduced the liver glycogen concentration to normal*.

Similar treatment with α-glucosidase was attempted in the terminal weeks in a child with type 4 glycogen storage disease and again the liver content of glycogen was dramatically reduced*.

In parallel with these studies in polysaccharide storage diseases, enzyme replacement has been examined in acatalasia in mice where subcutaenous injection of catalase protected these animals against an otherwise lethal dose of hydrogen peroxide[14]. Uricase, again of fungal origin, has been used to reduce the uricaemia and to abort acute attacks in patients with tophaceous gout, but one patient showed an allergic reaction to the enzyme and another sustained an acute attack immediately after cessation of treatment[15].

PLASMA AND LEUCOCYTE INFUSIONS

Whatever the mode of action of enzymes placed in the peritoneal cavity might be, there is experimental evidence that proteins injected into the circulation can reach parenchymal liver cells and be metabolised by, and perhaps enter into, the lysosomes of these cells. In contrast, denatured protein and non-enzymic proteins such as haemoglobin are preferentially removed by reticuloendothelial cells[16]. Such a situation is more than could have been hoped for by those making the first attempts at enzyme replacement therapy and only studies in which the accumulated substrate was small enough to diffuse towards the enzymes could have been embarked upon with any confidence[14,15].

An early attempt to treat two patients with lecithin–cholesterol acyltransferase deficiency by infusions of plasma resulted in only a slight and transient increase in the concentration of cholesterol esters, but the evidence indicated that these had been formed from lecithin*, and hence the transfused enzyme had been active. Fresh plasma infusions were given to two patients with Fabry's disease (angiokeratoma) with rather better effect. The enzyme persisted in the patient's plasma for 7 days and, 10 days after infusion, the concentration of the abnormal ceramide trihexoside was half that before treatment*.

The most frequent infusion studies and those with the most promising results have been with patients with a mucopolysaccharidosis. Infusions of plasma were made even before the specific enzyme defects associated with these diseases were known and studies have now been made in patients with the Hurler (*Mucopolysaccharidosis type 1), Hunter (*Mucopolysaccharidosis type 2) and Sanfilippo (*Mucopolysaccharidosis type 3) syndromes. Results were monitored in terms of the amount of urinary glycosaminoglycans excreted, and the proportions of these with high and low molecular weight. Where success was claimed the total amount sometimes increased and sometimes decreased, but the low molecular weight fragments were increased at the expense of the high. Observations on clinical improvement have not been well controlled, but sometimes there have been dramatic improvements in joint mobility and in the general mobility of the patient.

It is reasonable to suppose that enzyme administration in the more protected form of leucocyte infusions might have a greater or more lasting effect than that obtained with plasma. This has been studied in a child with mucopolysaccharidosis type 2[*], and some unpublished observations (Raine and Stephenson) in a patient with metachromatic leucodystrophy have shown that enzyme activity can be significantly increased for three weeks by infusions of separated leucocytes.

Encouraging and discouraging reports of infusion studies occur in about equal numbers but there is little point in reviewing these in detail, for two reasons. The first is a suggestion that any effects that have occurred depended not on enzymic but on osmotic changes following the infusions and that after an infusion of dextran 70 in a patient with mucopolysaccharidosis type 3, there resulted 'a remarkable decrease in the hepatosplenomegaly and the patient's behaviour is now more alert and quiet'[17]. Similar studies in a patient with mucopolysaccharidosis type 5, however, were less clear.

The second reason why judgment of these early trials may be premature is the study by Figura and Kresse[18] of the rate of uptake of enzyme by fibroblasts from a patient with Sanfilippo B disease. If the rates observed in the cultured cells are typical, these authors calculated that to increase the enzyme content of the deficient cells to half normal values requires 150 ml plasma, or 35×10^9 leucocytes per *gram* of cells. Although a marked therapeutic effect can be expected from only a 10% increase in enzyme activity, it is clear that insufficient enzyme has been administered in the clinical studies performed so far, and means of increasing this, perhaps by administering fractionated serum proteins[19], should be sought.

ENZYME ADMINISTRATION IN LIPOSOMES

Liposomes are droplets of phospholipid and cholesterol formed in the presence of water, and they consist of concentric lipid bilayers separated by water into which various solutes can be introduced. They were first used as models in studies of membrane transport[20]. The value of these particles for introducing into cells, by a process of pinocytosis, therapeutic agents which, otherwise, would not easily cross membranes, has been explored in the case of chelating agents in the treatment of heavy metal intoxication[21,22].

The use of liposomes to restore enzyme activity to cells with a genetic deficiency has been examined by Gregoriadis and Ryman and their colleagues[23,24]. A number of enzymes have been satisfactorily incorporated into liposomes and these injected intravenously into experimental animals. Subsequent examination of the organs radiochemically, immunochemically, and by study of enzyme activity, has shown that more than half of the injected enzymes reaches the liver and spleen within 12 hours, and thereafter declines only slowly over the next few days. It is probable that the enzyme becomes incorporated into the lysosomes as the structure of the injected liposomes is destroyed[25,26].

Experiments with cultured macrophages and fibroblasts, which lack invertase and which have been caused to incorporate sucrose, have shown that liposomes containing invertase can free these cells of the sucrose-induced vacuoles within 24 hours[27]. Such studies demonstrate that enzymes can be introduced into the very organelles normally responsible for preventing storage of metabolites, and the extent to which this principle can be applied to the treatment of storage disorders of the liver and perhaps of the brain in animals and man will be awaited with interest.

ENCAPSULATED AND ISOLUBILISED ENZYMES

Since 1956 Professor T. M. S. Chang[28] has been making artificial model cells in the form of microcapsules of collodion, nylon and other materials, containing mixtures of enzymes, haemoglobin and other agents of physiological significance. There are many possible applications of these capsules, the manufacture of which is now well standardised, and Chang and his colleagues have used capsules containing catalase to treat a strain of mice with a genetic form of acatalasaemia[29] and have treated uraemic dogs over many months with capsules containing urease.

The capsules can be placed in the peritoneal cavity or incorporated in an extra-corporeal unit placed between an artery and vein. Even intravenous injection has been tried but this has not been satisfactory, although even here it is clear that alteration of the membrane material could lead to significant improvement. There are still substantial problems, however, although these are mainly mechanical, and problems relating to coagulation and platelet survival have proved less serious than expected. Applications are being explored in adults, where the mechanics of maintaining an arterio-venous shunt have been partly overcome but this is likely to delay the application of this form of enzyme therapy in children.

The same problems may reduce the extent to which another form of extracorporeal enzyme therapy will be utilised, namely enzymes bound to a solid matrix. These can exist in several forms, the first of which was granules of resin, but now enzymes have been bound to plastic sheets[30] and it is conceivable that these could be placed in the peritoneum and renewed at intervals. Already a wide range of enzymes have been insolubilised in this way, and their stability is sometimes greater than that of unbound enzymes placed in the same environment. Because these materials have industrial uses it is likely that their further development will be active and their potential in the treatment of a number of metabolic disorders has been reviewed by Cederholm-Williams[31].

ENZYME INDUCTION BY VIRUSES

In the course of experiments with the Shope papilloma virus it was noted that in some workers exposed to the virus the concentration of arginine in the plasma was diminished and that this was associated with an increase in the arginase activity of the blood[32]. This phenomenon is believed to be brought about by a mechanism analogous to that by which bacteriophage causes bacteria to produce bacteriophage protein rather than bacterial protein, that is the viral RNA or DNA in preference to the cells own RNA and DNA, influences the ribosomes synthesising the enzyme protein—a process known as transduction.

Transduction with natural nuclear material is well established, but the possibility of combining genetic information in the form of synthetic nucleotide sequences with natural nucleic acid has also been achieved by Rogers and Pfuderer[33]. These workers added poly-adenine (A) to tobacco mosaic virus RNA and from plants infected with this material they were able to isolate poly-lysine, the genetic code for which is (AAA).

This process was taken a stage further when Merril, Geier and Petricciani[34] infected cultured fibroblasts from a patient with galactosaemia with a virus containing the genetic information for the synthesis of the missing galactose-1-phosphate uridyl transferase. Activity of this enzyme could barely be detected in the galactosaemic cells whereas after infection nearly normal activity was achieved over 4 days, and after treatment with viral DNA instead of whole virus the activity was even greater.

An attempt has been made to utilise this concept in the treatment of argininaemia using the Shope virus, with which the original observations were made, by Van Sande and his colleagues[35].

GENETIC ENGINEERING

The concept of manipulating the genome is a highly emotive one that is well treated in the Sunday Press and it would be a pity to emphasise in this Chapter a topic that many believe impossible, or if possible, one they would rather be without. However, many new developments have passed through a phase that bordered on science fiction, and it remains to be seen what will happen with this one. Suffice it to say that there is sufficient awareness of the dangers of such developments to ensure that a great deal of effort will be made to minimise them, and it is doubtful if potential dangers have ever wholly prevented developments from which some good could be anticipated. Indeed there are natural mechanisms for the repair of damaged genetic material, and it is probable that the cutaneous and the neurological forms of xeroderma pigmentosum are consequences of different deficiencies of an enzyme essential for the repair of DNA[36].

Apart from such natural repair processes, the possibility that DNA can be incorporated into cells and the altered genome transmitted to daughter cells clearly exists in mammals[37] as well as in more primitive species. Even if such direct intervention with the genome is not utilised it is possible that a patient's own deficient cells may be corrected in this way before being reintroduced into the patient, thereby overcoming the immunological problems that at present cause the greatest difficulty in correcting genetic defects by transplantation of normal tissues.

CELL AND BONE-MARROW TRANSPLANTS

The possibility of treating inherited deficiencies of either enzymes or other functional proteins by transplanting normal tissue was appreciated more than 10 years ago, and because experiments with cellular infusions could be made more easily and were, perhaps, less hazardous to the patient, these took precedence over whole organ transplants which could be expected to be just as feasible and equally beneficial.

Immunological deficiency diseases were the first models. Hitzig, Kay and Cottier[38] treated two infants with the severe Swiss form of agammaglobulinaemia by transplanting whole thymus tissue with various combinations of infusions of bone marrow, thymus cells and liver cells and obtained clear, but brief, evidence of a functional response. Bone-marrow infusion into a similar infant in Kentucky was unsuccessful[39] but another in Boston responded to bone-marrow infusions for a few weeks[40]. Greater attention to the histocompatability of the transfused bone marrow gave better results in the sex-linked form of this disease[41] and the Wiskott–Aldrich syndrome[42].

The possibility of transplanting cells of other types by intravenous infusion, after which it is reported, the cells can recognise their histogenetic type, has been explored by Desai[43] in haemophilia A and von Willebrand's disease (factor VIII deficiency) and in haemophilia B (factor IX deficiency) and again early reports are encouraging. The appropriate coagulation factors increased to a functional extent and the amount of treatment required prior to cell infusion was significantly reduced for at least 6 months.

Whatever the outcome of whole organ transplant studies, further work on cellular transplantation will be justified by the fact that this form of treatment is technically more simple, likely to be more available, and can be repeated with less disturbance to the recipient, provided the remaining immunological problems can be satisfactorily overcome.

ORGAN TRANSPLANTS

Treatment of enzyme deficiency diseases by organ transplant may involve one or both of two principles. In the first, if the deficient enzyme is normally confined to one organ, as in phenylketonuria, replacement of the defective organ by one from a normal subject can be expected to cure the disease. However, the second is demonstrated by the discovery that patients with Fabry's disease, in whom renal transplantation was performed because the disease had advanced to the point of chronic renal failure, the transplanted kidney functioned not only as an excretory organ but also as a reservoir of enzyme activity preventing further deposition of the abnormal lipid in tissues that were still devoid of the enzyme. This concept of an implanted functional source of enzyme activity is clearly of widespread application.

Some of the earliest organ transplants in man aimed at correcting an inherited deficiency disease were those patients with immune deficiency diseases already referred to, in whom thymus tissue was transplanted into skeletal muscle. Two patients, with aplasia of the thymus and parathyroid glands (DiGeorge's syndrome) showed immunological competence after a thymus transplant[44,45].

Extension of organ transplants beyond the thymus has been encouraged by the results of experimental work in animals. Thus spleen and liver transplants in haemophilic dogs have resulted in restoration of the clotting factors[46-48] and preparations of the islets of Langerhans have been successfully transplanted beneath the renal capsule in rat and rabbit[49]. Similar preparations injected intraperitoneally have restored the blood sugar of alloxan diabetic rats to normal for one month[50]. Liver has been transplanted into Gunn rats deficient in bilirubin uridine diphosphate glucuronyl transferase: 3 months later plasma bilirubin was normal and the enzyme activity was substantial, not only in the transplanted lobe but also in the residual lobe which previously had been shown to be devoid of enzyme activity[51].

Liver transplantation has been performed in an 11-year-old boy with Wilson's disease in terminal hepatic failure. Seventeen months later there was no abnormal accumulation of copper in the transplanted organ[52]. Following the encouraging experiments with spleen transplants in animals, a patient with Gaucher's disease has been treated in this way, but without success[53].

The results of renal transplantation in patients and an affected heterozygote with Fabry's disease have been the most satisfactory so far. A 38-year-old man in chronic renal failure has survived transplantation for 2 years. The activity of α-galactosidase previously absent from the plasma has increased to a tenth of normal, sufficient to lower the plasma concentration of trihexoside to normal. Clinically the patient was relieved from attacks of pain, had more energy and, previously anhidrotic, began to sweat normally[54]. In an affected female heterozygote (the disease is sex-linked) a kidney was transplanted at the same time as splenectomy was performed: her own kidneys were retained. A male hemizygote who was being maintained on dialysis following bilateral nephrectomy also received a successful transplant. Both patients, when reported on 6 months later, were relieved of the excruciating pain associated with this disease, and the abnormal lipid in plasma and desquamated cells from the renal tract was restored to normal concentrations[55]. However, before generalising too far from these early results, it is interesting to note that the plasma concentration of ceramide trihexoside had been reduced to normal in one patient by a period of renal dialysis[55], and a careful study in a fourth patient has shown that not only the concentration of ceramide trihexoside but also that of its precursor, globoside, is reduced by renal transplantation[56]. This allows the possibility that the improvement may be partly due to diminished formation of the abnormal lipid and not entirely due to the effects of the transplanted enzyme.

Renal transplantation has been performed in at least five children with cystinosis* with relief of the amino aciduria. The extra-renal components of the disease, such as cystine deposits in the cornea and other tissues, were not improved, however, and cystine deposits were later found to have occurred in the allograft, although their distribution in the transplanted kidney differed from that seen in the patient's own organ. Transplantation in a patient with idiopathic Fanconi syndrome also resulted in the disease recurring in the allograft[57].

CONCLUSION

There are more than sufficient approaches to treatment already being made, quite apart from any new ones that may be devised to justify an optimistic view, and it can be confidently expected that in a generation the question 'what is the use of looking for them if you cannot do anything to treat them?' still voiced although, even now, no longer relevant, will have long since ceased to be asked of inherited metabolic disease and will refer to some other developing branch of medicine.

REFERENCES

* To avoid duplication, references for statements marked with an asterisk are listed in the section *Treatment of Other Inherited Metabolic Diseases*, page 265, and can be recognised by their titles under the heading of the disease to which they relate.

1. Scriver, C. R., Clow, C. L. and Lamm, P. (1973). On the screening, diagnosis and investigation of hereditary amino acidopathies. *Clinical Biochemistry*, **6**, 142

2. Raine, D. N. (1974). The need for a national policy for the management of inherited metabolic disease. *Molecular Variants in Disease*. Supplement to *Journal of Clinical Pathology*, to be published.

3. Franklin, A. W., Porter, A. M. W. and Raine, D. N. (1973). Research investigations in children. *Brit. Med. J.*, **2**, 402

4. Lie, S. O., McKusick, V. A. and Neufeld, E. F. (1972). Simulation of genetic mucopolysaccharidoses in normal human fibroblasts by alteration of medium pH. *Proc. Nat. Acad. Sci. U.S.A.*, **69**, 2361

5. Schafer, I. A., Sullivan, J. C., Svejcar, J., Kofoed, J. and Robertson, W. van B. (1966). Vitamin C induced increase of dermatan sulfate in cultured Hurler's fibroblasts. *Science*, **153**, 1008

6. Kofoed, J. A. and Robertson, W. van B. (1966). Ascorbic acid and the synthesis of chondroitin sulphate. *Biochim. Biophys. Acta*, **124**, 86

7. Bates, C. J., Levene, C. I. and Kodicek, E. (1969). The effect of scurvy on hexosamine-containing substances in healing wounds of guinea pigs. *Biochem. J.*, **113**, 783

8. Strauss, W. (1958). Colorimetric analysis with *N,N*-dimethyl-*p*-phenyl-enediamine of the uptake of intravenously injected horseradish peroxidase by various tissues of the rat. *J. Biophys. Biochem. Cytol.*, **4**, 541

9. Miller, F. (1962). Acid phosphatase localisation in renal protein absorption droplets in *Proc. 5th Int. Cong. Electron Microscopy*, Vol. 2, p. Q-2 (New York: Academic Press)

10. Jacques, P. (1963). Endocytose dune protéine étrangère par le foie du rat. *Arch. Int. Physiol. Biochem.*, **71**, 306

11. Straus, W. (1963). Comparative observations on lysosomes and phago-somes in kidney and liver of rats after administration of horseradish peroxidase in *Ciba Foundation Symposium on Lysosomes*, p. 151 (London: J. & A. Churchill)

12. Baudhuin, P., Hers, H. G. and Loeb, H. (1964). An electron microscopic and biochemical study of type II glycogenosis. *Lab. Invest.*, **13**, 1139

13. Cuthbertson, W. F. J., Fleming, I. D. and Rice, M. S. (1967). Effect of glucamylase on tissue glycogen and tissue glucamylase in the rat. *Biochem. J.*, **103**, 307

14. Feinstein, R. N., Braun, J. T. and Howard, J. B. (1966). Reversal of H_2O_2 toxicity in the acatalasemic mouse by catalase administration: suggested model for possible replacement therapy of inborn errors of metabolism. *J. Lab. Clin. Med.*, **68**, 952

15. Kissel, P., Lamarche, M. and Royer, R. (1968). Modification of uricaemia and the excretion of uric acid nitrogen by an enzyme of fungal origin. *Nature (London)*, **217**, 72

16. Gregoriadis, G., Morell, A. G., Sternlieb, I. and Scheinberg, I. H. (1970). Catabolism of desialylated ceruloplasmin in the liver. *J. Biol. Chem.*, **245**, 5833

17. Rostenberg, I., Hernandez-Tellez, A., Romero-Villasenor, G., Mora, G., Guizar-Vazquez, J. and Cantu, J. M. (1973). Effects of dextran 70 (Macrodex) in a type III mucopolysaccharidosis. *Ann. Genet.*, **16**, 121

18. Figura, K. von, and Kresse, H. (1974). Quantitative aspects of pinocytosis and the intracellular fate of N-acetyl-α-D-glucosaminidase in Sanfilippo B fibroblasts. *J. Clin. Invest.*, **53**, 85

19. Coppa, G. V., Singh, J., Nichols, B. L. and DiFerrante, N. (1973). Urinary excretion of disulfated disaccharides in Hunter syndrome: correction by infusion of a serum fraction. *Analyt. Lett.*, **6**, 225

20. Bangham, A. D., Standish, M. M. and Watkins, J. C. (1965). Diffusion of univalent ions across the lamellae of swollen phospholipids. *J. Molec. Biol.*, **13**, 238

21. Rahman, Y. E., Rosenthal, M. W. and Cerny, E. A. (1973). Intracellular plutonium: removal by liposome-encapsulated chelating agents. *Science*, **180**, 300

22. Rahman, Y. E., Rosenthal, M. W., Cerny, E. A. and Moretti, E. S. (1974). Preparation and prolonged tissue retention of liposome-encapsulated chelating agents. *J. Lab. Clin. Med.*, **83**, 640

23. Gregoriadis, G., Leathwood, P. D., and Ryman, B. E. (1971). Enzyme entrapment in liposomes. *FEBS Lett.* **14**, 95

24. Gregoriadis, G. and Ryman, B. E. (1972). Fate of protein-containing liposomes injected into rats. *Eur. J. Biochem.*, **24**, 485

25. Gregoriadis, G. and Ryman, B. E. (1972). Lysosomal localisation of β-fructofuranosidase-containing liposomes injected into rats. *Biochem. J.*, **129**, 123

26. Gregoriadis, G. and Ryman, B. E. (1973). Possible use of liposomes in enzyme replacement therapy. (J. W. T. Seakins, R. A. Saunders and C. Toothill, editors) *Treatment of Inborn Errors of Metabolism*, p. 203 (Edinburgh: Churchill Livingstone)

27. Gregoriadis, G. and Buckland, R. A. (1973). Enzyme-containing liposomes alleviate a model for storage disease. *Nature (London)*, **244**, 170

28. Chang, T. M. S. (1972) *Artificial Cells.* (Springfield: Charles C. Thomas)

29. Chang, T. M. S. and Poznansky, M. J. (1968). Semipermeable micro-capsules containing catalase for enzyme replacement in acatalasaemic mice. *Nature (London)*, **218**, 243

30. Wilson, R. J. H., Kay, G. and Lilly, M. D. (1968). The preparation and properties of pyruvate kinase attached to porous sheets and the operation of a two-enzyme continuous-feed reactor. *Biochem. J.*, **109**, 137

31. Cederholm-Williams, S. A. (1973). Insoluble enzymes: therapeutic potential. (J. W. T. Seakins, R. A. Saunders and C. Toothill, editors) *Treatment of Inborn Errors of Metabolism*, p. 195 (Edinburgh: Churchill Livingstone)

32. Rogers, S. (1966). Shope papilloma virus: a passenger in man and its significance to the potential control of the host genome. *Nature (London)*, **212**, 1220

33. Rogers, S. and Pfuderer, P. (1968). Use of viruses as carriers of added genetic information. *Nature (London)*, **219**, 749

34. Merril, C. R., Geier, M. R. and Petricciani, J. C. (1971). Bacterial virus gene expression in human cells. *Nature (London)*, **233**, 398

35. van Sande, M., Terheggen, H. G., Clara, R., Leroy, J. G. and Lowenthal, A. (1971). Lysine-cystine pattern associated with neurological disorders. (N. A. J. Carson and D. N. Raine, editors) *Inherited Disorders of Sulphur Metabolism*, p. 85 (London: Churchill Livingstone)

36. Patterson, M. C., Lohman, P. H. M., Westerveld, A. and Sleuyter, M. L. (1974). DNA repair monitored by an enzymatic assay in multinucleate xeroderma pigmentosum cells after fusion. *Nature (London)*, **248**, 50

37. Petricciani, J. C. and Patterson, R. M. (1974). Incorporation of exogenous DNA into mammalian chromosomes. *Nature (London)*, **249**, 649

38. Hitzig, W. H., Kay, H. E. M. and Cottier, H. (1965). Familial lymphopenia with agammaglobulinaemia: an attempt at treatment by implantation with foetal thymus. *Lancet*, **ii**, 151

39. Hathaway, W. E., Brangle, R. W., Nelson, T. L. and Roeckel, I. E. (1966). Aplastic anemia and alymphocytosis in an infant with hypogamma-globulinemia: graft-versus-host reaction? *J. Ped.*, **68**, 713

40. Rosen, F. S., Gotoff, S. P., Craig, J. M., Ritchie, J. and Janeway, C. A. (1965). Further observations of the Swiss type of agammaglobulinaemia (alymphocytosis). The effect of synergic bone marrow cells. *New Eng. J. Med.*, **274**, 18

41. Gatti, R. A., Meuwissen, H. J., Allen, H. D., Hong, R. and Good, R. A. (1968). Immunological reconstitution of sex-linked lymphopenic immuno-logical deficiency, *Lancet*, **ii**, 1366

42. Bach, F. H., Albertini, R. J., Joo, P., Anderson, J. L. and Bortin, M. M. (1968). Bone-marrow transplantation in a patient with the Wiskott-Aldrich syndrome. *Lancet*, **ii**, 1364

43. Editorial (1969). Hemophilia treated with spleen cells. *J. Amer. Med. Ass.*, **207**, 1267

44. August, C. S., Rosen, F. S., Filler, R. M., Janeway, C. A., Markowski, B. and Kay, H. E. M. (1968). Implantation of a foetal thymus restoring immunological competence in a patient with thymic aplasia (DiGeorge's syndrome). *Lancet*, **ii**, 1210

45. Cleveland, W., W., Fogel, B. J., Brown, W. T. and Kay, H. E. M. (1968). Foetal thymic transplant in a case of DiGeorge's syndrome. *Lancet*, **ii**, 1211

46. Webster, W. P., Penick, G. D., Peacock, E. E. and Brinkhous, K. M. (1967). Allo-transplantation of spleen in hemophilia. *North Carolina Med. J.*, **28**, 505

47. Norman, J. C., Covelli, V. H. and Sise, H. S. (1968). Transplantation of the spleen: experimental cure of hemophilia. *Surgery*, **64**, 1

48. Marchioro, T. L., Hougie, C., Ragde, H., Epstein, R. B. and Thomas, E. D. (1969). Hemophilia: role of organ homografts. *Science*, **163**, 188

49. Thomas, D. R., Fox, M. and Grieve, A. A. (1973). Isolation of the islets of Langerhans for transplantation. *Nature (London)*, **242**, 258

50. Younoszai, R., Sorenson, R. L. and Lindall, A. W. (1970). Homotransplantation of isolated pancreatic islets. *Diabetes*, 19, Suppl. 1, 406

51. Mukherjee, A. B. and Krasner, J. (1973). Induction of an enzyme in genetically deficient rats after grafting of normal liver. *Science*, **182**, 68

52. DuBois, R. S. *et al.* (1971). Orthotopic liver transplantation for Wilson's disease. *Lancet*, **i**, 505

53. Groth, C.G., Hagenfeldt, L., Dreborg, S., Löfström, B., Öckerman, P. A., Samuelsson, K., Svennerholm, L., Werner, K. and Westberg, G. (1971). Splenic transplantation in a case of Gaucher's disease. *Lancet*, **i**, 1260.

54. Philipart, M., Franklin, S. S. and Gordon, A. (1972). Reversal of an inborn sphinoglipidosis (Fabry's disease) by kidney transplantation. *Ann. Intern. Med.*, **77**, 195

55. Desnick, R. J., Simmons, R. L., Allen, K. Y., Woods, J. E., Anderson, C. F., Najarian, J. S. and Krivit, W. (1972). Correction of enzymatic deficiencies by renal transplantation, Fabry's disease. *Surgery*, **72**, 203

56. Clarke, J. T. R., Guttmann, R. D., Wolfe, L. S., Beaudoin, J. G. and Morehouse, D. D. (1972). Enzyme replacement therapy by renal allo-transplantation in Fabry's disease. *New Eng. J. Med.*, **287**, 1215

57. Briggs, W. A., Kominami, N., Wilson, R. E. and Merrill, J. P. (1972). Kidney transplantation in Fanconi syndrome. *New Eng. J. Med.*, **286**, 25

MANUFACTURED PRODUCTS USEFUL IN THE TREATMENT OF INHERITED METABOLIC DISEASE

The information in this table is intended to help those unfamiliar with the products to obtain them with a minimum of delay. Inclusion of a product should not be interpreted as a recommendation either of the product itself or of its suitability for the treatment of the disease under which it is listed. Almost all require supplementing in some way and the manufacturer's literature or some other guide should be studied carefully.

The list is revised from that first published in Raine, D. N. Management of Inherited Metabolic Disease, *Brit. Med. J.*, **2** (1972), 329, but even now it is incomplete and unrepresentative of certain parts of the world. The Editor would appreciate any information that would make the list more useful.

Disorder	Preparation	Manu-facturer
Galactosaemia	Comminuted Chicken Meat	U
	Galactomin 17 or 18	U
	Gerber MBF	MG
	Lactostrict	CCF
	Nutri-Soja	N
	Promine-D	N
	Similac-Isomil	AL
	Velactin	W
Galactose–glucose intolerance	Galactomin 19	U
Glycinaemia, nonketotic	GPS-AM	MG
Histidinaemia	Albumaid Histidine Low	SHS
	Formula HF(2)	U
	H-AM	MG
	Histidon	N
Homocystinuria	Albumaid X Methionine	SHS
	Cystinex	N
	Nutri-Soja	N
	Promine-D	N
Isovaleric acidaemia	ILV-AM	MG

Disorder	Preparation	Manufacturer
Lactose intolerance	Comminuted Chicken Meat	U
	Galactomin 17 or 18	U
	Gerber MBF	MG
	Lactalac M	CCF
	Lactalac V	CCF
	Nutri-Soja	N
	Nutrilose	N
	Nutricid	N
	Similac-Isomil	AL
	Velactin	W
Maple syrup urine disease	Formula VLIF (1)	U
	ILV-AM	MG
	Leucidon	N
	MSUD Aid	SHS
Methioninaemia	Albumaid X Methionine	SHS
	Cystinex	N
	Fomula LPTM (2)	U
	Nutri-Soja	N
	Promine-D	N
β–Methyl-crotonyl-glycinuria	ILV-AM	MG
Methylmalonic aciduria	IMTV-AM	MG
Phenylketonuria	Albumaid XP	SHS
	Aminogran	AH
	Cymogran	AH
	Minafen	U
	P-AM	MG
	PK Aid No. 1	SHS
	Phenistrict A	CCF
	Phenistrict B	CCF
	Phenistrict C	CCF
	Phenyldon	N
Prolinaemia	MP 1 HPD	SHS
	Pro-AM	MG
Propionic acidaemia	ILV-AM	MG
Tyrosinaemia	Albumaid X Phenylalanine and Tyrosine	SHS
	Formula LPT (1)	U
	Formula LPTM (2)	U
	PT-AM	MG
	Tyrosidon	N
	Tyrostrict	CCF
Valinaemia	ILV-AM	MG

Other Preparations of Value

Preparation		Manufacturer
Fat emulsion	Prosparol	DF
Glucose polymers	Caloreen	SHS
	Fantomalt	N
	Gastrocaloreen	SHS
	Hycal	B
	Nutrical	N
Gluten-free products	Aglutella Gentili	DFS
	Aproten Anellini	CE
	Aproten Crispbread	CE
	Aproten Flour	CE
	Aproten Gluten-free Semolina	CE
	Aproten Rigatini	CE
	Aproten Tagliatelle	CE
	Glutenex	L
	Nutregen Special Wheat Starch★	E
	Rite-Diet Bread Mix	WF
	Rite-Diet Gluten-free Protein-free Canned Bread	WF
	Rite-Diet Flour	WF
	Rite-Diet Savoury Biscuits	WF
	Rite-Diet Sweet Biscuits	WF
Low-calcium products	Locasol	U
Low-protein foods	Aglutella Gentili	DFS
	Aminex Biscuits	L
	Aproten Anellini	CE
	Aproten Crispbread	CE
	Aproten Flour	CE
	Aproten Rigatini	CE
	Aproten Tagliatelle	CE
	Azeta Biscuits	DFS
	Nutregen Special Wheat Starch★	E
	Rite-Diet Gluten-free Protein-free Canned Bread	WF
	Rite-Diet Protein-free Flour	WF
Low-protein and low lactose foods	Outline Low-fat Spread†	VDB
	Tomor Kosher Margarine†	VDB

★ A booklet *Special Wheat Starch Recipes for Gluten Free Diets* is available without charge from the manufacturers

† The composition of these products varies through the year and in different countries and should be checked with the manufacturers

Preparation		*Manu-facturer*
Low-sodium products	Edosol	U
	Rite-Diet Salt-free Canned Bread	WF
Medium-chain	Alembical D	LK
triglycerides	Caprilac	N
	Capricid	N
	Caprilon	N
	MCT (1)	U
	MCT Oil	SHS, U
Mineral supplements	Metabolic Mineral Mix	SHS

Attention is drawn to the existence in Canada of the National Food Distribution Centre for the Treatment of Hereditary Metabolic Disease, 1500 Atwater Avenue (15th Floor), Montreal H3Z 2W2. Quebec, Canada. This holds stocks of more than 20 products of different manufacturers (catalogue available) and acts through a network of 15 regional centres in Canada and has supplied other countries in emergency. The project is nationally co-ordinated and is advised by Dr. C. R. Scriver and Carol L. Clow.

Manufacturers—United Kingdom Offices

AH   Allen and Hanburys Ltd., Bethnal Green, London E2 6LA. (Tel: 01-739 4343)

AL   Abbott Laboratories Ltd., Queenborough, Kent ME11 5EL. (Tel: 079 56 3371)

B   Beecham Pharmaceuticals, Beecham House, Brentford, Middx. TW8 9BD (Tel: 01-560 5151)

DF   Duncan Flockhart & Co. Ltd., Birkbeck Street, London E2 6LA. (Tel: 01-739 3451)

E   Energen Foods Co., Ashford, Kent. (Tel: 0233 23411)

DFS   Carlosta Ltd., 33 Ermine Road, London SE13 7JY. (Tel: 01-692 3949)

CE   Carlo Erba (U.K.) Ltd., 28–30 Great Peter Street, London SW1P 2BX. (Tel: 01-799 2876)

L   Liga Infant Food Ltd., Liga House, 23 Saxby Street, Leicester LE2 0NL. (Tel: 0533 57748)

LK   E. J. R. Lovelock, Oaklands House, Oaklands Drive, Sale, Manchester M33 1WS. (Tel: 061-962 4423)

MJ   Bristol Laboratories, Langley, Slough SL3 6EB. (Tel: 0753 43261)

SHS   Scientific Hospital Supplies Ltd., 38 Queensland Street, Liverpool L7 3JG. (Tel: 051-709 3588)

U   Unigate Foods Ltd., Cow and Gate Baby Foods, 40–42 Stoke Road, Guildford, Surrey GU1 4HS. (Tel: 0483 68181)

VDB   Van den Berghs, Kildare House, Dorset Rise, London EC4P 4DY. (Tel: 01-353 3060)

W   Wander Ltd., Pharmaceutical Division, 98 The Centre, Feltham, Middx. TW13 4EP. (Tel: 01-890 1366)

WF   Welfare Foods (Stockport) Ltd., 63–65 Higher Hillgate, Stockport, Cheshire SK1 3HE. (Tel: 061-480 9408)

AH   *International*—Marketing Services Division, Glaxo Holdings Ltd., Graham Street, London, N1 8JZ, England. (Tel: 01-253 3060)

AL   *Angola*—Abbott Laboratories (Pty.) Ltd., P.O. Box 5307, Luanda, Angola, Portuguese West Africa

Australia—Abbott Australasia Pty. Ltd., P.O. Box 101, Cronulla, N.S.W 2230, Australia

Bahrain—Wael Pharmacy and Drug Store, Post Box No. 648, Bahrain, Arabian Gulf. (Tel.: 54886)

Belgium—Abbott S.A., Rue Defacqz 113-115, B-1050 Brussels, Belgium

Bolivia—Abbott Laboratories de Bolivia, Casilla 255, La Paz, Bolivia

Canada—Abbott Laboratories Ltd., P.O. Box 6150, Montreal H3C 3K6, Quebec, Canada

Costa Rica—Abbott Laboratories, Apartado 2338, San Jose, Costa Rica

Dominican Republic—Abbott Laboratories International Co., Apartado No. 846, San Domingo, Dominican Republic

Ecuador—Abbott Laboratories del Ecuador, S.A., Apartado Postal 3423, Guayaquil, Ecuador. (Cables: Abbottlab)

Egypt—Abbott Laboratories S.A., P.O. Box 2350, Cairo, Egypt, U.A.R. (Tel: 55417)

El Salvador—Abbott Laboratories International Co., Apartado No. 352, San Salvador, El Salvador (Tel: 23-4019)

Ethiopia—International Pharmaceutical Private Limited Company (INTERPHARM), P.O. Box 2466, Addis Ababa, Ethiopia (Tel: 15-63-48)

Germany—Chemische Fabrik von Heyden GmbH, Volkartstrasse 83, 8000 München 19, West Germany. (Tel: 120755)

Ghana—Ghana National Trading Corporation, P.O. Box 67, Ghana House, High Street, Accra, Ghana. (Cables: Gnatcorp)

Greece—Abbott Laboratories (Hellas) S.A., 194 Syngrou Avenue, Kallithea, Athens, Greece. (Cables: Abbottlab-Athens)

Guatemala—Abbott Laboratorios, S.A., Apartado Postal No. 37, Guatemala, Guatemala

Haiti—Abbott Laboratories, 29 rue Cheriez, P.O. Box 703, Port-au-Prince, Haiti

Honduras—Abbott Laboratories, Apartado Postal 957, San Pedro Sula, Honduras and Abbott Laboratories, Apartado Postal 58, Tegucigalpa, Honduras

Hong Kong—Abbott Laboratories Ltd., G.P.O. Box 14402, North Point, Hong Kong. (Cables: Abbottlab-Hong Kong)

Iran—Pharmaceutical Industries Development Ltd., P.O. Box 879, Tehran, Iran

Iraq—Iraq Stores Co., P.O. Box 26, Baghdad, Iraq

Israel—Tazziz Drug Store, P.O. Box 78, Jerusalem, Israel. (Tel: 2040) and Nissen Preminger Ltd., P.O. Box 29001, 9 Montefiore Street, Tel Aviv, Israel. (Tel: 53027)

Italy—Abbott S.p.A., I64010 Campoverde di Aprilia, (Latina), Italy

Jamaica—Kongs Commercial Agencies Ltd., P.O. Box 195, 7 West Street, Kingston, Jamaica, West Indies. (Tel: 922-1885)

Jordan—Tazziz Drug Store, P.O. Box 921, Amman, Jordan. (Tel: 37860)

Kuwait —Al-Mojil Drug Establishment, P.O. Box No. SAFAT-2761, Kuwait, Arabian Gulf

Lebanon—Abbott Laboratories, S.A., P.O. Box 112940, Beirut, Lebanon. (Tel: 233851)

Libya—Abdullah A. Muftah, P.O. Box 3940, Tripoli, Libya, U.A.R. (Tel: 31273) and Abdullah A. Muftah, P.O. Box 1564, Benghazi, Libya, U.A.R. (Tel: 92390)

Mozambique—Abbott Laboratories, S.A. (Pty.) Ltd., P.O. Box 1958, Lourenco Marques, Mozambique

Netherlands—M & R Laboratoria B.V., Postbus 626, Zwolle, Holland. (Tel: 05200-12626)

Nigeria—G. B. Ollivant, P.O. Box 144, Wilberforce House, 182/184, Yakubu Gowon Street, Lagos, Nigeria. (Tel: 26841-225)

Panama—Abbott Laboratories International Co., Apartado Postal No. 4543, Panama 5, Panama

Peru—Abbott Laboratories del Peru S.A., Apartado No. 2402, Lima, Peru. (Tel: 61-4791)

Philippines—Abbott Laboratories (Philippines), P.O. Box 29, Commerical Center, Post Office, Makati, Rizal D-708, Philippines

Puerto Rico—Abbott Laboratories, P.O. Box 21184, Rio Piedras, Puerto Rico 00928 (Cables: Abbottlab, San Juan, Puerto Rico)

Saudi Arabia—Al Kamal Import Office, P.O. Box 405, Jeddah, Saudi Arabia

Singapore—Abbott Laboratories (Singapore) Private Ltd., G.P.O. Box No. 1016, Singapore 7. (Tel: 320876)

South Africa—Abbott Laboratories South Africa (Pty.) Ltd., P.O. Box 1616, Johannesburg 2000, South Africa. (Tel: 942-3100)

Sudan—Khartoum Commercial Agency, P.O. Box 646, Khartoum, Sudan. (Tel: 80197)

Surinam—Abbott laboratories, c/o Chephfasu N.V., P.O. Box 788, Paramaribo, Surinam

Taiwan—The Great Wealth Co., Post Box 55134, Taipei, Taiwan

Thailand—The Borneo Company (Thailand) Ltd., 1041, Silom Road, Bangkok, Thailand. (Tel: 31090)

U.S.A.—Abbott Laboratories, 14th Street and Sheridan Road, North Chicago, Illinois, 60064, U.S.A. (Tel: 688-6100)

Zaire—Abbott Laboratories, P.O. Box 8244, Kinshasa, Republic of Zaire

Zambia—Abbott Laboratories, S.A. Geneva, P.O. Box 3931, Lusaka, Zambia. (Tel: Lusaka 74974, Ext. 35)

CE *Argentina*—Carlo Erba Argentina S.A.C.eI, Maipù 521, Buenos Aires, Argentina. (Tel: 392-9091)

Australia—D.H.A. Pharmaceuticals Pty. Ltd. (inc. in NSW), Manufacturing Division, Cherry Lane, Laverton North, Victoria, Australia. (Tel: 399 2311)

Austria—Aesca G.m.b.H., Schönbrunner Strasse 213-215, A-1121, Wien, Austria. (Tel: 0222-831621)

Belgium—P.C.B. Therapeutica, Division PCB s.a., Rue de Genève 512, 1030 Bruxelles, Belgium. (Tel: (02) 418690)

Denmark—Astra-Sjuco, Roskildevej 22, DK-2620, Albertslund, Denmark. (Tel: 01-647755)

Eire—T. P. Mullen, T. P. Mullen & Co. Ltd., 23B Dublin Industrial Estate, Finglas Road, Dublin, 11, Eire. (Tel: Dublin 306255)

Finland—Astra-Sjuco, Pl 6, SF-02671, Hämevaara, Finland. (Tel: 90-84 82 11)

France—Laboratoires Carlo Erba S.A., 105 Bureaux de la Colline, 92, St. Cloud, France

Germany—Aponti Kindernährmittel G.m.b.H., Postfach 10 01 88, Holzmarkt 59/65, 5, Köln, 1, West Germany. (Tel: 0221-21 92 62)

Iran—Sa'id Tabiti & Co., P.O. Box 14/1551, 69, Shah Reza Avenue, Mabeine Pahlavi Va Kaledj, Tehran, Iran. (Tel: 661 437)

Japan—Nippon Montedison K.K., Montedison Building, 1-3-2, Aobadai, Meguro-ku, Tokyo 153, Japan. (Tel: 462-0551)

Libya—The Libyan Co. for Cosmetics and Perfumes, P.O. Box 1743, Benghazi, Libya. (Tel: 87322)

Netherlands—Multi-Pharma B.V., Posthus 4171, Linnaeusparkweg 220, Amsterdam-0, Netherlands. (Tel: 020-947164)

New Zealand—Dental & Medical Supply Co. Ltd., P.O. Box 1994, Wellington, New Zealand

Norway—Astra-Sjuco, Postboks 1, N-1473 Skårer, Norway. (Tel: 02-70 15 90)

Sweden—Astra-Sjuco AB, Fack, S-402 20 Götebörg 5, Sweden. (Tel: 031-87 02 00)

Switzerland—Unipharma S.A., 6903 Lugano, Switzerland. (Tel: 091-601433)

Tunisia—Henriette Taieb, 8 rue d'Alger, Tunis, Tunisia

U.S.A.—General Mills Chemicals Inc., 4620 West 77th Street, Minneapolis, Minnesota 55435, U.S.A. (Tel: 612-540-4269)

CCF *Netherlands*—Coöperatieve Condensfabriek Friesland, P.O. Box 226, Pieter Stuyvesantweg 1, Leeuwarden, Netherland. (Tel: 05100-41041)

DFS	*Italy*—Ditta Federico Salza, Via Sottoborgo 46, Pisa, Italy

E	*Italy*—Ditta Federico Salza, Via Sottoborgo 46, Pisa, Italy *Malta*—Francis Busuttil and Sons Ltd., Busuttil Buildings, Venera Square, St. Venera, Malta

L	*Australia*—Tomasetti & Son Pty. Ltd., 634 Graham Street, Port Melbourne 3207, Australia. (Tel: 64.4221) Tomasetti & Son Pty. Ltd., 2 Marjorie Street, Sefton, New South Wales, Australia. (Tel: 6448333) Tomasetti & Son Pty. Ltd., 213 West Beach Road, Richmond, South Australia, Australia. (Tel: 3521188) Tomasetti & Son Pty. Ltd., 34 Douglas Street, Milton, Queensland, Australia. (Tel: 360277) Tomasetti & Son Pty. Ltd., 90 Guildford Road, Mount Lawley, Western Australia, Australia. (Tel: 717200) *Belgium*—Betterfood S.A., Kapelsesteenweg 753, 2070 Ekeren 2, Belgium. (Tel: 031-64.25.50) *Canada*—Messrs. TOP's Importing Ltd., Box 190, Grimsby, Ontario, Canada. (Tel: 416-945.4141) *Eire*—Liga Ireland Ltd., 61 Middle Abbey Street, Dublin 1, Eire. (Tel: 48956) *France*—Codime S.à.r.l., 4 Rue Guillaume Lefèbvre, 59100 Roubaix, France. (Tel: (20) 75.25.66) *Germany*—Liga Nährungsmittel G.m.b.H., Beethovenstrasse 3, 4072 Wickrath, Germany *Italy*—Ditta Annoni S.A.S., Via Nicolò Bettoni 2, 20125 Milano, Italy. (Tel: 02-690.801) *Netherlands*—Liga Fabrieken B.V., Postbus 27, Laan van Brabant 48, Roosendaal, Netherlands. (Tel: 01650–34940) *South Africa*—Prima Vera Trading Co., P.O. Box 49, Pretoria, South Africa. (Tel: 70-9134) *Sweden*—Famaco AB, Post Box 9007, S-102 71, Stockholm 9, Sweden. (Tel: 08-1858 40)

LK	*Italy*—Alembic Oil Italiana s.r.l., Piazza Della Vittoria 4, 16121 Genoa, Italy. (Tel: 566570, Genoa)

MG	*Germany*—Maizena Gesellschaft m.b.H., Pharm.-wissenschaftliche Abteilung, Postfach 1000, Spaldingstrasse 218, 2 Hamburg 1, West Germany. (Tel: 040-2884-1)

MJ	*Argentina*—Mead Johnson International Ltd., Casilla Correo No. 7, Sucursal 46B, Buenos Aires, Argentina. (Tel: 38-3095) *Australia*—Mead Johnson, Post Office Box 530, 345 Pacific Highway, Crows Nest, N.S.W. 2065, Australia. (Tel: 02-929-8366)

Austria—Frika, Pharmazeutische Fabrik G.m.b.H., Postfach 43, A-1091, Vienna, Austria
Belgium—Mead Johnson Benelux S.A.-N.V., Chaussee de la Hulpe 185-187, Bruxelles 1170, Belgium. (Tel: 02-660.00.37)
Brazil—Mead Johnson S.A., Caixa Postal 8700, 01000 Sao Paulo, S.P. Brazil
Canada—Mead Johnson Canada, 231 Dundas St. East, Belleville, Ontario, Canada
Colombia—Mead Johnson International Ltd., Apartado Aereo 12375, Bogota D.E., Colombia
Cyprus—George Petrou Ltd., P.O. Box 1232, Nicosia, Cyprus. (Tel: 021-72857)
Eire—Bristol-Myers Co. Ltd., Robinhood Industrial Estate, Clondalkin, Co. Dublin, Eire. (Tel: 508047)
France—Laboratoires Allard S.A., 10 Avenue de Messine, 75008 Paris, France. (Tel: 522-62-50)
Greece—Bristol Hellas, Ltd., P.O. Box 711, 226, Piraeus Street, Athens 310/1, Greece. (Tel: 358-211/5)
Iran—Bristol (Iran) S.A., P.O. Box 11-1435, Tehran, Iran
Mexico—Mead Johnson de Mexico, S.A. de C.V., Apartado Postal 21-979, Mexico 21, D.F. Mexico. (5-49-30-85)
Netherlands—Mead Johnson Nederland, Spaklerweg 53, Amsterdam, Netherlands
New Zealand—Bristol-Myers (New Zealand) Ltd., P.O. Box 9175, 234 Khyber Pass Road, Newmarket, Auckland 1, New Zealand (Tel: 33-972)
Philippines—Mead Johnson Philippines, Inc., P.O. Box 1234, Commercial Center Post Office, Makati, Rizal, Philippines
South Africa—The B-M Group (Pty.) Ltd., Post Office Box 9706, Johannesburg, South Africa
Sri Lanka—J. L. Morison, Son & Jones (Ceylon) Ltd., P.O. Box 430, Colombo, Sri Lanka
Sweden—Bristol Laboratorier A.B., Hufvodsta Gård, Box 4100, 17104 Solna, Sweden (Tel: 08-82 04 30)
U.S.A.—Mead Johnson Laboratories, Evansville, Indiana 47721, U.S.A. (Tel: 812-426-6000)
Venezuela—Mead Johnson de Venezuela, S.A., Apartado 62469, Caracas, Venezuela. (Tel: 34/94/50)

N   *Netherlands*—Nutricia Verkoop Nederland B.V., Postbus 1, Zoetermeer, Netherlands. (Tel: 079-163900)

SHS   *Austria*—C. H. Knorr G.m.b.H., Postfach 168, Nährungsmittelfabriken, A-4600 Wels, Austria. (Tel: 072 42-5346)
Australia—Muir and Neil Pty. Ltd., Box 1562 G.P.O., 479 Kent Street, Sydney, N.S.W. 2000, Austrlia. (Tel: 26-2644)
and Muir and Neil Pty. Ltd., 46 Cliff Street, South Yarra, Melbourne, Victoria 3141, Australia. (Tel: 24-4959)

Canada—Food Bank, National Food Distribution Centre, 1500 Atwater Avenue, (Floor 15), Montreal, Quebec H3Z 2W2, Canada. (For products other than 'Caloreen')
Abbott laboratories Ltd., P.O. Box 6150, Montreal, Quebec H3C 3K5, Canada ('Caloreen' only)
Denmark—Mecobenzon A/S, Halmtorvet 29, 1503 Copenhagen V, Denmark. (Tel: (01) 310194)
Eire—T. P. Mullen, T. P. Mullen & Co. Ltd., 23B Dublin Industrial Estate, Finglas Road, Dublin, 11, Eire. (Tel: Dublin 306255)
France—Société des Produits du Mais, 379 Avenue du Général-de-Gaulle, 92 140 Clamart, France. (Tel: 736-55-00)
Germany—Maizena Gesellschaft m.b.H., Postfach 1000, Spaldingstr. 218, 2 Hamburg 1, West Germany
New Zealand—Muir and Neil Pty. Ltd., 105-107, Wellesley Street West, Auckland C.1, New Zealand. (Tel: 378 765)
Norway—Norsk Medisinaldepot, Box 100, Veitvedt, Oslo 5, Norway
Switzerland—Dr. Bender & Dr. Hobein AG, Reidlistrasse 15a, 8042 Zurich, Switzerland. (Tel: 01-26 17 77)

U International—Unigate International Division—Bythesea Road, Trowbridge, Wilts, U.K. (Tel: 02214 3611)
Australia—Muir and Neil Pty. Ltd., Box 1562, G.P.O., 479 Kent Street, Sydney, N.S.W. 2000, Australia. (Tel: 26-2644) and Muir and Neil Pty. Ltd., 46 Cliff Street, South Yarra, Melbourne, Victoria 3141, Australia. (Tel: 24-49 59)
Canada—Cow and Gate (Canada) Ltd., 27 Apple Street, Brockville, Ontario, Canada K6V 4X7. (Tel: 613-345-1431)
Iran—Iran-Behdasht Co. Ltd., P.O. Box 12-1144, 118-122, West Takhte Jamshid Ave., Tehran, Iran. (Tel: 52956)
Italy: Medifood, S.R.L., Via Balbi 31/1, 16126, Genoa, Italy
Lebanon—Société d'Entreprises Vita, POB 6063, Rue de Damas, Imm. Al-Kamal, Beirut, Lebanon. (Tel: 295891)
New Zealand—Muir and Neil Pty. Ltd., P.O. Box 5105, 105-7 Wellesley Street West, Auckland, C.1, New Zealand. (Tel: 37-8765)
South Africa—Cow and Gate South Africa (Pty.) Ltd., 171 Jacob Maré St., Pretoria, South Africa. (Tel: 484148)
Spain—Dieteticos Ordesa S.A., Hospitalet, Barcelona, Spain
Yugoslavia—Belje-Trufood, Savjetovalište za djécju prehranu, Pik Belje, Darda, Yugoslavia

WF Eire—T. P. Mullen, T. P. Mullen & Co. Ltd., 23B Dublin Industrial Estate, Finglas Road, Dublin 11, Eire. (Tel: Dublin 306255)

TREATMENT OF OTHER INHERITED METABOLIC DISEASES

This table is intended as an index to the book, as a reminder of diseases to be considered in diagnosis and as a source of further information on the treatment of some of these. The presence of a literature citation does not imply recommendation and some failures are listed so that these may be modified or avoided.

The alphabetical system is that of McKusick *Mendelian Inheritance in Man* 3rd Ed. (1971), modified to accord with British spelling. Prefixes indicating quantity—for example hypo–, hyper–, a–, and Greek letters—are ignored for indexing purposes. The number in brackets is that used by McKusick: those starting with 2 or 3 are recessive and sex-linked respectively.

The table includes under:

> **S**—An assessment of the severity of the disease graded 1–4. 1 = totally benign; 2 = benign in the absence of a precipitating agent such as a drug; 3 = mild to moderate; 4 = severe to lethal.
>
> **T**—An assessment of the extent to which the disease is at present treatable within the categories; Established, Promising, Experimental and, where no treatment has been proposed, Symptomatic.
>
> **D**—The deficient enzyme, where this is known.

Such a table can be neither complete nor wholly accurate and the Editor would appreciate any information that would improve or extend it.

Acanthocytosis; *see aβ*-Lipoproteinaemia (20010)
Acid phosphatase deficiency (20095) **S** 4 **T** Symptomatic **D** *Acid phosphatase*
Nadler, H. L. (Editors; H. G. Hers and F. Van Hoof). *Lyosomes and Storage Diseases* (New York; Academic Press.) (*Prednisolone increased serum and lymphocyte enzyme activity*)
Acrodermatitis enteropathica (20110) **S** 4 **T** Established **D**—
Moynahan, E. J. Acrodermatitis enteropathica. *Proc. Roy. Soc. Med.*, **55**, (1962), 240. (*Di-iodohydroxyquinoline cleared skin lesions*)
Javett, S. N. Regrowth of hair during penicillamine treatment of acrodermatitis enteropathica. *Lancet*, **i**, (1963), 504. (*Pencillamine produced rapid healing of skin lesions following earlier slow response to di-iodohydroxyquinoline*)
Addison's disease and spastic paraplegia (20150) **S** 3 **T** Symptomatic **D**—
Penman, R. W. B. Addison's Disease in association with spastic paraplegia. *Brit. Med. J.*, **1**, (1960), 402. (*Addisonian crisis responded to conventional therapy*)
Adenylate kinase deficiency (20160) **S** 4 **T** Symptomatic **D** *Adenylate kinase*
Szeinberg, A. *et al.* Hereditary deficiency of adenylate kinase in red blood cells. *Acta Haemat.*, **42**, (1969), 111. (*Severe haemolytic anaemia treated with transfusions*)
Adrenal hyperplasia type I (20170) **S** 4 **T** Established **D** *Steroid 21-hydroxylase*
Bongiovanni, A. M. and Root, A. W. The adrenogenital syndrome. *New Eng. J. Med.*, **268**, (1963), 1391

Raiti, S. and Newns, G. H. Linear growth in treated congenital adrenal hyperplasia. *Arch. Dis. Childhood*, **46**, (1971), 376

Hamilton, W. and Moodie, T. The treatment of congenital adrenal hyperplasia with aminoglutethimide. *Develop. Med. Child. Neurol.*, **12** (1970), 618

hyper β-**Alaninaemia** (23740) **S** 4 **T** Symptomatic **D**—

Scriver, C. R. *et al.* Hyper-β-alaninemia associated with β-amino-aciduria and γ-amino butyric aciduria, somnolence and seizures. *New Eng. J. Med.*, **274**, (1966), 635. (*Biochemical but no clinical improvement with pyridoxine hydrochloride*)

Alaninuria with microcephaly, dwarfism, enamel hypoplasia, diabetes mellitus (20290) **S** 3 **T** Symptomatic **D**—

Stimmler, L. *et al.* Alaninuria associated with microcephaly, dwarfism, enamel hypoplasia, and diabetes mellitus in two sisters. *Arch. Dis. Childhood*, **45**, (1970), 682. (*Diabetes treated with insulin*)

Aldosterone deficiency due to defect in 18-hydroxylase or 18-dehydrogenase (20340) **S** 4 **T** Established **D**—

Visser, H. K. A. and Cost, W. S. A new hereditary defect in the biosynthesis of aldosterone. Urinary C(21)—corticosteroid pattern in three related patients with a salt-losing syndrome, suggesting an 18-oxidation defect. *Acta Endocr.*, **47**, (1964), 589. (*Effective treatment with DOCA and salt supplements*)

Alkaptonuria (20350) **S** 3 **T** Promising **D** *Homogentisate oxidase*

(*Diets low in phenylalanine and tyrosine are being tried in some centres*)

Amauriotic family idiocy; *see* Gangliosidosis GM2 type 1 (27280)

Amaurotic family idiocy, juvenile (20420) **S** 3 **T** Symptomatic **D**—

β-Aminoisobutyric aciduria (21010) **S** 1 **T** Not required **D**—

*hyper***Ammonaemia type 1** (23720) **S** 4 **T** Promising **D** *Ornithine carbamoyltransferase*

Campbell, A. G. M. *et al.* A cause of lethal neonatal hyperammonemia in males. *New Eng. J. Med.*, **288**, (1973), 1. (*No response to protein restriction, dialysis or exchange transfusion*)

Hopkins, I. J. *et al.* Hyperammonaemia due to ornithine transcarbamylase deficiency. *Arch. Dis. Childhood*, **44**, (1969), 143. (*Responded to protein restriction*)

Herrin, J. T., and McCredie, D. A. Peritoneal dialysis in the reduction of blood ammonia levels in a case of hyperammonaemia. *Arch. Dis. Childhood*, **44**, (1969), 149

Corbeel, L. M. *et al.* Periodic attacks of lethargy in a baby with ammonia intoxication due to a congenital defect in ureogenesis. *Arch. Dis. Childhood*, **44**, (1969), 681. (*Low protein diet*)

Levin, B. *et al.* Hyperammonaemia: a variant type of deficiency of liver ornithine transcarbamylase. *Arch. Dis. Childhood*, **44**, (1969), 162

Kang, E. S. *et al.* Ornithine transcarbamylase deficiency in the newborn infant. *J. Pediat.*, **82**, (1973), 642. (*Temporary improvement after exchange transfusions*)

*hyper***Ammonaemia type 2** (23730) **S** 4 **T** Promising **D** *Carbamoylphosphate synthase*

Freeman, J. M. *et al.* Ammonia intoxication due to a congenital defect in urea synthesis. *J. Pediat.*, **65**, (1964), 1039. (*Low protein diet*)

Hommes, F. A. *et al.* Carbamylphosphate synthetase deficiency in an infant with severe cerebral damage. *Arch. Dis. Childhood*, **44**, (1969), 688. (*Low protein diet*)

Amylopectinosis; *see* Glycogen storage disease type 4 (23250)

Anaemia, hypochromic (30130) **S** 4 **T** Exp **D** δ-*Aminolaevulinic acid synthetase*
Bishop, R. C., and Bethell, F. H. Hereditary hypochromic anaemia with transfusion hemosiderosis treated with pyridoxine. *New Eng. J. Med.*, **261**, (1959), 486. (*Responded to pyridoxine*)

Anderson's disease; *see* Glycogen storage disease type 4 (23250)

Angiokeratoma, diffuse (30150) **S** 3 **T** Symptomatic **D** *Ceramide trihexoside* α-*galactosidase*
Philippart, M. *et al.* Reversal of an inborn sphingolipidosis (Fabry's disease) by kidney transplantation. *Ann. Int. Med.*, **77**, (1972), 195
Desnick, R. J. *et al.* Correction of enzymatic deficiencies by renal transplantation: Fabry's disease. *Surgery*, **72**, (1972), 203
Clarke, J. T. R. *et al.* Enzyme replacement therapy by renal allotransplantation in Fabry's disease. *New Eng. J. Med.*, **287**, (1972), 1215
Mapes, C. A. *et al.* Enzyme replacement in Fabry's disease, an inborn error of metabolism. *Science*, **169**, (1970), 987

Antitrypsin deficiency (20740) **S** 3 **T** Symptomatic **D**—
Editorial. Antitrypsin deficiency in chronic obstructive lung disease. *Lancet*, **i**, (1970), 71. (*Avoid lung irritants and smoking: early treatment of infections*)

Antopol's disease; *see* Glycogen storage disease limited to heart (23210)

Argininaemia (20780) **S** 3 **T** Symptomatic **D** *Arginase*
Terheggen, H. G. *et al.* Argininaemia with arginase deficiency. *Lancet*, **ii**, (1969), 748. (*Low protein diet*)

Argininosuccinic aciduria (20790) **S** 3 **T** Experimental **D** *Argininosuccinate lysase*
Westall, R. G. Treatment of arginosuccinic aciduria. *Amer. J. Dis. Child.*, **113**, (1967), 160
Levin, B. Arginosuccinic aciduria. *Amer. J. Dis. Child.*, **113**, (1967), 162. (*Restricted protein intake*)
Levin, B. *et al.* Argininosuccinic aciduria. *Arch. Dis. Childhood*, **36**, (1961), 622. (*Diets of different protein and arginine content*)

Aspartyl-glycosaminuria (20840) **S** 3 **T** Symptomatic **D** 2-*Acetamido-1-(β-L-aspartamido)-1,2-dideoxy-glucosidase*

Ataxia, intermittent (20880) **S** 3 **T** Symptomatic **D** *Pyruvate decarboxylase*

Batten's disease; *see* Amaurotic family idiocy, juvenile (20420)

*hyper***Bilirubinaemia type 2 (Dubin–Johnson)** (23750) **S** 3 **T** Experimental **D**—
Dubin, I. N. Chronic idiopathic jaundice: A review of 50 cases. *Amer. J. Med.*, **24**, (1958), 268

*hyper***Bilirubinaemia-shunt** (23780) **S** 2 **T** Symptomatic **D**—
Israels, L. G. *et al.* Hyperbilirubinaemia due to an alternate path of bilirubin production. *Amer. J. Med.*, **27**, (1959), 693. (*Plasma bilirubin reduced by splenectomy in several cases*)

*hyper***Bilirubinaemia, transient familial neonatal** (23790) **S** 2 **T** Established **D**—

The Treatment of Inherited Metabolic Disease

Arias, I. M. *et al.* Transient familial neonatal hyperbilirubinemia. *J. Clin. Invest.*, **44**, (1965), 1442. (*Exchange transfusions in neonatal period*)
Blue diaper syndrome (21100) S 4 T Symptomatic **D—**
Byler's disease (21160) S 4 T Symptomatic **D—**
Carnosinaemia (21220) S 4 T Symptomatic **D** *Aminoacyl-histidine dipeptidase*
*a***Catalasaemia, Japanese** (20020) S 3 T Symptomatic **D** *Catalase*
*a***Catalasaemia, Swiss** (20020) S 3 T Symptomatic **D** *Catalase*
Cerebral cholesterinosis (21370) S 4 T Symptomatic **D—**
Salen, G. and Meriweather, T. W. Chenodeoxycholic acid inhibits sterol biosynthesis in cerebrotendinous xanthomatosis. *Clin. Res.*, **20**, (1972), 465. (*Chenodeoxycholic acid decreased synthesis of cholesterol and cholestanol in 3 subjects*)
Salen, G. and Grundy, S. M. The metabolism of cholestanol, cholesterol and bile acids in cerebrotendinous xanthomatosis. *J. Clin. Invest.*, **52**, (1973), 2822. (*Clofibrate reduced plasma concentration and excretion of cholestanol and increased bile acid production in two cases*)
Cerebrotendinous xanthomatosis; *see* Cerebral cholesterinosis (21370)
Chloride diarrhoea (21470) S 4 T Experimental **D—**
Evanson, J. M. and Stanbury, S. W. Congenital cholridorrhoea or so-called congenital alkalosis with diarrhoea. *Gut*, **6**, (1965), 29. (*Corrects potassium deficiency by low chloride diet and potassium supplements*)
Launiala, K. *et al.* Familial chloride diarrhoea–chloride malabsorption. *Mod. Probl. Pediat.*, **11**, (1967), 137. (*Clinical improvement and biochemical 'normality' with excess KCl*)
Cholesterol ester storage disease of liver (21500) S 3 T Symptomatic **D—** *Acid lipase*
(*May be a milder variant of Wolman's disease*)
Citrullinuria (21570) S 4 T Experimental **D—***Argininosuccinate synthetase*
McMurray, W. C. *et al.* Citrullinuria. *Pediat.*, **32**, (1963), 347. (*Effect of varying protein intake*)
Morrow, G. Citrullinemia. *Amer. J. Dis. Child.*, **113**, (1967), 157. (*Low protein diet*)
Cori's disease; *see* Glycogen storage disease type 3 (23240)
Crigler–Najjar syndrome (21880) S 4 T Symptomatic **D** *UDP-glucuronyl-transferase*
Arias, I. M. *et al.* Chronic nonhemolytic unconjugated hyperbilirubinemia with glucuronyl transferase deficiency. *Amer. J. Med.*, **47**, (1969), 395. (*Some patients, thought to have a partial deficiency, responded to phenobarbitone, others who may have a total deficiency do not*)
Gorodischer, R. *et al.* Congenital nonobstructive nonhemolytic jaundice—effect of phototherapy. *New Eng. J. Med.*, **282**, (1970), 375. (*Phototherapy lowered bilirubin*)
Cystathioninuria (21950) S 1 T Not required **D—***Homoserine dehydratase*
Berlow, S. Studies in cystathioninemia. *Amer. J. Dis. Child.*, **112**, (1966), 135. (*Clinical improvement with pyridoxine*)
Frimpter, G. W. *et al.* Cystathioninuria: management. *Amer. J. Dis. Child.*, **113**, (1967), 115. (*No clinical improvement with pyridoxine*)
Cystinosis type 1 (21980) S 4 T Experimental **D—**

Goldman, H. *et al.* Use of dithiothreitol to correct cystine storage in cultured cystinotic fibroblasts. *Lancet*, **i**, (1970), 811. (*Biochemical improvement in one case in an advanced state*)

Aaron, K. *et al.* Cystinosis; new observations 1. Adolescent (type III) form 2. Correction of phenotypes in vitro with dithiothreitol. *Inherited Disorders of Sulphur Metabolism* (Editors: N. A. J. Carson and D. N. Raine). (1971), p. 150. (Edinburgh; Churchill Livingstone)

Mahoney, C. P. *et al.* Renal transplantation for childhood cystinosis. *New Eng. J. Med.*, **283**, (1970), 397. (*Four cases followed up for 14 to 32 months*)

Briggs, W. A. *et al.* Kidney transplantation in Fanconi syndrome. *New Eng. J. Med.*, **286**, (1972), 25. (*One case with cystinosis*)

Clayton, B. E. and Patrick, A. D. Use of dimercaprol or penicillamine in the treatment of cystinosis. *Lancet*, **ii**, (1961), 909

Cystinosis type 2 (21990) **S** 3 **T** Experimental **D**—; *see* Cystinosis type 1

Cystinosis type 3 (22000) **S** 1 **T** Not required **D**—

Cystinuria type 1 (22010) **S** 2 **T** Established **D** *Renal tubular transport of four amino acids*

Zinneman, H. H. and Jones, J. E. Dietary methionine and its influence on cystine excretion in cystinuric patients. *Metabolism*, **15**, (1966), 915. (*No significant reduction of urinary cystine achieved*)

Dent, C. E. *et al.* Treatment of cystinuria. *Brit. Med. J.*, **1**, (1965), 403. (*High fluid regime and alkali*)

Stephens, A. D. and Watts, R. W. E. The treatment of cystinuria with N-acetyl-D-penicillamine a comparison with the results of D-penicillamine treatment. *Quart. J. Med.*, **40**, (1971), 355

Roesel, R. A. and Coryell, M. E. Determination of cystine excretion by the nitroprusside method during drug therapy of cystinuria. *Clinica Chimica Acta*, **52**, (1974), 343. (*Test useful for penicillamine but not for mercaptopropionyl glycine*)

Cystinuria type 2 (22010) **S** 2 **T** Established **D**—; *see* Cystinuria type 1

Cystinuria type 3 (22010) **S** 2 **T** Established **D**—; *see* Cystinuria type 1

Diabetes insipidus, nephrogenic (30480) **S** 3 **T** Established **D**—

Lant, A. F. The antidiuretic effect of diuretics in diabetes insipidus. *J. Roy. Coll. Phys. London*, **2**, (1968), 298. (*Long-term diuretic therapy*)

Crawford, J. D. *et al.* Clinical results of treatment of diabetes insipidus with drugs of the chlorothiazide series. *New Eng. J. Med.*, **262**, (1960), 737

Diabetes insipidus, neurohypophyseal type (30490) **S** 3 **T** Established **D**—

Lant, A. F. The antidiuretic effect of diuretics in diabetes insipidus. *J. Roy. Col. Phys. London*, **2**, (1968), 298

Crawford, J. D. *et al.* Clinical results of treatment of diabetes insipidus with drugs of the chlorothiazide series. *New Eng. J. Med.*, **262**, (1960), 737. (*Vasopressin and diuretics*)

Dibasic aminoaciduria type 1 (12600) **S** 1 **T** Not required **D**—

Dibasic aminoaciduria type 2 (22270) **S** 4 **T** Experimental **D**—

Kekomäki, M. *et al.* Familial protein intolerance with deficient transport of basic amino acids. *Acta Paed. Scand.* **56**, (1967), 617. (*Dietary treatment with arginine supplements*)

Diphosphoglycerate mutase deficiency of red cells (22280) **S** 3 **T** Symptomatic **D** *Diphosphoglyceromutase*

Schröter, W. Kongenitale nichtsphärocytäre hämolytische Anämie bei 2,3-Diphosphoglyceratmutase-mangel der Erythrocyten im frühen Säuglingsalter. *Klin. Wochen.*, **43**, (1965), 1147. (*Very severe haemolytic disease treated with multiple transfusions*)

Disaccharide intolerance type 1 (22290) **S** 4 **T** Established **D** *β-Fructofuranosidase*
Anderson, C. M. *et al.* Intestinal sucrase and isomaltase deficiency in two siblings. *Pediatrics*, **31**, (1963), 1003. (*Sucrose-free diet*)

Disaccharide intolerance type 2 (22300) **S** 4 **T** Established **D** *β-Gala...osidase*
Launiala, K. *et al.* Disaccharidases and histology of duodenal mucosa in congenital lactose malabsorption. *Acta Paed. Scand.*, **55**, (1966), 257. (*Symptoms and intestinal mucosa improved on lactose-free diet*)

Disaccharide intolerance type 3 (22310) **S** 3 **T** Established **D** *β-Galactosidase*
Ferguson, A. and Maxwell, J. D. Genetic aetiology of lactose intolerance. *Lancet*, **ii**, (1967), 188. (*Lactose-free diet relieved symptoms*)

Dubin–Johnson syndrome; *see hyper* Bilirubinaemia type 2 (23750)

Dyggve–Melchior–Clausen disease (22380) **S** 3 **T** Symptomatic **D**—

Dysautonomia (22390) **S** 3 **T** Symptomatic **D**—

Enterokinase deficiency (22620) **S** 3 **T** Promising **D** *Enterokinase*
Hadorn, B. *et al.* Intestinal enterokinase deficiency. *Lancet*, **i**, (1969), 812. (*Improved on pancreatic extract*)

Fabry's disease; *see* Angiokeratoma, diffuse (30150)

Farber's lipogranulomatosis (22800) **S** 4 **T** Symptomatic **D**—

Fatty metamorphosis of viscera (22819) **S** 4 **T** Symptomatic **D**—
Reye, R. D. K. *et al.* Encephalopathy and fatty degeneration of the viscera: a disease entity in childhood. *Lancet*, **ii**, (1963), 749. (*Hydrocortisone and intravenous glucose*)
Utian, H. L. *et al.* White liver disease. *Lancet*, **ii**, (1964), 1043. (*Steroids and other drugs and intravenous glucose*)

Forbes' disease; *see* Glycogen storage disease type 3 (23240)

Formimino transferase deficiency (22910) **S** 3 **T** Symptomatic **D** *Formimino transferase*
Arakawa, T. *et al.* Formimino transferase deficiency syndrome associated with megaloblastic anaemia responsive to pyridoxine or folic acid. *Tohoku J. Exp. Med.*, **94**, (1968), 3

Fructose and galactose intolerance (22950) **S** 3 **T** Established **D**—
Dormandy, T. L. and Porter, R. J. Familial fructose and galactose intolerance. *Lancet*, **i**, (1961), 1189. (*Improved on diet low in fructose and galactose*)

Fructose intolerance (22960) **S** 4 **T** Established **D** *Ketose-1-phosphate aldolase*
See Chapter 6, page 151

Fructose 1,6-diphosphatase deficiency (22970) **S** 3 **T** Symptomatic **D** *Hexose diphosphatase*
Greene, H. L. *et al.* Ketotic hypoglycemia due to hepatic fructose-1,6-diphosphatase deficiency. Treatment with folic acid. *Amer. J. Dis. Child.*, **124**, (1972), 415. (*Folic acid increased enzyme activity and prevented hypoglycaemia*)

Fructosidosis (23000) **S** 3 **T** Symptomatic **D** α-L-*Fucosidase*
Galactokinase deficiency (23020) **S** 3 **T** Established **D** *Galactokinase*
   See Chapter 4, page 92
   Sidbury, J. B. Some inferences from galactokinase deficiency. *Pediatrics,*
   53, (1974), 309
   Olambiwonnu, N. O. *et al.* Galactokinase deficiency in twins: clinical and
   biochemical studies. *Pediatrics,* **53**, (1974), 314
Galactosaemia, classical (23040) **S** 4 **T** Established **D** *Galactose-1-phosphate*
uridyltransferase
   See Chapter 4, page 91
Galactosaemia, Duarte (23040) **S** 1 **T** Not required **D** *Galactose-1-phosphate*
uridyltransferase
Galactosaemia, Negro (23040) **S** 3 **T** Experimental **D** *Galactose-1-phosphate*
uridyltransferase
   See Chapter 4, page 91
Gangliosidosis generalised GM1 type 1 (23050) **S** 4 **T** Symptomatic **D**
GM1 ganglioside β-galactosidase isoenzymes A B and C
Gangliosidosis generalised GM1 type 2 (23060) **S** 4 **T** Symptomatic **D**—
GM1 ganglioside β-galactosidase isoenzymes B and C
Gangliosidosis GM2 type 1 (27280) **S** 4 **T** Symptomatic **D**β- *Acetylglucos-*
aminase A
Gangliosidosis GM2 type 2 (26880) **S** 4 **T** Symptomatic **D** *β-Acetylglucos-*
aminase A and B
Gangliosidosis GM2 type 3 (23070) **S** 3 **T** Symptomatic **D** *β-Acetylglucos-*
aminase A
Gangliosidosis GM3 (24550) **S** 4 **T** Symptomatic **D** *Lactosylceramide β-*
galactosidase
Globoid leucodystrophy; *see* Krabbe disease (24520)
Glucose-galactose malabsorption (23160) **S** 4 **T** Established **D**—
   Meeuwisse, G. W. and Melin, K. Glucose-galactose malabsorption. *Acta*
   Paed. Scand. Suppl., **188**, (1969), 3. (*Dietary carbohydrates replaced by fructose*)
   Schneider, A. J. *et al.* Glucose-galactose malabsorption. Report of a case with
   autoradiographic studies of a mucosal biopsy. *New Eng. J. Med.*, **274**, (1966),
   305. (*Carbohydrate-free diet for 3 months: then introduced gradually*)
Glucose-6-phosphate dehydrogenase deficiency (30590) **S** 2 **T** Promising
D *Glucose-6-phosphate dehydrogenase*
   Carson, P. E. *et al.* Enzymatic deficiency in primaquine-sensitive erythrocytes.
   Science, **124**, (1956), 484. (*Therapeutic concentrations of primaquine can cause*
   haemolysis)
   Dern, R. J. *et al.* The haemolytic effect of primaquine: V primaquine-
   sensitivity as a manifestation of a multiple drug sensitivity. *J. Lab. Clin. Med.*,
   45, (1955), 30. (*Many drugs in addition to primaquine cause haemolysis*)
   Keller, D. F. *G-6-PD Deficiency* (1971), p. 30. (London; Butterworths).
   (*Current list of drugs to be avoided*)
Glutathione peroxidase deficiency (23170) **S** 2 **T** Not required **D** *Gluta-*
thione peroxidase
   Necheles, T. F. *et al.* Erythrocyte glutathione-peroxidase deficiency and
   hemolytic disease of the newborn infant. *J. Ped.* **72**, (1968), 319.

(Hyperbilirubinaemia may require exchange transfusion but mild haemolytic process ceased by third month)

Glutathione reductase, haemolytic anaemia due to deficiency of in red cells (23180) **S** 3 **T** Experimental **D** *Glutathione reductase*
Carson, P. E. *et al.* Decreased glutathione reductase with susceptibility to hemolysis. *J. Lab. Clin. Med.,* **58**, (1961), 804. *(Avoid drugs which induce haemolytic anaemia)*

Glutathione synthetase deficiency (23190) **S** 3 **T** Symptomatic **D** *Glutathione synthetase*
Mohler, D. N. *et al.* Glutathione synthetase deficiency as a cause of hereditary haemolytic disease. *New Eng. J. Med.,* **283**, (1970), 1253. *(Mild compensated haemolytic disease relieved by splenectomy although reticulocytosis remained)*

Glycogen storage disease limited to heart (23210) **S** 3 **T** Symptomatic **D—**

Glycogen storage disease type 1 (23220) **S** 3 **T** Promising **D** *Glucose-6-phosphate*
See Chapter 5, page 115

Glycogen storage disease type 2 (23230) **S** 3 **T** Symptomatic **D** α-1,4-*glucosidase*
See Chapter 5, page 115
Hug, G. and Schubert, W. K. Hepatic lysosomes in Pompe's disease: disappearance during glucosidase administration. *J. Clin. Invest.,* **46**, (1967), 1073

Glycogen storage disease type 3 (23240) **S** 3 **T** Experimental **D** *Amylo-1,6-glucosidase Debrancher enzyme)*
See Chapter 5, page 115

Glycogen storage disease type 4 (23250) **S** 4 **T** Symptomatic **D** α-*glucan branching glycosyl-transferase*
See Chapter 5, page 115
Fernandes, J. and Huijing, F. Branching enzyme deficiency glycogenosis: studies in therapy. *Arch. Dis. Childhood,* **43**, (1968), 347 *(Intravenous α-glucosidase reduced liver glycogen)*

Glycogen storage disease type 5 (23260) **S** 3 **T** Experimental **D** *Muscle glycogen phosphorylase*
McArdle, B. Skeletal muscle glycogenoses other than type 2. *Some Inherited Disorders of Brain and Muscle* (Editors; J. D. Allan and D. N. Raine). (1969), p. 46. (Edinburgh; Churchill Livingstone). *(Trials with isoprenaline and other agents)*

Glycogen storage disease type 6 (23270) **S** 3 **T** Promising **D** *Glycogen phosphorylase*
See Chapter 5, page 115

Glycogen storage disease type 7 (23280) **S** 2 **T** Symptomatic **D** *Muscle phosphofructokinase*
Tarui, S. *et al.* Phosphofructokinase deficiency in skeletal muscle. A new type of glycogenosis. *Biochem. Biophys. Res. Comm.,* **19**, (1965), 517. *(Avoid excessive exercise)*

Glycogen storage disease type 8 (30600) **S** 3 **T** Experimental **D** *Liver phosphorylase kinase*
See Chapter 5, page 115

Glycoprotein storage disease (23290) **S** 3 **T** Symptomatic **D—**

Gout (30620) **S** 3 **T** Promising **D** *Hypoxanthine-guanine phosphoribosyltransferase*
  Kelley, W. N. *et al.* Hypoxanthine-guanine phosphoribosyltransferase deficiency in gout. *Ann. Int. Med.*, **70**, (1969), 155. (*Allopurinol lowers uric acid concentration*)
Hartnup disease (23450) **S** 3 **T** Experimental **D** *Renal tubular transport of neutral amino acids*
  Halvorsen, K. and Halvorsen, S. Hartnup disease. *Pediatrics*, **31**, (1963), 29. (*Treatment with nicotinamide*)
  Wong, P. W. K. *et al.* Observations on nicotinic acid therapy in Hartnup disease. *Arch. Dis. Childhood*, **42**, (1967), 642
Hepatolenticular degeneration; *see* Wilson's disease (27790)
Her's disease; *see* Glycogen storage disease type 6 (23270)
Hexokinase deficiency (23570) **S** 3 **T** Symptomatic **D** *Hexokinase*
  Valentine, W. N. *et al.* Hereditary haemolytic anaemia with hexokinase deficiency. Role of hexokinase in erythrocyte aging. *New Eng. J. Med.*, **276**, (1967), 1. (*Haemolytic anaemia improved by splenectomy*)
Hexose phosphate isomerase deficiency (23575) **S** 3 **T** Symptomatic **D** *Glucose phosphate isomerase*
  Paglia, D. G. *et al.* Occurrence of defective hexosephosphate isomerisation in human erythrocytes and leukocytes. *New Eng. J. Med.*, **280**, (1969), 66. (*Anaemia improved by splenectomy*)
Histidinaemia (23580) **S** 3 **T** Promising **D**—*Histidine ammonia-lysase*
  Griffiths, M. Clinical aspects of the dietary treatment of histidinaemia. A report of four cases. *Treatment of Inborn Errors in Metabolism* (Editors; J. W. T. Seakins, R. A. Saunders and C. Toothill). (1973), p. 87. (Edinburgh; Churchill Livingstone)
  Wadman, S. K. *et al. Clinica Chimica Acta*, **49**, (1973), 377. (*Special problems of dietary correction in older children*)
  Neville, B. G. R. *et al.* Histidinaemia: study of relation between clinical and biological findings in 7 subjects. *Arch. Dis. Childhood*, **47**, (1972), 190
  Popkin, J. S. *et al.* Is hereditary histidinaemia harmful? *Lancet*, **i**, (1974), 721
  Editorial. Histidinaemia: to treat or not to treat? *Lancet*, **i**, (1974), 719
Hooft's disease (23630) **S** 3 **T** Symptomatic **D**—
Homocystinuria (23620) **S** 3 **T** Promising **D** *L-serine dehydratase*
  See Chapter 2, page 33
Hunter syndrome; *see* Mucopolysaccharidosis type 2 (30990)
Hurler syndrome; *see* Mucopolysaccharidosis type 1 (25280)
β-Hydroxy-isovaleric aciduria and β-methyl crotonylglycinuria (21020) **S** 3 **T** Experimental **D** *β-Methylcrotonyl-CoA carboxylase*
  See Chapter 8, page 209
Hydroxykynureninuria (23680) **S** 4 **T** Symptomatic **D** *Kynureninase*
  Komrower, G. M. and Westall, R. Hydroxykynureninuria. *Amer. J. Dis. Child.*, **113**, (1967), 77. (*Some improvement with pyridoxine and nicotinic acid*)
Hydroxylysinuria (23690) **S** 3 **T** Symptomatic **D**—
Hydroxyprolinaemia (23700) **S** 3 **T** Experimental **D** *Hydroxyproline oxidoreductase*
  See Chapter 9, page 224

The Treatment of Inherited Metabolic Disease

Hypoxanthine-guanine phosphoribosyl transferase deficiency (30800)
S 4 T Symptomatic D *Hypoxanthine-guanine phosphoribosyl transferase*
Watts, R. W. E. *et al*. Clinical and biochemical studies on the treatment of
the Lesch Nyhan syndrome. *Arch. Dis. Childhood*, **49**, (1974), 693. (*Allopurinol
lowers serum uric acid but neurological state unaffected*)
I-cell disease; *see* Mucolipidosis type 2 (25250)
Iminoglycinuria (24260) S 1 T Not required D *Transport of Gly Pro and Hyp*
Indolyl-acroyl-glycinuria with mental retardation (24290) S 3 T Sympto-
matic D—
   Mellman, W. J. *et al*. Indolylacroyl glycine excretion in a family with mental
   retardation. *Clinica Chimica Acta*, 8, (1963), 843. (*Neomycin cleared metabolite
   from urine*)
Isovaleric acidaemia (24350) S 4 T Symptomatic D *Isovaleric acid–CoA
dehydrogenase*
   See Chapter 8, page 192
Kinky hair disease; *see* Menkes syndrome (30940)
Krabbe disease (24520) S 4 T Symptomatic D *Galactocerebroside β-galactosidase*
Lactic acidosis (24540) S 4 T Experimental D—
   Brunette, M. G. *et al*. Thiamine-responsive lactic acidosis in a patient with
   deficient low-Km pyruvate carboxylase activity in liver *Pediatrics*, **50**, (1972),
   702
   For general maintenance see Chapter 8, page 164
Lactose intolerance; *see* Disaccharide intolerance type 2 (22300) and type 3
(22310)
Lactosyl ceramidosis; *see* Gangliosidosis GM3 (24550)
Leber's optic atrophy (30890) S 3 T Symptomatic D—
   Wilson, J. Leber's hereditary optic atrophy: some clinical and aetiological
   considerations. *Brain*, **86**, (1963), 347. (*Improved when smoking avoided*)
Lecithin-cholesterol acetyl-transferase deficiency (24590) S 3 T Sympto-
matic D *Lecithin cholesterol acyltransferase*
   Norum, K. R. and Gjone, E. G. The effect of plasma transfusion on the
   plasma cholesteryl esters in patients with familial plasma lecithin-cholesterol
   acyltransferase deficiency. *Scan. J. Clin. Lab. Invest.*, **22**, (1968), 339. (*Bio-
   chemical but no clinical improvement over 2 weeks*)
Leigh's encephalopathy; *see* Necrotizing encephalopathy (25600)
Lesch–Nyhan syndrome; *see* Hypoxanthine-guanine phosphoribosyl transferase
deficiency (30800)
Limit dextrinosis; *see* Glycogen storage disease type 3 (23240)
Lipase, congenital absence of pancreatic (24660) S 3 T Experimental D
Lipase
   Sheldon, W. Congenital pancreatic lipase deficiency. *Arch. Dis. Childhood*,
   39, (1964), 268. (*Pancreatic extract improved but did not relieve steatorrhoea*)
Lipidosis, juvenile dystonic (24680) S 3 T Symptomatic D—
Lipomucopolysaccharidosis; *see* Mucolipidosis type 1 (25240)
an α-**Lipoproteinaemia** (20540) S 3 T Experimental D α-*Lipoprotein*
a β-**Lipoproteinaemia** (20010) S 4 T Experimental D β-*Lipoprotein*
   Kayden, H. J. Abetalipoproteinemia. *Ann. Rev. Med.*, **23**, (1972), 285. (*Fat
   restricted diet and iron and vitamin supplements*)

Leyland, F. C. *et al.* Use of medium chain triglyceride diets in children with malabsorption. *Arch. Dis. Childhood*, **44**, (1969), 170. (*MCT corrected steatorrhoea*)

Kuo, P. T. and Bassett, D. R. Blood and tissue lipids in a family with hypo-β-lipoproteinaemia. *Circulation*, **26**, (1962), 660. (*Improvement when natural fat replaced by corn oil*)

Lowe's oculo-cerebro-renal syndrome (30900) **S** 4 **T** Experimental **D**—
Lowe, C. U. *et al.* Organic-aciduria, decreased renal ammonia production, hydrophthalmos and mental retardation. *Amer. J. Dis. Child.*, **83**, (1952), 164. (*Vitamin D and alkalis improved boney lesions*)

*hyper***Lysinaemia** (23870) **S** 3 **T** Symptomatic **D** *Lysine: α-ketoglutarate oxidoreductase*

Lysine intolerance (24790) **S** 4 **T** Promising **D** *L-lysine NAD oxidoreductase*
Colombo, J. P. *et al* Lysine intolerance with periodic ammonia intoxication. *Amer. J. Dis. Child.*, **113**, (1967), 138. (*Low-lysine diet*)

McArdle's disease; *see* Glycogen storage disease type 5 (23260)

Mannosidosis (24850) **S** 4 **T** Symptomatic **D** α-*Mannosidase*

Maple-syrup-urine disease (24860) **S** 4 **T** Experimental **D** *keto-acid decarboxylase*
See Chapter 3, page 71

Maple-syrup-urine disease, intermittent (24860) **S** 3 **T** Experimental **D** *Keto acid decarboxylase*
See Chapter 3, page 71

Maroteaux–Lamy syndrome; *see* Mucopolysaccharidosis type 6 (25320)

Megaloblastic anaemia responsive to folic acid, ataxia, mental retardation and convulsions (24930) **S** 3 **T** Experimental **D**—

Menkes syndrome (30940) **S** 3 **T** Experimental **D**—
Danks D. M. *et al.* Menkes' kinky-hair syndrome. *Lancet*, **i**, (1972), 1100. (*Oral and intravenous copper*)

Metachromatic leucodystrophy (25010) **S** 4 **T** Symptomatic **D** *Cerebroside sulphate sulphatase (arylsulphatase A)*
Green, H. L. *et al.* Metachromatic leucodystrophy: treatment with arylsulfatase A. *Arch. Neurol.*, **20**, (1969), 147. (*No clinical improvement after i.v. administration of beef brain arylsulphatase A*)
Melchior, J. C. and Clausen, J. Metachromatic leucodystrophy in early childhood. Treatment with a diet deficient in vitamin A. *Acta Paed. Scand.*, **57**, (1968), 2. (*Biochemical but no clinical improvement in one case*)
Moosa, A. and Dubowitz, V. Late infantile metachromatic leucodystrophy: effect of low vitamin A diet. *Arch. Dis. Childhood*, **46**, (1971), 381. (*Arrest of disease over 2 years in one case*)
Dubowitz, V. Therapeutic possibilities in metachromatic leucodystrophy. *Treatment of Inborn Errors in Metabolism* (Editors; J. W. T. Seakins, R. A. Saunders and C. Toothill). (1973), p. 253. (Edinburgh; Churchill Livingstone)

Metachromatic leucodystrophy, adult (25000) **S** 3 **T** Symptomatic **D**—

Metachromatic leucodystrophy and amaurotic idiocy, combined features of (24980); *Probably identical with* Metachromatic leucodystrophy with mucopolysacchariduria (24990)

Metachromatic leucodystrophy, juvenile (250202) **S** 3 **T** Symptomatic **D**—
Metachromatic leucodystrophy with mucopolysacchariduria (24990)
S 4 **T** Symptomatic **D**—
Methaemoglobin reductase deficiency (NADH) (25080) **S** 3 **T** Experimental **D** *Methaemoglobin: NADH oxidoreductase*
   Tönz, O. *The Congenital Methaemoglobinaemias.* (1968), p. 72. (Basel and New York; S. Karger). (*Oral ascorbic acid and intravenous methylene blue*)
Methaemoglobin reductase deficiency (NADPH) (25070) **S** 2 **T** Not required **D** *Methaemoglobin: NADPH oxidoreductase*
Methionine malabsorption (25090) **S** 4 **T** Experimental **D**—
   Hooft, C. *et al.* Methionine malabsorption syndrome. *Annales Paediatrici (Basel)*, **205**, (1965), 73. (*Low-methionine diet*)
α-Methylacetoacetic and α-Methyl-β-hydroxybutyric aciduria (Unassigned) **S** 4 **T** Symptomatic **D**—
   See Chapter 8, page 192
Methylmalonic aciduria type 1 (25100) **S** 4 **T** Experimental **D** *Methylmalonyl-CoA mutase*
   See Chapter 8, page 205
Methylmalonic aciduria type 2 (25110) **S** 4 **T** Experimental **D** *Methylmalonyl-CoA isomerase*
   See Chapter 8, page 205
Morquio syndrome; *see* Mucopolysaccharidosis type 4 (25300)
Mucolipidosis type 1 (25240) **S** 3 **T** Symptomatic **D**—
Mucolipidosis type 2 (25250) **S** 4 **T** Symptomatic **D**—
Mucolipidosis type 3 (25260) **S** 4 **T** Symptomatic **D**—
Mucopolysaccharidosis type 1—Hurler (25280) **S** 4 **T** Experimental **D** *α-L-iduronidase*
   Danes, B. S. *et al.* Plasma infusions in the Hurler syndrome. *Amer. J. Dis. Child.*, **125**, (1973), 533. (*No clinical or biochemical effect*)
   Danes, B. S. *et al.* Treatment of Hurler syndrome. *Lancet*, **ii**, (1972), 883. (*No clinical or biochemical effect of weekly infusions of fresh frozen plasma*)
   Booth, C. W. and Nadler, H. L. Plasma infusions in an infant with Hurler's syndrome. *J. Pediat.*, **82**, (1973), 273. (*Conversion of high to low molecular weight urinary mucopolysaccharides but no clinical improvement in 8 months*)
   DiFerrante, N. *et al.* Induced degradation of glycosaminoglycans in Hurler's and Hunter's syndromes by plasma infusion. *Proc. Nat. Acad. Sci.*, **68**, (1971), 303
   Dekaban, A. S. *et al.* Effects of fresh plasma or whole blood transfusions on patients with various types of mucopolysaccharidosis. *Pediatrics*, **50**, (1972), 688
   DeJong, B. P. *et al.* Failure to induce scurvy by ascorbic acid depletion in a patient with Hurler's syndrome. *Pediatrics*, **42**, (1968), 889. (*Scorbutic diet for one year had no effect*)
   Danes, B. S. and Bearn, A. G. The effect of retinol (vitamin A alcohol) on urinary excretion of mucopolysaccharides in the Hurler syndrome. *Lancet*, **i**, (1967), 1029. (*Studies on three cases*)
   Madsen, J. A. and Linker, A. Vitamin A and mucopolysaccharidosis: a clinical and biochemical evaluation. *J. Pediat.*, **75**, (1969), 843. (*Clinical deterioration in two cases*)

Wolfson, S. L. *et al.* Biochemical and roentgenographic response to long-term corticosteroid therapy in the Hurler syndrome. *Amer. J. Dis. Child.*, **102**, (1961), 638. (*Clinical improvement with high doses*)

Mucopolysaccharidosis type 2—Hunter (30990) **S** 4 **T** Experimental **D**
Sulphoiduronate sulphatase
DiFerrante, N. *et al.* Induced degradation of glycosaminoglycans in Hurler's and Hunter's syndromes by plasma infusion. *Proc. Nat. Acad. Sci.*, **68**, (1971), 303

Erickson, R. P. *et al.* Inefficacy of fresh frozen plasma therapy of mucopolysaccharidosis II. *Pediatrics*, **50**, (1972), 693

Coppa, G. V. *et al.* Urinary excretion of disulfated disaccharides in Hunter syndrome: correction by infusion of a plasma fraction. *Analytical Letters*, **6**, (1973), 225. (*Disulphated disaccharides which characterise the disease disappeared from urine after protein fraction administered*)

Dekaban, A. S. *et al.* Effects of fresh plasma or whole blood transfusions on patients with various types of mucopolysaccharidosis. *Pediatrics*, **50**, (1972), 688

Knudson, A. G. *et al.* Effect of leukocyte transfusion in a child with type II mucopolysaccharidosis. *Proc. Nat. Acad. Sci.*, **68**, (1971), 1738

Danes, B. S. and Bearn, A. G. The effect of retinol (vitamin A alcohol) on urinary excretion of mucopolysaccharide in the Hurler syndrome. *Lancet*, **i**, (1967), 1029. (*Studies on three cases—despite title!*)

Madsen, J. A. and Linker, A. Vitamin A and mucopolysaccharidosis: a clinical and biochemical evalution. *J. Pediat.*, **75**, (1969), 843. (*Clinical deterioration in one case*)

Mucopolysaccharidosis type 3—Sanfilippo (25290) **S** 4 **T** Experimental **D**
It is now recognised that there are two types of this disease, type A due to heparan sulphate N-sulphatase deficiency and type B due to N-acetyl-α-D-glucosaminidase deficiency
Rostenberg, I. *et al.* Effects of dextran 70 (Macrodex) in a type III mucopolysaccharidosis. *Annales Genetique*, **16**, (1973), 121

Dekaban, A. S. *et al.* Effects of fresh plasma or whole blood transfusions on patients with various types of mucopolysaccharidosis. *Pediatrics*, **50**, (1972), 688

Dean, M. F. *et al.* Mobilization of glycosaminoglycans by plasma infusion in mucopolysaccharidosis type III—two types of response. *Nature New Biology*, **243**, (1973), 143. (*Results conform with being two types of Sanfilippo syndrome*)

Dean, M. F. *et al.* Treatment of the mucopolysaccharidoses. *Treatment of Inborn Errors of Metabolism* (Editors: J. W. T. Seakins, R. A. Saunders and C. Toothill). (1973), p. 277. (Edinburgh; Churchill Livingstone). (*Plasma infusion in three patients*)

Madsen, J. A. and Linker, A. Vitamin A and mucopolysaccharidosis: a clinical and biochemical evaluation. *J. Pediat.*, **75**, (1969), 843. (*Clinical deterioration in two cases*)

Mucopolysaccharidosis type 4—Morquio (25300) **S** 3 **T** Symptomatic **D**—
Madsen, J. A. and Linker, A. Vitamin A and mucopolysaccharidosis: a clinical and biochemical evaluation. *J. Pediat.*, **75**, (1969), 843. (*No effect in two cases*)

Mucopolysaccharidosis type 5—Scheie (25310) **S** 3 **T** Symptomatic **D** α-L-*iduronidase*
(*Now designated type 1S to distinguish it from type 1H, Hurler syndrome which has a more severe deficiency of the same enzyme*)
Mucopolysaccharidosis type 6—Maroteaux-Lamy (25320) **S** 3 **T** Symptomatic **D**—
Myeloperoxidase deficiency (25460) **S** 3 **T** Experimental **D** *Myeloperoxidase*
Necrotising encephalopathy (25600) **S** 4 **T** Experimental **D**—
Clayton, B.E., *et al.* Leigh's subacute necrotising encephalopathy: clinical and biochemical study, with special reference to therapy with lipoate. *Arch. Dis. Childhood*, **42**, (1967), 467
DeGroot, C. J. *et al.* The enzyme defect in Leigh's encephalopathy. *Enzymopenic Anaemias, Lysosomes and Other Papers* (Editors; J. D. Allan, K. S. Holt, J. T. Ireland and R. J. Pollitt). (1969), p. 77. (Edinburgh; E. & S. Livingstone Ltd.). (*Treatment with lipoic acid*)
Hommes, F. A. *et al.* Leigh's encephalomyelopathy: an inborn error of gluconeogenesis. *Arch. Dis. Childhood*, **43**, (1968), 423. (*Treatment with lipoic acid*)
Lonsdale D. *et al.* Intermittent cerebellar ataxia associated with hyperpyruvic acidemia hyperalaninemia and hyperalaninuria. *Pediatrics*, **43**, (1969), 1025. (*Treatment with thiamine*)
Pincus, J. H. *et al.* Subacute necrotising encephalomyelopathy. *Arch. Nerol.*, **24**, (1971), 511. (*Thiamine and thiamine propyl disulfide*)
Grover, W. D. *et al.* Biochemical studies and therapy in subacute necrotising encephalomyelopathy (Leigh's syndrome). *J. Pediat.*, **81**, (1972), 39
Murphy, J. V. Efficacy of recommended therapeutic regimens in Leigh's disease. *Devel. Med. Child. Neurol.*, **16**, (1974), 362. (*Glutamine and pyridoxine treatment*)
Neurovisceral storage disease with curvilinear bodies (25700) **S** 3 **T** Symptomatic **D**—
Niemann–Pick disease (25720) **S** 4 **T** Symptomatic **D** *Sphingomyelinase*
Crocker, A. C. and Farber, S. Niemann–Pick disease: A review of 18 patients. *Medicine*, **37**, (1958), 1
Norum's disease; *see* Lecithin-cholesterol acetyl-transferase deficiency (24590)
Oasthouse urine disease; *see* Smith–Strang disease (27050)
Orotic aciduria (25890) **S** 3 **T** Experimental **D** *Orotidylic decarboxylase*
Huguley, C. M. *et al.* Refractory megaloblastic anaemia associated with excretion of orotic acid. *Blood*, **14**, (1959), 615. (*Clinical improvement on yeast nucleotides orally but preparation poorly tolerated*)
Haggard, M. E. and Lockhart, L. H. Megaloblastic anaemia with orotic aciduria. *Amer. J. Dis. Child.*, **113**, (1967), 733. (*Prednisone increased but megaloblastic marrow unchanged. Oral uridine produced a rapid clinical and biochemical remission*)
Becroft, D. M. O. *et al.* Hereditary orotic aciduria—Long-term therapy with uridine and a trial of uracil. *J. Pediat.*, **75**, (1969), 885. (*Good results with oral uridine over several years. Uracil unsuccessful*)
Pentosuria (26080) **S** 1 **T** Not required **D** *Xylitol: NADP oxidoreductase*
Phenylketonuria (26160) **S** 3 **T** Established **D** *Phenylalanine-4-hydroxylase*
See Chapter 1, page 1

*hypo*Phosphatasia (14630) **S** 3 **T** Symptomatic **D** *Alkaline phosphatase*
*hypo*Phosphatasia (24150) **S** 3 **T** Symptomatic **D** *Alkaline phosphatase*
   Fraser, D. Hypophosphatasia. *Amer. J. Med.*, **22**, (1957), 730. (*Vitamin D not recommended*)
   Warshaw, J. B. *et al.* Serum alkaline phosphatase in hypophosphatasia. *J. Clin. Invest.*, **50**, (1971), 2137. (*Effect of long and medium chain triglycerides on serum enzyme activity*)
*pseudo-hypo*Phosphatasia (26440) **S** 3 **T** Experimental **D**—
   Scriver, C. R. and Cameron, D. Pseudohypophosphatasia. *New Eng. J. Med.*, **281**, (1969), 604. (*Low calcium diet and prednisolone for 4 months healed bone*)
*hyper*Phosphatasia with mental retardation (23930) **S** 3 **T** Symptomatic **D**—
   Phosphoethanolaminuria; *see Hypo*Phosphatasia (24150)
Phosphoglycerate kinase deficiency haemolytic anaemia (31180) **S** 3 **T** Symptomatic **D** *Phosphoglycerate kinase*
   Valentine, W. N. *et al.* Hereditary haemolytic anaemia associated with phosphoglycerate kinase deficiency in erythrocytes and leucocytes. *New Eng. J. Med.*, **280**, (1969), 528. (*Splenectomy markedly reduced frequency of transfusions required to correct severe anaemia*)
Phosphoglycerate kinase deficiency of erythrocyte (26170) **S** 2 **T** Not required **D** *Phosphoglycerate kinase*
   Krause, A. P. *et al.* Red cell phosphoglycerate kinase deficiency. *Biochem. Biophy. Res. Comm.*, **30**, (1968), 173. (*Mild life-long anaemia—no treatment required*)
hyper-**Pipecolataemia** (23940) **S** 4 **T** Symptomatic **D**—
   Gatfield, P. D. *et al.* Hyperpipecolatemia: a new metabolic disorder associated with neuropathy and hepatomegaly: a case study. *Canad. Med. Ass. J.*, **99**, (1968), 1215. (*No improvement after lysine restriction*)
Polysaccharide, storage of unusual (26360) **S** 3 **T** Symptomatic **D**—
   Pompe's disease; *see* Glycogen storage disease type 2 (23230)
Prolinaemia type 1 (23950) **S** 2 **T** Experimental **D** *L-Proline: NAD(P)5-oxidoreductase*
   See Chapter 9, page 221
Prolinaemia type 2 (23950) **S** 3 **T** Experimental **D**—*Δ¹ pyroline-5-carboxylate dehydrogenase*
   See Chapter 9, page 221
Propionic acidaemia (23200) **S** 4 **T** Experimental **D** *Propionyl-CoA carboxylase*
   See Chapter 8, page 221
Pseudo–Hurler disease; *see* gangliosidosis GM1 type 1 (23050)
Pseudo–Hurler polydystrophy; *see* Mucolipidosis type 3 (25260)
Pyruvate kinase deficiency (26620) **S** 4 **T** Experimental **D** *Pyruvate kinase* (*There are two varieties of this disease—designated A and B*)
   Necheles, T. F. *et al.* Red cell pyruvate kinase deficiency: the effect of splenectomy. *Arch. Inter. Med.*, **118**, (1966), 75
   Busch, D. *et al.* Kinetic properties of pyruvate kinase and the problems of therapy in different types of pyruvate kinase deficiency. *Red Cell Structure and Metabolism* (Editor; B. Ramot). (1969), p. 193. (London and New York; Academic Press). (*Good clinical response with intravenous adenine and inosine in type B patients, but not in the more common type A patients*)

Refsum's disease (26650) **S** 3 **T** Experimental **D** *Phytanic acid oxidase*
  Eldjarn, L. *et al.* Dietary effects on serum-phytanic-acid levels and on clinical
  manifestations in heredopathia atactica polyneuritiformis. *Lancet*, **i**, (1966),
  691. (*Improvement on chlorophyll-free diet*)
Riley–Day syndrome; *see* Dysautonomia (22390)
Rubinstein syndrome (26860) **S** 3 **T** Symptomatic **D**—
Saccharopinuria (26870) **S** 3 **T** Symptomatic **D** *Aminoadipic semialdehyde-glutamate reductase*
Sandhoff's disease; *see* Gangliosidosis GM2 type 2 (26880)
Sanfilippo syndrome; *see* Mucopolysaccharidosis type 3 (25290)
Sarcosinaemia (26890) **S** 3 **T** Symptomatic **D**—
Scheie syndrome; *see* Mucopolysaccharidosis type 5 (25310)
Sea-blue histiocyte syndrome (26960) **S** 3 **T** Symptomatic **D**—
*hyper*Serotoninaemia (23960) **S** 3 **T** Symptomatic **D**—
Smith–Strang disease (27050) **S** 4 **T** Symptomatic **D**—
Spielmeyer–Vogt disease; *see* Amaurotic family idiocy, juvenile (20420)
Sucrose intolerance; *see* Disaccharide intolerance type 1 (22290)
Sulphatidosis, juvenile, Austin type (27220); *Probably identical with* Meta-chromatic leucodystrophy with mucopolysacchariduria (24990)
Sulphite oxidase deficiency; *see* Sulphocysteinuria (27230)
Sulphocysteinuria (27230) **S** 4 **T** Symptomatic **D** *Sulphite oxidase*
Suxamethonium sensitivity, dibucaine type (27240) **S** 2 **T** Symptomatic **D**
Cholinesterase
  Lehmann, H. and Ryan, E. The familial incidence of low pseudocholinesterase
  level. *Lancet*, **ii**, (1956), 124. (*Avoid organophosphorus compounds and other
  anticholinesterases*)
  Katz, R. L. *et al.* The effects of alkalosis on the action of the neuromuscular
  blocking agents. *Anesthesiology*, **24**, (1963), 18. (*Correct alkalosis before
  administering suxamethonium*)
Suxamethonium sensitivity, fluoride type (27240) **S** 2 **T** Symptomatic **D**
Cholinesterase
Suxamethonium sensitivity, silent type (27240) **S** 2 **T** Symptomatic **D**
Cholinesterase
Sweaty-feet syndrome; *see* Isovaleric acidaemia (24350)
Tangier disease; *see* anα-Lipoproteinaemia (20540)
Tay–Sachs disease; *see* Gangliosidosis GM2 type 1 (27280)
Thyroid dyshormonogenesis type 1 (27440) **S** 4 **T** Established **D**—
  Stanbury, J. B. and Chapman, E. M. Congenital hypothyroidism with goitre:
  absence of an iodide concentrating mechanism. *Lancet*, **i**, (1960), 1162.
  (*Responded to potassium iodide*)
Thyroid dyshormonogenesis type 2A (27450) **S** 4 **T** Established **D**—
  Parker, R. H. and Beierwaltes, W. H. Inheritance of defective organifica-
  tion of iodine in familial goitrous cretinism. *J. Clin. Endocr.*, **21**, (1961), 21.
  (*Thyroxine*)
Thyroid dyshormonogenesis type 2B (27460) **S** 4 **T** Established **D**—
  Furth, E. D. *et al.* Familial goiter due to an organification defect in
  euthyroid siblings. *J. Clin. Endocr. Metab.*, **27**, (1967), 1137. (*Thyroxine*)
Thyroid dyshormonogenesis type 4 (27480) **S** 4 **T** Established **D**—

Harden, R. M. *et al.* The influence of the plasma inorganic iodine concentration on thyroid function in dehalogenase deficiency. *Acta Endocr.*, **55**, (1967), 361. (*Thyroxine and iodine*)

Triose phosphate isomerase deficiency (27580) **S** 3 **T** Symptomatic **D** *Triosephosphate isomerase*

Trypsinogen deficiency (27600) **S** 3 **T** Experimental **D** *Trypsinogen*
Townes, P. L. Trypsinogen deficiency disease. *J. Pediat.*, **66**, (1965), 275
Morris, M. D. and Fisher, D. A. Trypsinogen deficiency disease. *Amer. J. Dis. Child.*, **114**, (1967), 203
Townes, P. L. *et al.* Further observations on trypsinogen deficiency disease: report of a second case. *J. Pediat.*, **71**, (1967), 220. (*Diet of protein hydrolysate in infancy successful and pancreatin granules when solids introduced*)

Tryptophanuria (27610) **S** 3 **T** Symptomatic **D**—
T-substance anomaly (27620) **S** 3 **T** Symptomatic **D**—
Tyrosinaemia (27670) **S** 4 **T** Experimental **D** *p-Hydroxyphenyl pyruvate hydroxylase*
Halvorsen, S. Dietary treatment of tyrosinosis. *Amer. J. Dis. Child.*, **113**, (1967), 38
Gentz, J. *et al.* Dietary treatment in tyrosinemia (tyrosinosis). *Amer. J. Dis. Child.*, **113**, (1967), 31
Harries, J. T. *et al.* Recovery after dietary treatment of an infant with features of tyrosinosis. *Arch. Dis. Childhood*, **44**, (1969), 258

Tyrosine transaminase deficiency (27660) **S** 3 **T** Experimental **D**—*Tyrosine aminotransferase*
Kennaway, N. G. and Buist, N. R. M. Metabolic studies in a patient with hepatic cytosol tyrosine aminotransferase deficiency. *Pediat. Res.*, **5**, (1971), 287. (*Dietary restriction of tyrosine and phenylalanine*)

Tyrosinosis (Medes) (27680) **S** 3 **T** Symptomatic **D**—
hyper\u200bUricaemia, ataxia, deafness (30720) **S** 3 **T** Symptomatic **D**—
hyper\u200bUricaemia, infantile, with abnormal behaviour and normal hypoxanthine guanine phosphoribosyl transferase (24000) **S** 3 **T** Experimental **D**—
Nyhan, W. L. *et al.* A new disorder of purine metabolism with behavioural manifestations. *J. Paediat.*, **74**, (1969), 20. (*Allopurinol decreased uric acid concentration*)

hyper\u200bUricaemia, lipodystrophy and neurologic defect (24010) **S** 3 **T** Symptomatic **D**—

Valinaemia (27710) **S** 3 **T** Experimental **D** *Valine amino transferase*
Tada K. *et al.* Hypervalinemia: its metabolic lesion and therapeutic approach. *Amer. J. Dis. Child.*, **113**, (1967), 64. (*Low valine diet and pyridoxine*)

Vogt–Spielmeyer's disease; *see* Amaurotic family idiocy, juvenile (20420)
Von Gierks's disease; *see* Glycogen storage disease type 1 (23220)

Wilson's disease (27790) **S** 3 **T** Established **D** *Caeruloplasmin* (*p-phenylene diamine oxidase*)
See Chapter 7, page 171

Wolman's disease (27800) **S** 4 **T** Symptomatic **D** *Acid lipase*
Wolman's disease with hypolipoproteinaemia and acanthocytosis (27810) **S** 4 **T** Symptomatic **D**—

Xanthinuria (27830) **S** 2 **T** Symptomatic **D** *Xanthine oxidase*
  Dent, C. E. and Philpot, G. R. Xanthinuria: an inborn error (or deviation) of
  metabolism. *Lancet*, **i**, (1954), 182. (*High fluid intake and alkali*)
Xanthurenic aciduria (27860) **S** 3 **T** Experimental **D** *Kynureninase*
  Tada, K. *et al.* Vitamin B_6 dependent xanthurenic aciduria. *Tohoku J. Exp.
  Med.*, **93**, (1967), 115. (*Biochemical improvement with pyridoxine in large doses*)
Xeroderma pigmentosum (27870) **S** 3 **T** Symptomatic **D** *Nucleic acid repair
  enzyme*
Xylosidase deficiency (27890) **S** 3 **T** Symptomatic **D** *β-Xylosidase*

Index

A

Astrocytosis, 76
Ataxia
  intermittent, 265
  maple syrup urine disease, 82
  Wilson's disease, 173
Aversion to sweet taste, 154, 158, 159, 163, 166
Azeta biscuits, 57, 255

B

Bacteriophage protein, 243
Basic amino acids, 220, 221
Behaviour problems after diet termination, 21
Betaine-homocysteine methyltransferase (BH methyltransferase), 38–40
Betaine supplementation, 38, 47, 48
Beutler's test (galactosaemia), 94
Bilirubinaemia, 265, 266
Bilirubin retention, 97, 98, 100
Bilirubin uridine diphosphate glucuronyl transferase, 246
Biochemistry
  homocystinuria, 33–35
  isovaleric acidaemia, 211
  maple syrup urine disease, 73–76
  propionic acidaemia, 202
  Wilson's disease, 173, 174
Biotin, 191, 193, 195, 203, 204, 209, 210
Biscuits, low protein, 63, 64
Bleeding tendency
  glucose-6-phosphate deficiency, 119, 120
  hereditary fructose intolerance, 162
Block, enzyme (hereditary fructose-intolerance), 152, 153
Block, metabolic
  homocystinuria, 34, 35
  maple syrup urine disease, 72, 73, 76, 86, 192
  organic acidaemias, 192
Blood sampling, 13
  cobalamin measurement, 206, 207
  galactosaemia, 94, 95
  Guthrie blood spot test, 13
  homocystinuria, 43
  methylmalonic aciduria, 206
  organic acidaemia, 200, 201
  penicillamine treatment, 179
Blue diaper syndrome, 266
Body weight (maple syrup urine disease treatment), 78

Bone marrow transplants, 245
Brain damage (homocystinuria), 35, 49
  see also Mental retardation
Brain development, 2, 22, 23
Branched chain amino acids, 72–74, 76–79, 81
  degeneration, 192, 198
Branched chain ketoaciduria; see Maple syrup urine disease
Branching enzyme deficiency, 115, 116
Bread
  galactose restricted diet, 102
  low protein, 62
British anitlewistle (BAL), 175
Byler's disease, 266

C

Caeruloplasmin, 173, 176, 187
Caesarian section (Wilson's disease), 186
Cakes, low protein, 63
Calcium, 5, 18
  disodium versenate, 172, 184
  glucose-6-phosphatase deficiency, 124, 125
  milk substitutes, 104
Caloreen, 255
Calories (maple syrup urine disease), 79, 86
Capricid, 256
Caprilac, 256
Caprilon, 256
Carbohydrate
  debranching enzyme deficiency, 135
  glucose-6-phosphatase deficiency, 124, 125, 128
  hereditary fructose intolerance, 163
  manufactured products, 52, 53
  organic acidaemias, 201
  phosphorylase system deficiency, 142
Carcinoma of the liver, 130–132
Carnosinaemia, 266
Carrier detection
  hereditary fructose intolerance, 154
  maple syrup urine disease, 72
Carrier, dietary restriction (galactokinase deficiency), 95
Catalasaemia, 266
Catalase, 240
Cataract formation
  galactosaemia, 93, 95, 96, 98, 106
  Wilson's disease, 172
Cell culture techniques, 238, 241

282

Irritability (maple syrup urine disease), 82
Islets of Langerhans transplants, 246
Isoluecine, 73–75, 78, 82–84, 88
  metabolism, 211
Isolubilised ensymes, 242, 243
Isomil, 102
Isovaleric acidaemia, 192, 193, 210, 211, 212, 253, 272
Isovaleryl CoA, 210
Isovalerylglycine, 211

J

Jaundice
  haemolytic, 171
  transferase deficiency, 96, 100
  Wilson's disease, 173
Joseph's syndrome, 221

K

Kayser Fleischer corneal pigment, 173, 174, 188
Keto acid
  derivatives (maple syrup urine disease), 73, 74, 76
  tests for 77
α–Ketoisocaproic acid, 72–74, 76, 78
α–Ketomethylvaleric acid, 72–74, 76
Ketones, 129, 198, 200, 203, 204, 206, 209
Ketonuria, 128, 138, 196, 198, 201, 202, 204, 207, 209, 212
Ketosis, 119, 129, 137–139, 142–144, 196, 199, 201, 202, 204, 205, 210–212
β–Ketothiolase deficiency, 212
Ketotic hyperglycaemia syndrome, 198, 205, 212
Ketovite, 16, 24, 26, 57, 228
Kidney transplantation, 246, 247
Kinky hair disease, 272
Krabbe disease, 272

L

Laboratory diagnosis (galactosaemia) 94, 95
Lactalac, 254
Lactate, 117, 121, 122, 129
Lacticacidaemia, 121, 123
Lactic acidosis, 164–166, 272

Lactic aciduria, 123, 124
Lactose, 101, 121, 122, 126
  hydrolysis of, 91, 92
  intolerance, 254, 272
Lactostrict, 253
Lactosyl ceramidosis, 272
Lead poisoning, 184
Leaky mutations (vitamin B_{12}), 195
Leber's optic atrophy, 272
Lecithin–cholesterol acetyl–transferase deficiency, 240, 272
Legumes (galactose restricted diet), 102, 104
Leigh's encephalopathy, 272
Leloir pathway (galactose metabolism), 91–93
Lemon sago, low protein, 66
Lenticular opacities (transferase deficiency), 98
Lesch–Nyhan syndrome, 277
Leucidon, 254
Leucine, 72–76, 79, 82–84, 88
  degradation, 195, 209, 210
Leucocyte infusions, 241
Leucopoenia, 183
Limit dextrinosis, 272
Lipaemia retinalis, 126
Lipase, 272
Lipidosis, juvenile dystonic, 272
Lipomucopolysaccharidosis, 272
Liponeogenesis, 126–128, 136, 142
Lipoproteinaemia, 272, 273
Lipoprotein lipase, 127
Liposomes, enzyme administration of, 241, 242
Listlessness (maple syrup urine disease), 71
Liver
  biopsy, 156–158, 161
  cholesterol ester storage disease, 266
  copper (Wilson's disease), 171
  dysfunction, 96–99
  function tests, 97, 116
  hepatic aldolase, 151–153
  hepatitis, 173
  hepatolenticular degeneration, 271
  hepatoma, 130, 131, 145
  hepatomegaly, 116, 139, 165, 166
  transplant, 246
Load tests (maple syrup urine disease), 72
Locasol, 255
Lofenalac, 5, 79
Los Angeles genetic variant, 99
Low calcium products, 255

288